FEBS Congress, Part B

Proceedings of the 16th
FEBS CONGRESS

Part B

25–30 June 1984, Moscow, USSR

Edited by
YU. A. OVCHINNIKOV

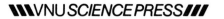 VNU *SCIENCE PRESS* ///   UTRECHT, THE NETHERLANDS

VNU Science Press BV
P.O. Box 2073
3500 GB Utrecht
The Netherlands

© 1985 VNU Science Press BV

First published 1985

ISBN 90-6764-046-8 Part B
ISBN 90-6764-044-1 set of three parts

Printed in Great Britain by J. W. Arrowsmith Ltd, Bristol

PREFACE

The investigation of the chemical nature of cell processes plays a key role in the study of living matter; the present advances in biochemistry, bioorganic chemistry, molecular biology, genetic engineering, etc. are widely known. Practically every day we are witnessing the revelation of new facts, the discovery of new bioregulators and the deciphering of new structures. The new direction in science, which is often called physico-chemical biology, not only strikes our imagination, but also has a considerable influence on the improvement of health care, efficiency in agricultural production and the development of new technologies.

In the summer of 1984, Moscow was the venue of the 16th Meeting of the Federation of European Biochemical Societies (FEBS). More than 4000 participants gathered in Moscow; this included not only Europeans, but also researchers from America, Asia and other parts of the world.

The scientific programme of the 16th FEBS meeting was very wide and covered practically all major aspects of the study of living matter on a molecular level. The lectures and posters presented at the meeting were devoted to the structure and function of biopolymers, the questions of the cell and membrane biology, the pressing problems of immunology, enzymology, neurobiology and modern directions of biotechnology.

The scientific level of all symposia organized within the framework of the meeting was extremely high and has reflected the latest achievments in each particular branch of science.

This three-part publication of the Proceedings of the 16th FEBS Congress includes the lectures that are of particular interest. We unfortunately could not publish all of the contributions—this would be hardly practicable.

On behalf of the organizing committee I should like to express my sincere gratitude to all attendants of the meeting for their active participation in this outstanding biochemical forum. I hope that the spirit of cooperation, mutual understanding and friendship which has marked the Moscow FEBS meeting will contribute to future progress in the study of living matter, to the well being of all nations and to peace and happiness on Earth.

Professor Yu. A. Ovchinnikov
Moscow

ORGANIZING COMMITTEE

Chairman	Professor Yu. A. Ovchinnikov
Vice-chairman	Professor S. E. Severin
Secretary-general	Professor V. F. Bystrov

Members

I. G. Atabekov	P. G. Kostyuk
A. A. Bayev	A. A. Krasnovsky
I. V. Berezin	E. M. Kreps
A. E. Braunstein	W. L. Kretovich
E. I. Chazov	R. V. Petrov
V. A. Engelhardt	E. S. Severin
G. P. Georgiev	V. P. Skulachev
G. R. Ivanitsky	A. S. Spirin
V. T. Ivanov	I. V. Torgov
M. N. Kolosov	Yu. M. Vasiliev

CONTENTS

BIOCHEMISTRY OF PHOTOSYNTHESIS

PIGMENTS AND ELECTRON TRANSFER COMPONENTS OF PHOTOSYNTHETIC BACTERIA

J. AMESZ
Department of Biophysics, University of Leiden,
The Netherlands

INTRODUCTION

Traditionally, the photosynthetic bacteria have played a very important role in the study of photosynthesis. This is especially true for the purple bacteria. For a long time the green bacteria have been relatively ignored, but recently important advances have been made in elucidating their electron transport and membrane organization.

The antenna of purple bacteria varies in size between about 50 and 200 bacteriochlorophyll (BChl) molecules per reaction center. By use of detergents it is possible to solubilize the pigment-protein complexes of the photosynthetic membrane and to obtain pure antenna and reaction center complexes. The green bacteria, especially the 'classical' green sulfur bacteria (Chlorobiaceae) have a much larger antenna. Most of the antenna is contained in the chlorosomes, oval-shaped bodies that are adjacent to the cytoplasmic membrane. The chlorosomes contain BChl $\underline{c}$ or the related pigments BChl $\underline{d}$ or $\underline{e}$. BChl $\underline{a}$ and the reaction center are contained in the cytoplasmic membrane. This membrane does not appear to contain separate reaction center-protein complexes. The smallest complex obtained so far (the 'core' complex) contains about 20 BChl $\underline{a}$ molecules and it seems likely that the reaction center is an intrinsic part of this complex.

The gliding green bacteria (Chloroflexaceae) occupy an intermediary position. They have chlorosomes that contain BChl $\underline{c}$, but their membrane organization is similar to that of purple bacteria, and isolated reaction centers, with properties similar to those of purple bacteria, have recently been obtained.

Proceedings of the 16th FEBS Congress
Part B, pp. 3–8
© 1985 VNU Science Press

For a comprehensive review of various aspects of bacterial photosynthesis we refer to ref. 1.

ELECTRON TRANSPORT IN GREEN BACTERIA

Recent studies have shown that the reaction center of green sulfur bacteria is in many respects similar to that of system I of green plants. The primary electron donor is called P840. Optical and ESR measurements [2] provided evidence that two iron-sulfur centers function as secondary electron acceptors, with midpoint potentials of approximately -560 mV and > -400 mV, respectively. Photoaccumulation experiments at still lower redox potential indicated the reduction of BChl $\underline{a}$ absorbing at 814 nm [3]. Optical difference spectra in the nanosecond and picosecond region (ref. 4 and A.M. Nuijs et al., unpublished) indicate that the primary electron acceptor is bacteriopheophytin $\underline{c}$. In about 500 ps. the electron is transferred to a secondary acceptor, but so far there is no flash spectroscopic evidence that this acceptor would be BChl $\underline{a}$.

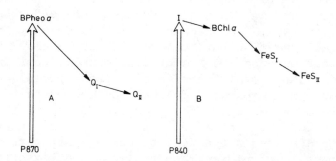

Fig. 1. Schemes for electron transport. A: purple bacteria and Chloroflexaceae; B: green sulfur bacteria. P870, P840: primary electron donors (in Chloroflexaceae denoted P865). Q_I and Q_{II}: quinones; FeS_I and FeS_{II}: iron-sulfur centers; BPheo $\underline{a}$: bacteriopheophytin $\underline{a}$; I: primary electron acceptor, probably bacteriopheophytin $\underline{c}$. The function of BChl $\underline{a}$ as electron acceptor is uncertain.

4

The electron acceptor chain of Chloroflexus has been found to be very similar to that of purple bacteria (see fig. 1A). Menaquinone functions as secondary electron acceptor [5], whereas the primary electron acceptor has been identified as bacteriopheophytin a [6]. The properties of the primary electron donor, P865, are similar to those of P870 of purple bacteria [6-8].

ANTENNA COMPLEXES

In addition to the reaction center, the photosynthetic membrane of purple bacteria contains antenna pigment-protein complexes (see ref. 1 for a review). The antenna complexes of Rhodopseudomonas sphaeroides have been most extensively investigated. Information about the orientation of the pigments was obtained by measurement of linear dichroism and fluorescence polarization, while in some cases the distances between the pigment molecules could be estimated from measurements of energy transfer.

The B800-850 complex contains BChl a absorbing at 850 nm and at 800 nm in a ratio of 2 : 1. A negative polarization for BChl a 850 fluorescence was observed upon excitation in the Q_x band at 600 nm (as for BChl in vitro) and a relatively small positive value of 0.14 upon excitation at 800 or 850 nm. This can be explained by an arrangement of the porphyrin rings of BChl 850 in such a way that the Q_y transitions (850 nm) are all approximately in one plane, while the Q_x transitions are perpendicular to that plane. However, upon measurement of the weak BChl 800 fluorescence at low temperature, a positive p-value upon excitation in the Q_x band is observed [9]. This can be explained by an arrangement with at least two BChl 800 molecules in one subunit. The porphyrin rings of these BChl 800 molecules are approximately in one plane, with the Q_y (and thus also the Q_x) transitions perpendicular to each other. Energy transfer between the BChl 800 molecules must be fast enough as to obtain equilibrium before energy transfer to BChl 850 takes place. These and other optical studies, together with the data on the primary structure result in the model [9] for B800-850 shown in fig. 2.

5

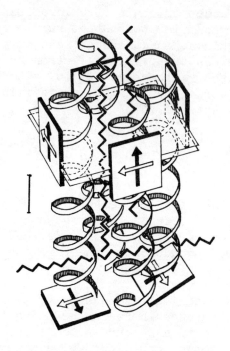

Fig. 2. Model of the B800–850 complex. The upper squares
are the porphyrin rings of BChl 850, the lower ones of
BChl 800. Open and solid arrows: Q_y and Q_x transitions,
respectively. Zig-zag lines are carotenoids (spheroidene)
and the spirals are the α-helices of the peptides. The
plane of the membrane is horizontal. The bar represents
5 Å.

   In the other complex of Rps. sphaeroides, B875, the arrangement of the BChl molecules is probably roughly the
same as of BChl 850. However, the fluorescence polarization shows characteristics that were not encountered in
B800–850. As can be seen in fig. 3, on the short-wave side
of the B875 band the p-value is close to that of BChl 850,
but it increases sharply across the band to a value of
0.4. In membranes of Rps. sphaeroides (wild type and R-26),
and of Rhodospirillum rubrum the effect is only observed
at low temperature [10]. Computer simulation shows that
it can be explained by assuming that one of the six BChl
molecules that are thought to form the basic unit (R.A.

6

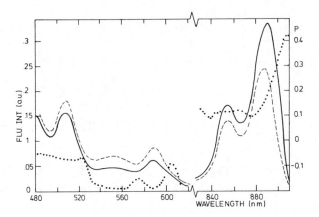

Fig. 3. Excitation spectra (4 K) of membranes from Rps. sphaeroides with the fluorescence measured parallel (solid line) or perpendicular (dashed line) to the polarization of the excitation beam. Detection at 915 nm. Right-hand scale: degree of polarization, p (dotted line).

Niederman et al., unpublished) absorbs at 12 nm longer wavelength [10]. At room temperature, the fluorescence is depolarized by energy transfer, but this energy transfer does not occur at low temperature. A heterogeneity of the B875 complex of R. rubrum was recently also suggested by others. For a discussion we refer to ref. 10.

The investigations were supported by the Netherlands Organization for the Advancement of Pure Research (ZWO) via the Foundations for Chemical Research (SON) and for Biophysics.

REFERENCES

1. Amesz, J. and Knaff, D.B. (1985). Molecular mechanisms of bacterial photosynthesis. In: Environmental Micro- biology of Anaerobes, A.J.B. Zehnder (ed.). John Wiley, New York, to be published.
2. Swarthoff, T., Gast, P., Hoff, A.J. and Amesz, J. (1981). An optical and ESR investigation of the ac-

ceptor side of the reaction center of the green photo-synthetic bacterium <u>Prosthecochloris aestuarii</u>. FEBS Lett. 130, 93-98.

3. Swarthoff, T., Gast, P., van der Veek-Horsley, K.M., Hoff, A.J. and Amesz, J. (1981) Evidence for photo-reduction of monomeric bacteriochlorophyll <u>a</u> as an electron acceptor in the reaction center of the green photosynthetic bacterium <u>Prosthecochloris aestuarii</u>. FEBS Lett. 131, 331-334.

4. Van Bochove, A.C., Swarthoff, T., Kingma, H., Hof, R.M., van Grondelle, R., Duysens, L.N.M. and Amesz, J. (1984). A study of the primary charge separation in green bacteria by means of flash spectroscopy. Biochim. Biophys. Acta 764, 343-346.

5. Vasmel, H. and Amesz, J. (1983). Photoreduction of menaquinone in the reaction center of the green photo-synthetic bacterium <u>Chloroflexus aurantiacus</u>. Biochim. Biophys. Acta 724, 118-122.

6. Kirmaier, C., Holten, D., Mancino, L.J. and Blanken-ship, R.E. (1984). Picosecond photodichroism studies on reaction centers from the green photosynthetic bac-terium <u>Chloroflexus aurantiacus</u>. Biochim. Biophys. Acta 765, 138-146.

7. Vasmel, H., Meiburg, R.F., Kramer, H.J.M., de Vos, L.J. and Amesz, J. (1983). Optical properties of the photosynthetic reaction center of <u>Chloroflexus auran-tiacus</u> at low temperature. Biochim. Biophys. Acta 724, 333-339.

8. Den Blanken, H.J., Vasmel, H., Jongenelis, A.P.J.M., Hoff, A.J. and Amesz, J. (1983). The triplet state of the primary donor of the green photosynthetic bacteri-um <u>Chloroflexus aurantiacus</u>. FEBS Lett. 161, 185-189.

9. Kramer, H.J.M., van Grondelle, R., Hunter, C.N., Wes-terhuis, W.H.J. and Amesz, J. (1984). Pigment organi-zation of the B800-850 antenna complex of <u>Rhodopseudo-monas sphaeroides</u>. Biochim. Biophys. Acta 765,156-165.

10. Kramer, H.J.M., Pennoyer, J.D., van Grondelle, R., Westerhuis, W.H.J., Niederman, R.A. and Amesz, J. (1984). Low-temperature optical properties and pigment organization of the B875 light-harvesting bacterio-chlorophyll-protein complex of purple photosynthetic bacteria. Biochim. Biophys. Acta, in press.

8

PROTEIN–PROTEIN AND PROTEIN–LIPID INTERACTIONS AND THE REGULATION OF ELECTRON FLOW IN PHOTOSYNTHESIS

J. BARBER
Department of Pure & Applied Biology, Imperial College,
London, SW7 2BB, U.K.

INTRODUCTION

During the past two or three years we have witnessed a
considerable growth in our understanding of the relationship between the structure of the chloroplast thylakoid
membrane and its function as an energy converting system.
This recent knowledge has come from improved techniques in
protein and nucleic acid biochemistry but the detailed
application of optical and resonance spectroscopy has also
played an important role. No longer do we have to discuss
electron flow in photosynthesis just in terms of redox potentials as depicted in the Z-scheme (1). We can now define
discrete structural units embedded in the thylakoid membrane which together act as a water–NADP oxidoreductase
and ATP synthetase. Five different super-molecular protein
complexes have been identified; photosystem one (PS1),
photosystem two (PS2), cytochrome b_6-f (cyt b_6-f), light
harvesting chlorophyll a/b protein closely associated with
PS2 (LHCP2) and the coupling factor (CF_0-CF_1) complexes (2).

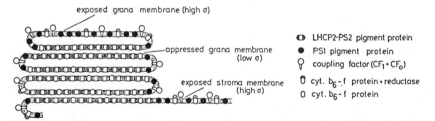

exposed grana membrane (high σ)

appressed grana membrane (low σ)

exposed stroma membrane (high σ)

◖ LHCP2-PS2 pigment protein
● PS1 pigment protein
♀ coupling factor ($CF_1 \cdot CF_0$)
◘ cyt. b_6-f protein + reductase
○ cyt. b_6-f protein

FIG.1 A diagrammatic representation of the possible distribution of super-molecular complexes in the thylakoid
membrane. It is proposed that the structure is maintained
by an asymetric distribution of electrical charge density
(σ) on the outer membrane surface as shown (3,4).

Several lines of evidence suggest that the five super-

Proceedings of the 16th FEBS Congress
Part B, pp. 9–20
© 1985 VNU Science Press

molecular complexes are not randomly distributed in the plane of the membrane (see Fig.1). Both from consideration of surface electrical charge distribution (3,4) and from membrane fragmentation studies (5-8) a model has emerged suggesting that LHCP2 and PS2 complexes are preferentially localized in the appressed thylakoid membranes which form the partition of the grana while PS1 and CF_o-CF_1 complexes are located in the non-appressed membranes which constitute the stromal and end-granal lamellae and have their external surfaces directly exposed to the stromal phase. The location of the cyt b_6-f complex is less certain and could be: (i) evenly distributed in both membrane regions (9,10), (ii) preferentially arranged at the interface between appressed and non-appressed regions, often called margins (2,11) or (iii) located only in the non-appressed regions (12). The recent finding that the cyt b_6-f complex can have NADP-ferredoxin associated with it (13) may indicate that there are two populations of this complex which give rise to its apparent even distribution between appressed and non-appressed membranes as suggested in refs. 9, 10 and as illustrated in Fig.1. In this case it is proposed that the partitioning between the two membrane regions would be governed by the difference in the exposed surface properties of the two populations.

CONSEQUENCES OF LATERAL SEPARATION

a) Electron transport and phosphorylation
The super-molecular protein complexes shown in Fig.1 must co-operate together to extract electrons and protons from water and pass them to NADP while at the same time bringing about the net synthesis of ATP. Because of the lateral separation of the major complexes, long range electron/proton transfer must occur. As shown in Fig.2, PS2 acts as a H_2O-plastoquinone (PQ) oxido-reductase. The reduced plastoquinone molecules (PQH_2) are able to diffuse laterally to their site of oxidation on the cyt b_6-f complex. It is highly likely that, because of their hydrophobicity and long isoprenoid side chain, PQH_2 and PQ partition into the midplane of the lipid matrix of the membrane (14). At the bilayer midplane the resistance to lateral motion is

at its minimum and the diffusion coefficient could be as high as 10^{-6} to 10^{-7} cm^2 s^{-1}.

FIG.2

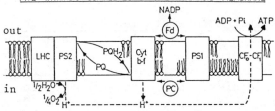

FIVE INTRINSIC COMPLEXES OF THE THYLAKOID MEMBRANE

According to Einstein's equation $<x^2> = 4Dt$ (where $<x>$ is the mean distance of diffusion in time (t) when the coefficient is D) PQ and PQH$_2$ could diffuse over very large distances in 1 or 2 ms and therefore satisfy the known kinetics of PQH$_2$ oxidation (t$_\frac{1}{2}$ 15 to 20 ms) even if there are many hundreds of nm between PS2 and the cyt b_6-f complex (14). These considerations, and also direct spectroscopic measurements (15), seem to suggest that under physiological conditions photosynthetic electron flow is not rate limited by PQ/PQH$_2$ diffusion but rather by the oxidation of PQH$_2$. The oxidation of PQH$_2$ occurs at a quinol/ quinone binding site within the cyt b_6-f complex and electrons are then passed to plastocyanin (PC), which is an extrinsic protein assumed to diffuse laterally along the membrane inner surface to an oxidation site on the PS1 complex generated by the photoactivation of P700, the reaction centre chlorophyll. The reduced stabilised product of PS1 is soluble ferredoxin (Fd) which can either reduce NADP or act as an electron source for cyclic electron flow via the cyt b_6-f complex. Since under normal conditions the diffusion of PQ/PQH$_2$, PC or Fd seems not to be rate limiting (15) then the separation of PS2 and PS1 into discrete domains has no serious consequences on the kinetics of electron flow. However, under certain conditions the situation could change, for example, at low temperatures the lateral diffusional processes will be slowed and may well become dominating in the control of electron flow.

   As shown in Fig.2 the oxidation of water and PQH$_2$ at the inner thylakoid membrane surface results in the release of protons. As a consequence of this, protons may become delocalized so that the free energy due to the establishment of an electrochemical potential gradient becomes available to synthesise ATP at the CF_0-CF_1 complex, as visualized in Mitchell's chemiosmotic hypothesis (16).

b) Energy transfer and regulation of electron transport
It seems very likely that the lateral separation of PS2 and PS1, and therefore the existence of appressed and non-appressed membrane regions, is the basis for finely controlling the efficiency of photosynthetic electron flow. Bonaventura and Myers (17), showed for the first time many years ago that a mechanism existed in the green alga *Chlorella* to optimise photosynthesis in response to changing light conditions. The phenomenon is now known as the State 1-State 2 transition and can also be detected in higher plants (18). State 2 is a 'low Emerson enhancement state' whereby some of the light absorbed by the pigments normally associated with PS2 is redirected in favour of PS1 so that a better balance is struck between the turn-over of the two photosystems. State 1 is a 'high Emerson enhancement state' which is created in excess PS1 light. It now seems clear that the State transitions are controlled by phosphorylation/dephosphorylation of the exposed outer surface of the LHCP2 complex (19-21). In excess PS2 light over-reduction of the PQ pool induces the activation of a membrane bound kinase and subsequent phosphorylation of LHCP2. As a result of this there is a change in energy distribution in favour of PS1, a reoxidation of the PQ pool and an increase in the quantum efficiency of PS1 reactions (22). Thus, the phosphorylation of LHCP2 leads to the State 2 condition which is more efficient when the incident radiation is preferentially absorbed by PS2. If the PQ pool becomes over-oxidised, for example, in excess PS1 light, kinase activity is inhibited and dephosphorylation of LHCP2 occurs via a membrane bound phosphatase. This is now the State 1 condition where any PS2 light is preferentially directed to P680 and a significant imbalance between PS2 and PS1 would be detected when terminating the additional PS1 light. Such a control mechanism clearly has important implications for light absorption by plants and algae where light quality and intensity changes occur at different depths in the vegetation canopy and algal bloom.

It seems that surface electrical charge changes due to
the phosphorylation/dephosphorylation of LHCP2 alters the
coulombic and Van der Waals forces acting between the surfaces of adjacent protein complexes and membranes (21,23).
The consequence of this is to induce lateral diffusion of
phosphorylated LHCP2 complexes from the appressed to non-
appressed regions so that they become more intimate with
PS1 (see Fig.3)

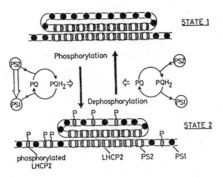

FIG.3 A diagrammatic representation of how phosphorylat-
ion/dephosphorylation of LHCP2 controls its spatial relationship with PS1 so as to optimise electron flow.

Thus the movement of LHCP2 would be expected to be accompanied by some membrane unstacking as shown in Fig.3.
Because the phosphorylation induced conformational changes
seem to be under the control of electrostatics, then the
degree of intermixing of LHCP2, LHCP2-PS2 and PS1 complexes, and also the change in the ratio of area of appressed
to non-appressed membranes, would be expected to depend on
the background level of cations. We have shown this to be
the case for isolated thylakoids both for changes in energy distribution (24) and for thylakoid stacking changes
(25). When electrostatic screening is high (e.g. $|Mg^{2+}|$ >
5 mM), protein phosphorylation induces very little unstacking and energy transfer changes involve mainly alterations in absorption cross-sections of the two photosystems
due to lateral diffusion of LHCP2. With lower levels of
screening cations (e.g. $|Mg^{2+}|$ <5 mM), the effect of phos-
phorylation is to induce significant unstacking with sufficient intermixing of PS2, LHCP2 and PS1 complexes to increase energy transfer between PS2 and PS1, as well as

changes in absorption cross-sections. It has yet to be determined how the interplay of background cations and LHCP2 phosphorylation relate precisely to the *in vivo* State 1-State 2 transition.

PROTEIN COMPLEXES

In the space available it is not possible to discuss in detail the structure and properties of each super-molecular complex. Fig.4 is an attempt, however, to diagrammatically summarise our present day understanding of the organisation of the individual complexes. With the exception of LHCP2 which is a major thylakoid protein, each complex is composed of several different polypeptides, some of which are encoded for in the nuclear genome and some in the chloroplast genome (see Fig.4 below).

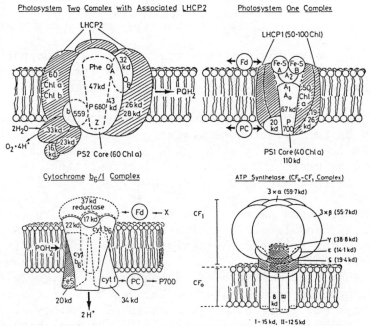

FIG.4 Diagrammatic representation of the structure of the super-molecular complexes of the thylakoid membrane. Shaded polypeptides are nuclear encoded while the others are products of the chloroplast genome.

14

The PS2 complex contains at least three polypeptides involved directly with water oxidation; 16,23 and 33 kd (26), a 47 kd reaction centre protein containing the special chlorophyll P680, the primary acceptors, pheophytin (Phe) and bound quinone, Q_A, and the primary donor Z, also thought to be a quinone (27). The PS2 complex also contains cytochrome $b-559$ with a subunit size of 10 kd (28), a light harvesting core pigment protein of 43 kd and plastoquinone/ herbicide binding protein (Q_B protein) of 32 kd. The amino acid sequence of the 47 kd protein have recently been determined from molecular genetics (29,30) and folding patterns predicted. The cyt b_6-f complex also contains several polypeptides of molecular weights shown in Fig.4. The Reiski protein (FeS) is the site of PQH2 oxidation while the cytochrome f polypeptide acts as the electron donor to PC. The two cytochromes $b-563$ (cyt b_6) are probably involved in cyclic electron flow and/or 'Q-cycling' (31,32) while the 17 kd polypeptide seems to be an intimate associate to the 22 kd cyt b_6 protein (33). A fifth polypeptide of molecular weight 37 kd is suggested to be Fd-NADP oxido-reductase (13). The amino acid sequence of the 34, 22 and 17 kd proteins have been determined with the notable characteristics that the hydropathy plots of the 22 and 17 kd proteins match closely those of the cyt b protein of mitochrondia (31,33). The 23 kd cyt f polypeptide is unusual in having only one obvious transmembrane segment (34).

The PS1 complex has a 67 kd reaction centre polypeptide which contains P700 and primary acceptors of unknown identity. The reaction centre is served by several light harvesting pigment proteins, one of which contains a low level of chlorophyll b and is now termed LHCP1. Other main components are the secondary iron-sulphur containing acceptors (Fe-S) and a 20 kd protein which probably binds PC. Amino acid sequence of some of these polypeptides are being determined using recombinant DNA techniques (35). Like the other complexes the detailed structure of CF_0-CF_1 is being actively investigated and is envisaged as a combination of several sub-units as shown in Fig.4.

The LHCP2 complex is usually closely associated with PS2 as shown in Fig.4 and consists of polypeptides of about 26 and 28 kd which are coded for in the nucleus. The organisation of one of the polypeptides in the membrane has been predicted from its amino acid sequence (36) and from image reconstruction of serial electron microscopy (37).

POLAR LIPIDS

The polar lipids of the thylakoid membrane are dominated by the electroneutral galactolipids, monogalactosyldiacylglycerol (MGDG) and digalactosyldiacylglycerol (DGDG). The other polar lipids represent only 20% of the total and are mainly the acidic lipids, phosphatidylglycerol (PQ) and sulphoquinovosyldiacylglycerol (SQDG). The major lipid class is MGDG, which in its isolated state does not form bilayers but prefers the hexagonal type-II structure (38). This property is a consequence of its head group size and degree of unsaturation and it seems likely that its main role in the thylakoid membrane is to maintain optimal packing of the super-molecular complexes into the bilayer (38). Indeed, recently we have shown that MGDG is necessary to have maximum activity of the CF_0-CF_1 complex (39). Another striking characteristic of the polar lipids is their very high degree of unsaturation (approx. 80% of acyl chains with three double bonds). Such a high unsaturation level seems to give rise to a very fluid membrane according to fluorescence anisotropy measurements (40) and thus is a suitable environment for the lateral diffusion processes of electron transfer and the State 1-State 2 transitions.

CONCLUSIONS

Clearly the recent advances in our knowledge can now be used to describe the structural-functional relationships of the thylakoid membrane in the true spirit of the Fluid-Mosaic model of Singer and Nicolson (2). Within the last year or so, gene sequencing of key polypeptides has helped to predict tertiary structures within the intrinsic complexes. The recent crystallization of the isolated reaction centre from the photosynthetic bacterium *Rhodopseudomonas viridis* together with diffraction studies down to 2·5 Å resolution (41) also heralds a new era for obtaining structural information. An important concept which

16

has also emerged recently is the fact that the structure of the thylakoid membrane is not rigid as depicted in Fig. 1, but has dynamic organisation responding to changes in environmental conditions.

REFERENCES

1. Hill, R. and Bendall, F. (1960). Function of the two cytochrome components in chloroplasts: a working hypothesis. Nature 139, 136-137.
2. Barber, J. (1983). Photosynthetic electron transport in relation to thylakoid membrane composition and organization. Plant, Cell and Environment 6, 311-322. •
3. Barber, J. (1980). An explanation for the relationship between salt-induced thylakoid stacking and chlorophyll fluorescence changes associated with changes in spillover of energy from photosystem II to photosystem I. FEBS Lett. 118, 1-10.
4. Barber, J. (1980). Membrane surface charges and potentials in relation to photosynthesis. Biochim. Biophys. Acta 594, 253-308
5. Boardman, N.K. and Anderson, J.M. (1964). Isolation from spinach chloroplasts of particles containing different proportions of chlorophyll a and chlorophyll b and their possible role in the light reactions of photosynthesis. Nature 203, 166-167.
6. Vernon, L.P., Shaw, E.R., Ogawa, T. and Raveed, D. (1971). Structure of photosystem I and photosystem II of plant chloroplasts. Photochem. Photobiol. 14, 343-357.
7. Andersson, B. (1978). Separation of spinach chloroplast lamellae fragments by phase partition including isolation of inside-out thylakoids. Thesis, University of Lund, Sweden.
8. Anderson, J.M. and Andersson, B. (1982) The architecture of photosynthetic membranes: lateral and transverse organisation. Trends in Biochem. Sci. 7, 288-292.
9. Cox, R.P. and Andersson, B. (1981). Lateral and transverse organisation of cytochromes in the chloroplast thylakoid membrane. Biochem. Biophys. Res. Comm. 103, 1336-1341.

10. Anderson, J.M. (1982). Distribution of the cytochromes of spinach chloroplasts between the appressed membranes of grana stacks and the stroma-exposed thylakoid regions. FEBS Lett. 138, 62-66.
11. Ghirardi, M.L. and Melis, A. (1983). Localization of photosynthetic electron transport components in mesophyll and bundle sheath chloroplasts from Zea mays. Arch. Biochem. Biophys. 224, 19-28.
12. Henry, L.E.A. and Møller, B.L.(1981). Polypeptide composition of an oxygen evolving photosystem II vesicle from spinach chloroplasts. Carlsberg Research Comm. 46, 227-242.
13. Clark, R.D. and Hind, G. (1983). Isolation of a five-polypeptide cytochrome b-f complex from spinach chloroplasts. J. Biol. Chem. 258, 10348-10354.
14. Millner, P.A. and Barber, J. (1984). Plastoquinone as a mobile redox carrier in the photosynthetic membrane FEBS Lett. 169, 1-6.
15. Haehnel, W. (1984). Photosynthetic electron transport in higher plants. Ann. Rev. Plant Physiol. 35, 659-693.
16. Mitchell, P. (1961).Coupling of phosophorylation to electron and hydrogen transfer by a chemiosmotic type of mechanism. Nature 191, 144-148.
17. Bonaventura, C. and Myers, J. (1969).Fluorescence and oxygen evolution from Chlorella pyrenoidosa. Biochim. Biophys. Acta 189, 366-383.
18. Canaani, O., Barber, J. and Malkin, S. (1984). Evidence that phosphorylation and dephosphorylation regulates the distribution of excitation energy between the two photosystems of photosynthesis in vivo. Proc. Nat. Acad. Sci. U.S.A. 81, 1614-1618.
19. Allen, J.F., Bennett, J., Steinback, K.E. and Arntzen, C.J. (1981). Chloroplast protein phosphorylation couples plastoquinone redox state to distribution of excitation energy between photosystems. Nature, 291, 21-25.
20. Horton, P. and Black, M.T. (1980). Activation of adenosine 5'-triphosphate induced quenching of chlorophyll fluorescence by reduced plastoquinone. The basis of State 1-State 2 transitions in chloroplasts FEBS Lett. 119, 141-144.

21. Barber, J. (1983). Membrane conformational changes due to phosphorylation and the control of energy transfer in photosynthesis. Photobiochem. Photobiophys. 5, 181-190.
22. Telfer, A., Bottin, H., Barber, J. and Mathis, P. (1984). The effect of magnesium and phosphorylation of the light-harvesting chlorophyll a/b protein on the yield of P700-photooxidation in pea chloroplasts Biochim. Biophys. Acta 764, 324-330.
23. Barber, J. (1982) Influence of surface charges on thylakoid structure and function. Ann. Rev. Plant Physiol. 33, 261-295.
24. Telfer, A., Hodges, M. and Barber, J. (1983). Analysis of chlorophyll fluorescence induction curves in the presence of DCMU as a function of magnesium concentration and NADPH activated LHC phosphorylation. Biochim. Biophys. Acta 724, 167-175.
25. Telfer, A., Hodges, M., Millner, P.A. and Barber, J.(in press). The cation dependence of the degree of protein phosphorylation-induced unstacking of pea thylakoids. Biochim. Biophys. Acta.
26. Barber, J. (1984).Has the mangano-protein of the water splitting reaction of photosynthesis been isolated? Trends in Biochem. Sci. 9, 79-80.
27. O'Malley, P.J. and Babcock, G.T. (1984) The molecular origin of EPR signal II. Biochim. Biophys. Acta 765, 370-379.
28. Widger, W.R., Cramer, W.A., Herrmann, R.G. and Trebst, A. (1984). Sequence homology and structural similarity between cytochrome b of mitochrondrial complex III and the chloroplast b$_6$-f complex: position of the cytochrome b hemes in the membrane. Proc. Nat. Acad. Sci. U.S.A. 81, 674-678.
29. Zurawski, G., Bohnert, H.J., Whitfeld, P.R. and Bottomley, W. (1982). Nucleotide sequence of the gene for the Mr 32,000 thylakoid membrane protein from Spinacia oleracea and Nicotianna debneyi predicts a totally conserved primary translation product of Mr 38,950. Proc. Nat. Acad. Sci. U.S.A. 79, 7699-7703.
30. Morris, J. and Herrmann, R.G. (1984) Nucleotide sequence of the gene for the P680 chlorophyll apoprotein of the photosystm II reaction centre from spinach.

Nucleic Acid Res. 12, 2837–2850.

31. Barber, J. (1984). Further evidence for the common an-
cestry of cytochrome b–c complexes. Trends in Biochem. Sci. 9, 79–80.

32. Hauska, G., Hurt, E., Gabellini, N. and Lockau, W.
(1983).Comparative aspects of quinol-cytochrome c/
plastocyanin oxidoreductases. Biochim. Biophys. Acta
726, 97–133.

33. Metz, J.G., Ulmer, G., Brickes, T.M. and Miles, D.
(1983). Purification of cytochrome b–559 from oxyden
evolving photosystem II preparations from spinach
and maize. Biochim. Biophys. Acta 725, 203–209.

34. Willey, D.L. and Gray, J.C. (1983). Location and nucleotide sequence of the gene for cytochrome f in pea
and wheat chloroplast DNA. In Advances in Photosynthesis Res. C. Sybesma (ed) Martinus Nijhoff/Dr W.
Junk, The Hague. Vol.IV, pp. 567–570.

35. Herrmann, R.G., Alt, J., Westhoff, J.T., Morris, J.,
Olesch, B. and Nelson, N. (1984). Organisation and
expression of genes for thylakoid membrane polypeptides. NATO Advanced Studies. Instit. Molecular Form
and Function of the Plant Genome. Abst. L20.

36. Thornber, J.P. personal communication.

37. Kuhlbrandt, W. (1984). Three-dimensional structure of
the light-harvesting chlorophyll a/b-protein complex.
Nature 307, 478–480.

38. Gounaris, K. and Barber, J. (1983) Monogalactosyldiacylglycerol: The most abundant polar lipid in Nature.
Trends in Biochem. Sci. 8, 378–381.

39. Pick, U., Gounaris, K., Admon, A. and Barber, J.(1984).
Activation of the CF_0-CF_1, ATP synthase from spinach
chloroplasts by chloroplast lipids. Biochim. Biophys.
Acta 765, 12–20.

40. Ford, R.C. and Barber, J. (1983). Time dependent decay
and anisotropy of fluorescence from diphenyl hexatr-
iene embedded in the chloroplast thylakoid membrane.
Biochim. Biophys. Acta 722, 341–348.

41. Michel, H., Deisenhofer, J., Miki, K. and Epp, O.
(1984). High resolution X-ray structure of photosynthetic reaction centres from Rhodopseudomonas viridis
3rd Eur. Bioenerg. Conf. Hannover, Germany. 3A, 29–30

THE ROLE OF CHLORIDE IN OXYGEN EVOLUTION

W. COLEMAN AND GOVINDJEE
University of Illinois, 289 Morrill Hall
505 S. Goodwin Ave., Urbana, IL 61801 (U.S.A.)

INTRODUCTION

Almost exactly 40 years ago, Warburg and Lüttgens (1) published a report on the ability of various anions to stimulate photosynthetic oxygen evolution in dialyzed chloroplasts. They reported that Cl^-, Br^-, I^-, and NO_3^- were effective (although Cl^- was the most effective), whereas rhodanide, SO_4^- and PO_4^{3-} were ineffective in restoring the Hill reaction. Later, Warburg and Lüttgens (2) examined further the anion specificity and noted that the effect saturated at 7 mM KCl. Several years later, amid controversy concerning the importance of Cl^- to photosynthesis in vivo (see refs. 3-5 for a discussion), Gorham and Clendenning (6) demonstrated that Cl^- is directly involved in stimulating the water-splitting reaction, and that it does not simply overcome the injurious effects of exposure to light. Most important, they demonstrated that adding Cl^- to depleted chloroplasts shifts the pH optimum of the Hill reaction to the alkaline side. They also noted that the stimulatory effect of Cl^- is similar to that found for dialyzed α-amylase, and that these two processes might share a common physical basis. The conclusion of Warburg and Lüttgens that Cl^- is a necessary cofactor for O_2 evolution is now the foundation for intensive study of the O_2-evolving complex (OEC) of Photosystem II (PSII) (see refs. 5, 7-9). After 40 years of research, however, the mechanism by which Cl^- activates O_2 evolution still remains a mystery.

Proceedings of the 16th FEBS Congress
Part B, pp. 21–28
© 1985 VNU Science Press

There have been relatively few detailed suggestions about how Cl^- functions in the OEC. Any proposed mechanism for Cl^- function must also explain the following: (1) Inactivation by Cl^- depletion is reversible (10,11); (2) Cl^--depletion is accelerated by incubating the thylakoids at high pH (7) and by adding uncouplers (12); (3) Cl^--binding is pH-dependent and reversible (13); (4) activation of the Hill reaction by added Cl^- shows hyperbolic kinetics, indicating saturation (11); (5) activation of the Hill reaction by anions is relatively specific for Cl^-, but not exclusive (2,10,11,13); and (6) the pH optimum of the Hill reaction is shifted to more alkaline pH by Cl^--binding (6,10,14). There are several possible roles for Cl^- in the mechanism of the water-splitting reactions, some of which have already been described (see 7-9,15,16). However, because of the lack of information about Cl^- binding at the molecular level, most of these suggestions must be considered as merely working hypotheses.

The model described here involves a dual role for Cl^-: (1) indirect activation of base catalysis (activation of H^+ removal from water) at the active site of the OEC (33kD-Mn-containing polypeptide(s), referred to as "proteins" hereafter) (Fig. 1A); and (2) activation of H^+ binding at other sites (e.g., at 24 and 18 kD proteins) (Fig. 1B). This kind of role is consistent with the known action of Cl^- (and other anions) in soluble enzymes. The key to this model is the ability of anions to shift the pk_a's of essential reactive groups in enzymes by suppressing adjacent positive charges on other groups. This behavior has been suggested to explain the effect of anions on the velocity-pH curves of salivary amylase and fumarate hydratase (17).

The mechanism at the active site (Fig. 1A) involves two ionized groups on the protein, which is consistent

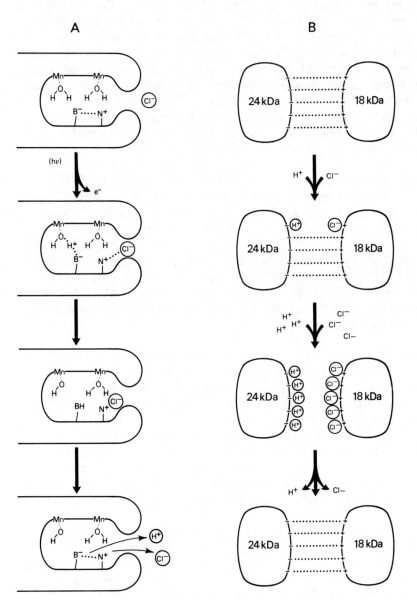

Figure 1. A Model for Cl^- Activation of O_2 Evolution in which Binding of the Anion Induces Shifts in the Apparent pk_a's of Reactive Groups on the Polypeptides of the O_2 Evolving Complex (see text for details).

with the bell-shaped velocity-pH curve for O_2 evolution. The group with the lower pK_a (the conjugate base of a weak acid) is labeled as B^-, and the group with the higher pK_a (for example, an amino group) is labeled as N^+. In its simplest form, the mechanism could operate as follows: a molecule of water is proposed to be bound to a Mn atom in the active site. The Mn serves to orient and polarize the water molecule, which facilitates removal of the protons (H^+s) (see ref. 18 for a discussion of Mn in yeast aldolase).

While the Mn (which is oxidized as a result of the light reaction) extracts an electron from water, B^- extracts a proton. We suggest that the group B^- would be able to temporarily bind this proton because the binding of Cl^- (or Br^-) to the positively charged group N^+ transiently raises the pK_a of B^-, and thus increases its affinity for the water proton. The Cl^- ion, therefore, would activate and control the rate of the water-splitting reaction by accelerating the removal of H^+s from water.

The net effect is similar to the model in ref. 8; here, Cl^- effectively stabilizes a "+" charge on the S states (preventing a back reaction) by moving it out onto the protein, even though Cl^- does not bind to the $Mn-H_2O$ complex directly. When the Cl^- unbinds from N^+ (either because its residence time is very short, as shown in 19, or because the incipient acidification of the lumen opens up new binding sites that draw the Cl^- away), the H^+ would be released from B^-, the salt bridge $B^-...^+N$ would re-form, and the cycle would be repeated.

Our model (Fig. 1A) explains the following: (1) the inactivation of O_2 evolution by Cl^--depletion is reversible (11), since the binding is electrostatic and does not require any complex architecture for the binding site; (2) Cl^- depletion is easier at high pH (7,12,20), since a pH > 8 would tend to deprotonate N^+; (3) the release of Cl^- is linked to the release of H^+s from the lumen (12,20); the coupling of Cl^- binding to H^+ binding is inherent in this model. This has also

been suggested to occur, for example, in ribonuclease
(21); (4) the stimulation of O_2 evolution by added Cl^-
(11) shows saturation kinetics, since Cl^- binding would
accelerate the catalysis of $2H_2O \longrightarrow O_2 + 4H^+$ until the
binding site becomes saturated and the turnover rate of
the OEC limits the reaction; (5) the effectiveness of
activation by an anion depends on its charge and ionic
radius (13); anions with a weak electric field (e.g., I^-)
would not effect the pk_a of B^- enough (by not supressing
N^+ sufficiently) to make the system reactive; those with
too strong a field (e.g., F^-) would tend not to unbind
as readily, and thus inhibit the turnover of the OEC;
(6) Cl^- is bound more tightly in the light, presumably
due to light-driven acidification of the lumen (12); the
lowering of the internal pH would tend to increase the
positive charge near N (cf. number 2) and thus increase
its affinity for Cl^-; and (7) the pH optimum of the Hill
reaction is shifted to more alkaline pH as more Cl^- is
added to Cl^--depleted thylakoids (6,10,14). In our
model, the alkaline shift would occur for two reasons:
(a) at a slightly acid pH in the presence of excess Cl^-,
the pK_a of BH is raised (relative to the Cl^- deficient
case) due to the neutralization of N^+ by Cl^-; this makes
B less reactive toward H_2O at slightly acid pH; and
(b) at slightly alkaline pH the binding of Cl^- to N^+
creates the more reactive species B^- (compared to the
unreactive B^-...N^+ which would prevail without Cl^-), and
stimulates the water-splitting reaction. The overall
effect is to shift the pH optimum for O_2 evolution to
the alkaline side in the presence of Cl^-.

There are several observations that the above model
alone cannot explain, and these exceptions have
interesting implications: First of all, there is
substantial Cl^- binding even in dark-adapted thylakoids.
Secondly, this binding appears to be associated with a
large, sequestered pool of bound H^+s, which remains even
in the dark, and which equilibrates with the bulk phase
only through the addition of uncouplers (20). Finally,
a plot of the Hill reaction rate vs. the concentration
of added Cl^- at low light intensity (W. Coleman, 1984
unpublished) does not give the smooth hyperbola that is

obtained at high light intensity, where it appears that a site (or sites) with a single binding affinity is saturated (11). Instead, the curve shows a "stair-step" dependence between 1 and 10 mM added Cl^-. Such a dependence has been observed for several enzymes (see e.g., refs. 17 and 22, for a discussion of this phenomenon). One hypothesis that has been proposed to explain this behavior is that these enzymes contain more than one binding site for the substrate, and these sites have different affinities (22). By analogy, therefore, we suggest that in spinach thylakoids there may be multiple Cl^- binding sites with different affinities. For this reason, we propose (Fig. 1B) that there may be a second set of Cl^- binding sites with a larger capacity and a slightly different function, namely, to assist in binding the protons released into the lumen (see ref. 12 for an earlier discussion). In this part of the model, Cl^- would promote the binding of H^+s at another site on the OEC. We suggest, as noted earlier, that this might involve binding to the 18 and 24 kD polypeptides. Here, again, Cl^- binds to amino groups and H^+ binds to negatively-charged groups (likely to be COO^- in this case).

The mechanism by which this system might operate (using, e.g., the 18 and 24 kD proteins) is as follows: At the slightly alkaline pH optimum for O_2 evolution, the two proteins would be oppositely charged based on measurements of their isoelectric points (see ref. 9 for a review). Thus, one could imagine that the excess positive charges on the 18 kD protein are at least partly neutralized by forming salt-bridges with the excess negative charges on the 24 kD protein. Discussion in (23) suggests that the 18 kD protein binds to the 24 kD protein. Light-driven H^+ pumping would tend to disturb this equilibrium by lowering the pH. The 24 kD protein would be able to bind the H^+s by breaking either some or all of the salt-bridges with the 18 kD protein, but in order to maintain charge balance, the 18 kD protein would be required to pick up a negatively charged counterion, such as Cl^-. As a result of this process, a considerable amount of "conformational" energy could be stored. This energy might also tend to stabilize the complex against denaturation. Such protection of the thylakoid membrane by Cl^- binding has been reported (see refs. 7,11,24). Binding of the H^+s would also tend to encourage H^+ pumping into the lumen, since the free $[H^+]$ would be kept at a minimum. As described earlier, activation of the ion binding is reciprocal: Cl^- stimulates the binding of H^+s and vice versa.

If the 18 and 24 kD proteins do have the role described above, it might not be as apparent in uncoupled thylakoids, and in PSII particles or inside-out vesicles, where the two proteins would not be operating in an enclosed space. However, the role of Cl^- at the OEC (Fig. 1A) would remain the same in all cases. Further research is needed to test our model.

REFERENCES

1   Warburg, O. and Lüttgens, W. (1944) Naturwiss. 32, 301.
2   Warburg, O. and Lüttgens, W. (1946) Biofizika 11, 303-321.
3   Rabinowitch, E.I. (1956) Photosynthesis and Related Processes, Vol. 2, part 2. Interscience Publishers, New York, see pp. 1549-1554.
4   Bové, J.M., Bové, C., Whatley, F.R. and Arnon, D.I. (1963) Z. Naturforsch. 18b, 683-688.
5   Critchley, C. (submitted, 1984) Biochim. Biophys. Acta, to be referred to as BBA hereafter.
6   Gorham, P.R. and Clendenning, K.A. (1952) Arch. Biochem. Biophys. 37, 199-223.
7   Izawa, S., Muallem, A. and Ramaswamy, N.K. (1983) In: The Oxygen-Evolving System of Photosynthesis, Y.Inoue, A.R. Crofts, Govindjee, N. Murata, G. Renger and K. Satoh (eds.). Academic Press, Tokyo, pp. 293-302.
8   Govindjee, Baianu, I.C., Critchley, C. and Gutowsky, H.S. (1983) See ref. 7 , pp. 303-315.

9   Govindjee, Kambara, T. and Coleman, W. (submitted, 1984) Photochem. Photobiol.
10 Hind, G., Nakatani, H.Y. and Izawa, S. (1969) BBA, 172, 277-289.
11 Kelley, P.M. and Izawa, S. (1978) BBA, 198-210.
12 Theg, S.M. and Homan, P.H. (1982) BBA, 679, 221-234.
13 Critchley, C., Baianu, I.C., Govindjee and Gutowsky, H.S. (1982) BBA, 682, 436-445.
14 Critchley, C. (1983) BBA, 724, 1-5.
15 Itoh, S., Yerkes, C.T., Koike, H., Robinson, H.H. and Crofts, A.R. (in press, 1984) BBA.
16 Theg, S.M., Jursinic, P. and Homann, P.H. (in press, 1984) BBA.
17 Dixon, M. and Webb, E.C. (1979) Enzymes, Third Edition. Academic Press, New York, pp. 395-407.
18 Horecker, B.L., Tsolas, O. and Lai, C.Y. (1972). In: The Enzymes, Third Edition, P.D. Boyer (ed.), Vol. 7, Academic Press, New York, pp. 213-258.
19 Baianu, I.C., Critchley, C., Govindjee and Gutowsky, H.S. (1984) Proc. Natl. Acad. Sci. U.S.A. 81, 3713-3717.
20 Theg, S.M., Johnson, J.D. and Homann, P.H. (1982) FEBS Lett. 145, 25-29.
21 Loeb, G.I. and Saroff, H.A. (1964) Biochem. 3, 1819-1826.
22 Lee, L.M.Y., Krupka, R.M. and Cook, R.A. (1973) Biochem. 12, 3503-3508.
23 Murata, N. and Miyao, M. (1983) See ref. 7, pp. 213-222.
24 Coleman, W.J., Baianu, I.C., Gutowsky, H.S. and Govindjee (1983). In: Advances in Photosynthesis Research, C. Sybesma, (ed.) Vol. I, Martinus Nijhoff/Dr. W. Junk Publishers, Den Haag, pp. 283-286.

THE MODELS OF PHOTOSYNTHETIC ELECTRON TRANSFER

A.A.KRASNOVSKY

A.N.Bakh Institute of Biochemistry, USSR
Academy of Sciences, Leninsky pr. 33,
Moscow, II707I, USSR

An attractive problem is the construction of
artificial solar energy convertors using the
knowledge of natural photosynthetic mechanisms.
As a result of excitation by light quantum of
pigment system electron is transferred from
donor to acceptor molecules thus solar energy
is converted and stored. The question arises
whether it is possible to use the energy of
charges separated in reaction centers of photosynthesis by short metabolic pathways with
minimal energy loss (I). For many years we were studying photo-redox reactions using various pigments, chlorophylls and analogs as pho-
tosensitizers, electron donors and electron
acceptors: NAD, NADP, methylviologen, ferredoxin possessing redox potential close to
hydrogen electrode. Photosensitized reduction
of electron acceptor coupled to oxydation of
electron donor was observed (review 2).

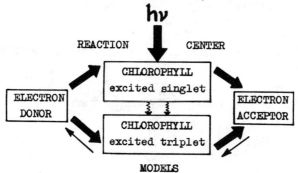

Proceedings of the 16th FEBS Congress
Part B, pp. 29–34
© 1985 VNU Science Press

If aqueous micelle solutions were used it was possible to employ a wide set of water soluble substances as electron donors and acceptors so as various chlorophyll analogues solubilized into detergent micelles. In systems outlined it is possible to introduce enzymes involved into action of short artificial electron-transfer chains. The first work in this field was performed in our laboratory: the construction of a system which composed of electron donor, solubilized chlorophyll, methylviologen as mediator and hydrogenase extracted from bacteria cells. In such a system under action of red light absorbed by chlorophyll it was possible to observe molecular hydrogen photoevolution (3).

The next system studied were liposomes containing lipophylic chlorophyllous pigments. The use of oxidized electron donor (ascorbic acid) inside liposome and reversible reduced acceptor (viologens) in outer space make it possible to compose charge-transfer systems having light energy storage (4). Into liposome membrane chlorophyll or pheophytin were introduced. Under action of light absorbed by pigments photoreduction of methylviologen was observed; in the case of pheophytin quantum yield was higher then with chlorophyll reaching up to 15%.

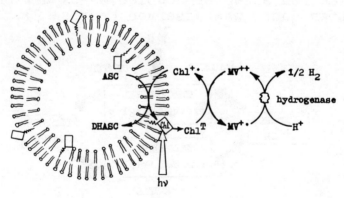

When sulfonated methylviologen was employed
(being dissolved in the form of negative ions)
the reaction efficiently was enhanced. Probably negative charged radical ion of sulfonated methylviologen is not able to penetrate
into membrane decreasing the speed of the
back reaction. Accumulation of reduced methylviologen (having redox potential close
to hydrogen electrode) is a prerequisite to
create photobiochemical systems evolving
molecular hydrogen. Really, when introducing
the enzyme hydrogenase it was possible to
observe hydrogen evolution. The hydrogenase
from sulfate reducing bacteria, having pronounced affinity to methylviologen was the
most active catalyst efficiently "pumping
out" reduced viologen in the course of its
formation. Probably it is possible to arrange
such a systems avoiding hydrogenase extraction when introducing bacterial cells into
liposomes as reduced viologen usually pene-
trates easilly through the cell walls.
    The next step on the way of complication
is to employ isolated chloroplasts. There
is a lot of works in this field when chloroplasts coupled to bacterial hydrogenase
evolved hydrogen in the presence of exogenous
electron donors (see review 5). It was revealed in our laboratory that a combination
of DTT and ascorbate in the presence of TMPD
makes possible to use practically full electron transfer capability of photosystem I in
chloroplasts.
    The main feature of the reaction mechanism
is probably that ascorbate donating electrones is maintained in reduced state by DTT
and TMPD is functions as a lipophylic intermediate carrying electron to the definite
site of electron transfer chain; viologen
accepts electron at the very end of photosystem I (6).

31

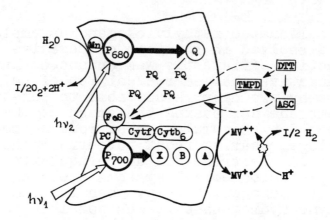

If photosystem I inside cloroplasts is
efficient a question inevitably arises whether
isolated particles of photosystem I would be
active as well. In such a preparation indeed
it was possible to observe viologen photoreduction and hydrogen evolution in the presence
of hydrogenase but the yield was low (7).
When a highly sensitive amperometric technique was used it was possible to reveal
hydrogen photoevolution by chloroplasts when
photosystem II was inhibited and electron
donor (hydroquinone) was introduced into the
site of photosystem II (8).
Coming back to creation of photobiochemical
models we should mention that for primary
charge separation inorganic photoreceptors
may serve as well. So, in our laboratory
a veriety of inorganic photocatalysts –
semiconductors – titanium dioxide, zink
oxide, tungsten trioxide and cadmium sulfide
were used. Under the action of light quantum
electron is shifted from the valence zone
into conduction zone and charge separated
may be localized on different active centers
of phase boundary of photocatalyst particles
suspended in the aqueous media. When introducing various water soluble electron donors
and acceptors into solution we managed to
realize a variety of redox reactions. So, in

our laboratory in I96I an inorganic model of
Hill reaction was created (9): as photocatalysts TiO_2, ZnO, WO_3 were used, as electron
acceptors ferrous compounds and quinones and
as electron donor - water milecules. Oxygen
was evolved and oxidants were reduced in
accord to stoichiometry of Hill reaction.
When methylviologen was introduced into water suspensions of photocatalysts under
anaerobic conditions illumination caused
viologen photoreduction even without exogenous electron donors which nevertheless enhanced reaction (IO). In any case in the
presence of exogenous electron donor photoevolution of hydrogen gas can be observed in
suspensions of TiO_2 and CdS as well (II).
Tris-buffer was a rather active electron
donor in this reaction (I2). Suspension of
TiO_2 in the presence of Tris-buffer, methylviologen and bacterial hydrogenase evolved
hydrogen under action of near UV (365 nm).
It was possible to simplify the system
using TiO_2 suspension in Tris-buffer with
Clostridia cells without exogenous electron
transfer mediator.

The question arises on the possible use of
photochemically induced electrons to reduce
not only hydrogen ions but also such stable
molecules as dinitrogen and carbon dioxide.

Hence another aspect of the problem considered here is to create model photobiochemical systems which could imitate ancient types
of solar energy transformation for the action
of primary selfreproducing molecular systems.

The final purpose of the studies presented
was firstly - to create efficient solar
energy convertors using the principles of
natural photosynthesis and secondly - to
get any information on possible pathways
of chemical and biological evolution of
solar energy conversion and storage (I3).

References:

1. Photochemical conversions. IOCD UNESCO.
   (1983). A.M.Braun (ed.). Lauzanne.
2. Krasnovsky, A.A. (1974). Light energy conversion in photosynthesis; molecular mechanisms. Nauka. Moskva (in Russian).
3. Krasnovsky, A.A., V.V.Nikandrov et al.
   (1975). Dokl. Akad. Nauk SSSR. 225, 711-
   713 (in Russian).
4. Krasnovsky, A.A., A.N.Semenova, V.V.Nikan-
   drov. (1982). Photobiochem. Photobiophys.
   4, 227-232.
5. Krasnovsky, A.A. (1979). Topics in photosynthesis. J.Barber (ed.). Elsevier,
   Amsterdam, pp. 281-298.
6. Krasnovsky, A.A., Chan-van-Ni, V.V.Nikan-
   drov, G.P.Brin. (1980). Plant Physiol.
   66, 925-930.
7. Nikandrov,V.V., A.I.Aristarchov, A.A.Kras-
   novsky. (1983). Biofizika. 28, 699-701
   (in Russian).
8. Maltzev, S.V., A.A.Krasnovsky. (1983). Fi-
   ziol. rast. 29, 951-958 (in Russian).
9. Krasnovsky, A.A., G.P.Brin. (1961). Dokl.
   Akad. Nauk SSSR. 139, 142-145 (in Russian).
10.Krasnovsky, A.A., G.P.Brin. (1973). Dokl.
   Akad. Nauk SSSR. 213, 1431-1434 (in Russian).
11.Krasnovsky, A.A., G.P.Brin, A.N.Luganskaya,
   V.V.Nikandrov. (1979). Dokl. Akad. Nauk
   SSSR. 249, 896-899 (in Russian).
12. Nikandrov, V.V., G.P.Brin, A.A.Krasnovsky.
   (1983). Photobiochem. Photobiophys. 6,
   101-107.
13.Krasnovsky, A.A. (1981). Biosystems. 14,
   81-87.

BIOSYNTHESIS, ASSEMBLY, REORGANIZATION AND PROPERTIES OF THE PIGMENT-PROTEIN COMPLEXES

GEORGE AKOYUNOGLOU
Biology Department, Nuclear Research Center "Demokritos",
Aghia Paraskevi, Attiki, Athens, Greece

INTRODUCTION

Chloroplasts of higher plants are comprised of a system of lamellae (thylakoids) which are embedded in the stroma matrix. The stroma contains many soluble proteins including the enzymes of the Calvin cycle which carry out the reduction of CO_2. In the thylakoids the reduction of $NADP^+$ by H_2O and the photophosphorylation of ADP to ATP, coupled to the electron flow, takes place by the generally accepted Z scheme. The reduction of $NADP^+$ is thought to be driven by light absorbed by two pigment assemblies, the photosystem (PS) I and PSII, consisting of proteins associated with chlorophyll (Chl), carotenoids (car), lipids and electron carriers. These assemblies are called "photosynthetic units". Each photosynthetic unit is supposed to be consisted of (a) the "core" of the unit which contains the reaction center (RC), i.e., the minimum components required to carry out the primary photochemical event, a small number of Chl$\underline{a}$ and b-car which act as antennae, and the enzymes and cofactors that stabilize the primary charge separation; (b) the light-harvesting pigments (Chl$\underline{a}$, Chl$\underline{b}$ and car) bound to protein. The reaction center communicates with the antenna and the light-harvesting pigments by utilizing the transfer of excitation energy. The chloroplast lamellae consist of lipids and proteins in about equal proportions; of the lipids 23% by weight are pigments (Chl and car). All of the pigments, together with lipids and proteins, are assembled into pigment-protein complexes which build up the two photosystems, PSI and PSII.

Isolation of the pigment-protein complexes.
Mild SDS-PAGE procedures (1,2) have allowed the separation of up to six major pigment-protein complexes, and three

Proceedings of the 16th FEBS Congress
Part B, pp. 35–46
© 1985 VNU Science Press

unidentified minor ones, from SDS-solubilized thylakoids of mature chloroplasts. These complexes, in order of increasing mobility, are the CPIa, CPI, LHCP[1], LHCP[2], CPa and LHCP[3]. Sucrose gradient centrifugation has been also used for the separation of the complexes (3). CPIa and CPI originate in PSI and the rest in PSII. CPIa is a highly organized form, and its polypeptide composition is identical to that of the Triton X-100 extracted PSI-110 particle (4), i.e., it contains the 69 kDa polypeptide (component of CPI), the 24, 23, 21 and 20 kDa, and the low molecular weight ones of 16, 15, 10.5 and 9 kDa. It also contains Chla, Chlb (Chla/Chlb=4.5), P700 (100 Chl/P700), b-car (18.5 moles/100 moles Chl), and lutein (3 moles/100 moles Chl). CPI is the P700-Chla-rich protein complex originating in the core of the PSI unit. It contains Chla, P700 (30 Chla/P700), b-car (12 moles/100 moles Chl) and a 69 kDa polypeptide. By rerunning the CPIa on a gel containing 100 mM Na^+ in the stacking gel, it can be dissociated into CPI and LHC-I, the light-harvesting complex of PSI (4). LHC-I contains Chla, Chlb (Chla/Chlb=3.4), xanthophylls (xanth; 11.5 moles/100 moles Chl) and a 21 kDa polypeptide (Fig. 1). In some cases a 24 kDa polypeptide, or two doublets, 24-23 and 21-20 kDa polypeptides were isolated. CPa originates in the core of the PSII unit. It contains Chla, the RC of PSII, b-car (10,2 moles/100 moles Chl), the 47 and 42 kDa polypeptides and a number of low Mr ones. LHCP[1] and LHCP[3] act as light-harvesting antennae of PSII (LHC-II). LHCP[3] is the monomeric form and LHCP[1] is an oligomeric form (trimer) of LHCP[3]. LHCP[2] is a mixture of LHC-I and of the dimer of LHC-II. A partial separation of LHCP[2] into LHC-I and LHC-II was achieved by rerunning the LHCP[2] on a gel containing 100 mM Na^+ in the stacking gel (4). The LHC-II complex contains Chla, Chlb (Chla/Chlb=1.2), xanth (24.3 moles/100 moles Chl) and a 25 kDa polypeptide .

Characteristics properties of the pigment-protein complexes: Effect of cations on the supramolecular structure and the 77K fluorescence emission spectra. Cations such as Mg^{2+} or Na^+ and low pH induce the dissociation of CPIa into CPI and LHC-I, and the oligomers of LHC-II into the monomeric form (4,5). This dissociation is closely fol-

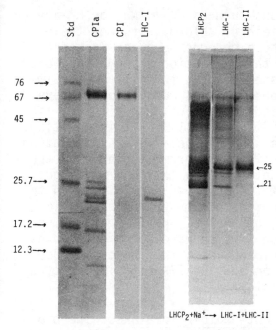

Fig.1. Polypeptide analysis by dissociating SDS-PAGE of the pigment-protein complexes bands excised from the gel, eluted in water, and lyophilized. CPI and LHC-I were separated from CPIa, and LHC-I and LHC-II from LHCP^2, by rerunning them on a gel containing 100mM Na$^+$ in the stacking gel. (Left) coomassie staining; (Right) silver nitrate staining.

LHCP$_2$+Na$^+$→ LHC-I+LHC-II

lowed by a drastic change in the 77K emission spectra (decrease in the F730/F685 ratio) in both the detergent solubilized thylakoids and the isolated complexes, especially those of the PSI unit (4,6,8). For example, CPIa emits in the absence of Mg^{2+} mainly at 735 nm, while in the presence of Mg^{2+} the emission shifts to 685 nm. Similarly, the isolated from CPIa LHC-I emits in the absence of Mg^{2+} mainly at 719 nm, and in its presence at 685 nm (see figs. 7 and 8 of ref. 4).

The dissociation of CPIa by cations, as well as the oligomer to monomer transformation of LHC-II, is a reversible process. For example, LHC-II precipitated by Mg^{2+} from SDS-solubilized thylakoids is in the monomeric form; removal of Mg^{2+} by Tricine washing induces the formation of the oligomeric forms (5). Similarly, treatment of thylakoids with phospholipase transforms the oligomeric forms of LHC-II into the monomeric one; addition of liposomes reconstitutes the oligomeric form (7).The reversibility has been also observed in the isolated CPIa complex; low pH induces a decrease in the F730/F685 ratio, which is restored by increasing the pH to 8.4(8,9).

It is known that cations such as Mg^{2+}, Na^+ or H^+ affect the fluorescence yield of chloroplasts and their 77K emission spectra. These changes were considered as being due to changes in the excitation energy transfer between the two photosystems, i.e., to spill-over. Similar effects have been observed, as we mentioned above, with detergent solubilized thylakoids, and with the isolated complexes of the PSI unit (4-6,8). It is tempting, therefore to suggest that the dissociation-reassociation of CPIa, and the changes in the supramolecular structure of the CPI and LHC-I, controlled by cations, may regulate the distribution of the absorbed energy between the two photosystems by changing the absorption properties, i.e., the cross section, of the PSI unit. It should be mentioned that Zn^{2+} or Cd^{2+} which have no effect on the fluorescence yield of chloroplasts, they have also no effect on the dissociation and the 77K emission spectra of the isolated CPIa complex (6).

Biosynthesis of the pigment-protein complexes. The biosynthesis of the pigment-protein complexes reflects in fact the biogenesis of the thylakoid, i.e., the differentiation of etioplasts into chloroplasts, which in angiosperms depends on light. The differentiation involves the biosynthesis of pigments, lipids and proteins, and it requires the close cooperation of the chloroplast and the cytoplasmic protein synthesizing systems. Similarly to mitochondria, most of the proteins are synthesized on cytoplasmic ribosomes, they are transported through the chloroplast envelope by a post-translational mechanism, processed inside the chloroplast by a soluble enzyme, inserted into the developing thylakoid and assembled into multi-enzyme complexes (9,10). The biosynthesis of the complexes is a step-wise process. This became evident from experiments with etiolated plants greened in intermittent light (2 min light - 98 min dark), and then transferred to continuous light (CL). Early in intermittent light (LDC) only Chla in limited amounts is synthesized, and only CPI and C̄Pa are formed. As the time in LDC increases one can detect the LHC-II, mostly in its monomeric form. Later during greening in CL the rest of the complexes are formed. It seems that the monomer of LHC-II is formed first which gradually gives rise to the ologomeric ones. At the same time the LHC-I is synthesized which is organized together with CPI into CPIa (9). The same trend is also observed when etiolated leaves are exposed directly to CL.

Studying the assembly of the pigment-protein complexes during thylakoid development, and especially the changes in their pigment content, it has been found that the relative concentration of the pigments in each complex is constant from the beginning of its formation; the pigment/protein ratio, however, increases as the duration in CL increases (see table I). This indicates that the assembly of the complex is a step-wise process, and that there are many pigment-binding sites on the apoprotein of each complex, which are filled gradually with pigments, but at a constant ratio. The step-wise assembly, therefore, of the complexes involves the organization of relatively simple components into organized supramolecular structures.

Parallel to the assembly of the pigment-protein complexes, and their organization into supramolecular structures, changes in the Chla fluorescence yield (Fmax/Chl) of the developing chloroplast takes place. It has been observed that there is a close correlation between the changes in the Fmax/Chl and the changes in the CPI/CPIa and LHCP[3]/LHCP[1+2] ratios. The Fmax/Chl is high when the CPI and LHCP[3] predominate, and low when the CPIa and LHCP[1+2] predominate (8,9). During the process of CPIa formation and the monomer to oligomer organization, changes in the absolute fluorescence yield at 77K, and a pronounced red-shift of the long wavelength peak takes place. In LDC the absolute intensity of the emission at 690 nm remains more or less constant, but the emission at 720-730 nm increases steadily, and so, the F690/F730 ratio decreases; at the same time the emission at 717 nm shifts to 725 nm. After transferring the plants to CL a sharp increase in both F690 and F730 emissions occurs, followed by a gradual decline as illumination is prolonged. The F690/F730 ratio, however, continuously declines and reaches the value of the green control, while the long wavelength peak shifts to 735 nm (8).

Table I. Changes in pigment content of the pigment-protein complexes isolated from thylakoids of etiolated leaves exposed to continuous light (CL)

Sample		Chl(a+b)	b-car	lut	nx	vx
		(mole/Mr of complex)				
CPI	18h CL	9.4	1.10	-	-	-
CPI	120h CL	19.8	2.70	-	-	-
CPIa	18h CL	22.2	4.30	0.60	-	-
CPIa	120h CL	33.5 ·	6.10	0.40	-	-
LHCP3	18h CL	1.8	0.04	0.26	0.05	0.04
LHCP3	120h CL	4.3	0.07	0.58	0.30	0.08
LHCP1+2	18h CL	1.9	0.02	0.29	0.14	0.05
LHCP1+2	120h CL	6.7	0.06	1.10	0.50	0.20

(From Antonopoulou, P. and Akoyunoglou, G. in preparation)

Reorganization of the pigment-protein complexes. The question that arises is whether the pigment-protein complexes after their assembly and organization into supramolecular structures are stable, or a reorganization can take place. It has been found (11-13) that during development, and under certain environmental conditions, a reorganization of the thylakoid components may take place. During this reorganization the following may happen: (a) dissociation of one or more pigment-protein complexes leading to liberation of Chla, which binds to newly synthesized polypeptides forming other pigment-protein complexes; (b) insertion of the newly synthesized polypeptides into the thylakoid, competition for the Chla already bound to another complex, removal of the Chla to form new complex and degradation of the old one.

The first case is observed in young etiolated leaves exposed to LDC for six days (86LDC), and then transferred to CL in the presence of the protein synthesis inhibitor chloramphenicol (CAP). Under these conditions destruction of a number of PSII units, i.e., dissociation of CPa, takes place and their Chla is reused for the formation of LHC-II (9). The second case is observed in young etiolated leaves exposed to CL for various durations, and then transferred to darkness (11-13). In this case the reorganization involves: disorganization of the LHC-I

and LHC-II, degradation of Chlb, digestion of their apoproteins, and reuse of their Chla for the formation of
more PSI and PSII units, mainly CPI and CPa. This is
demonstrated by (a) the increase in PSI/Chl, PSI/leaf,
P700/Chl, PSII/Chl and PSII/leaf during the dark incubation; (b) the decrease in LHC-I, LHC-II, CPIa and
Chlb/leaf; no change in Chla/leaf; and (c) the decrease
in the relative concentration of the 25, 24, 23 and 21
kDa polypeptides, and the increase of the 69, 47 and 42
kDa polypeptides. In addition, an increase in the concentration of a great number of other polypeptides is
also observed. That the synthesis of the polypeptides
continues in the dark is also supported from in vivo
^{14}C-labelling experiments shown in Table II. Parallel
to the formation of the new PSI and PSII units, an increase in the cyt/Chl and cyt/leaf is also observed,
indicating that the whole electron transfer chain between the newly synthesized PSII and PSI units is formed
in the dark. The reorganization taking place in the
dark transferred leaves depends on the developmental
stage of the chloroplast, in other words, it occurs
only in thylakoids still in the process of development,
which contain reduced amount of PS units, and not in
those which acquired the organization of the mature
chloroplast.
  Concerning the mechanism of the reorganization taking
place in the dark there are two possibilities: (a) the
apoproteins of the PSI and PSII reaction centers are
synthesized first, inserted into the developing thylakoid, compete for the Chla already bound to LHC-I and
LHC-II, remove it to form CPI and CPa, and then the
LHC-I and LHC-II are disorganized and their apoproteins
digested; or (b) the LHC-I and LHC-II are disorganized
first and then their Chla becomes available to bind to
the apoproteins of the PSI and PSII reaction centers.
In the first case the distruction of the LHC-I and
LHC-II will depend on the rate of synthesis of the reaction center polypeptides, while in the second case
it will not. Experiments with etiolated leaves exposed
first to LDC, then to CL for a short time and then to
darkness (13), as well as experiments with leaves transferred to darkness in the presence of CAP (Table III),

41

Table II. Thylakoid protein synthesis in bean leaves exposed to continuous light (CL) and then transferred to darkness (D) in the presence of ^{14}C-leucine

Sample	Chla/Chlb	cpm/ug Chl	cpm/mg protein
6d + 20h CL + (^{14}C-leucine+24h D)	4.37	127,000	584,000
6d + 72h CL + (^{14}C-leucine+24h D)	2.75	138	17,000

^{14}C-leucine was administered to the leaves by brushing 3 ml solution (0.08 mC, 342 uC/umole) to 60 leaves; the leaves were washed with water 2 hours prior to the isolation of the thylakoids.

Table III. Effect of chloramphenicol (CAP) on the reorganization of the thylakoid components of plants exposed to continuous light (CL) and then transferred to darkness.

	Sample	mg/leaf	Chla/leaf	Chlb/leaf	Chla/Chlb
CAP	6d+18h CL+6h D	47	14.88	3.04	4.97
CAP	6d+18h CL+26h D	52	15.70	2.36	6.60
H₂O	6d+18h CL+6h D	43	15.30	3.46	4.40
H₂O	6d+18h CL+26h D	52	14.40	0.53	27.00

Bean leaves with one cotyledon removed were exposed to CL for 18h, then they were dipped in CAP (1 mg/ml H$_2$0), or in H$_2$0 (control) for 20 min and placed in the dark. After 6h in the dark they were washed with water.

showed that the first hypothesis is correct.

Mechanism of complex assembly and thylakoid development. The experiments described above, as well as other experiments suggest the following mechanism operating on the assembly of the complexes and the development and growth of the thylakoid. According to this mechanism, in the early stages of etioplast development all thylakoid components are synthesized, but with a relatively low rate, except Chla which accumulates as PChlide a. From all

thylakoid components synthesized in darkness during etioplast development only a number of them accumulate, the
rest are digested, since in the absence of Chla they can
not be stabilized. As the age of the etiolated tissue increases a number of the thylakoid components stops to be
formed. Depending, therefore, on the age of the etiolated
tissue, i.e., on the developmental stage of the etioplast,
one may or may not observe the expression of some of these
components in the dark grown plants.Illumination of young
etiolated leaves transforms the PChlide a into Chlide a,
and stimulates also the synthesis of the other thylakoid
components. Moreover, in old etiolated leaves, light re-
induces the synthesis of those components, which have
been stopped to be synthesized in darkness.

The development of thylakoids depends on the rate by
which the different components are synthesized. If one,
or more of the components are synthesized at a low rate,
then their synthesis controls the way the thylakoid develops. The rate of Chla formation is a determining factor in thylakoid development, since most of the polypeptides are stabilized by forming with Chla pigment-
protein complexes. If Chla is formed at a low rate, then
its synthesis regulates the assembly of the pigment-protein complexes, and accordingly the development of the
thylakoid. This can be observed in experiments where etiolated leaves are exposed to LDC (16), or to ms flashes
(14), or to low intensity far-red light (15).

According to this mechanism we can explain the formation of the complexes in plants greened in LDC, and the
reorganization of the thylakoid components in plants
transferred to darkness after being exposed to CL, as
follows: (a) Complex assembly in plants exposed to LDC.
In the case of plants greened in LDC the Chla formed during the 2 min illumination of every cycle is very small,
and so the concentration of Chla becomes the limiting
factor. There is, therefore, a competition between the
different apoproteins of the complexes for the small a-
mount of Chla; it seems that the apoproteins of the reaction centers have a higher affinity for Chla than the
apoproteins of LHC-I and LHC-II, so they form CPI and CPa,
i.e., the core of the PSI and PSII units, while the apoproteins of LHC-I and LHC-II, not being able to be sta-

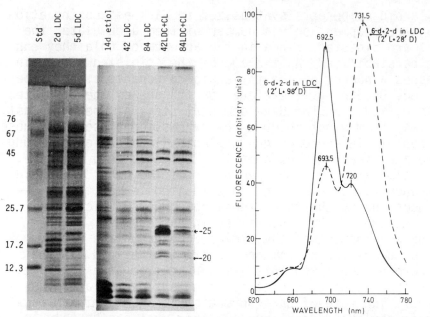

Fig.2. Slab gel electrophoresis of thylakoid polypeptides of 6-day etiolated bean leaves exposed to LDC.(Left):2 min light+28 min dark. (Right):2 min light+98 min dark.
Fig.3. Fluorescence spectra at 77K of 6-day etiolated bean leaves exposed to LDC (2 min light+28 or 98 min dark)

bilized, are digested. This explains the absence of LHC-II in the LDC-plants (1,16), even though the mRNA of the apo-protein is present and it is translated (17). If during the intermittent light the relative rate of Chla synthesis increases, either by shortening the dark period in the LDC or by decreasing the rate of synthesis of the reaction center apoproteins, then some Chla becomes available to bind on the LHC-I and LHC-II apoproteins forming the re-spective complexes. This is shown clearly in figs. 2-4. As it is obvious, when etiolated leaves are exposed to LDC which have shorter dark period (28 min), then the thyla-koids formed contain the apoproteins of LHC-I and LHC-II, in the form of their complexes. Moreover, the LHC-I is organized with CPI in the CPIa form, as the 77K fluores-cence spectra show (high 730 nm). Similarly, leaves ex-posed to LDC for 6-days (86LDC), where the rate of syn-

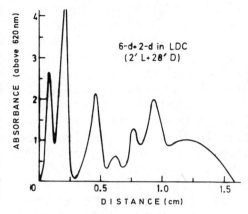

6-d+2-d in LDC
(2′ L+28′ D)

Fig. 4. SDS-PAGE profile of pigment-protein complexes of thylakoids isolated from 6-day etiolated bean leaves exposed to LDC (2 min light+28 min dark) for two days.

thesis of the reaction center polypeptides decreases,contains LHC-II in appreciable amounts (see fig.1 of ref.12). Reorganization of the complexes in plants transferred to darkness. During CL the rate of Chla synthesis is high, and all polypeptides are stabilized by forming complexes. After transfer to darkness the polypeptides continue to be synthesized. Since no Chla is formed in the dark, the reaction center polypeptides compete for the Chla already bound on LHC-I and LHC-II, remove it to form CPI and CPa. The removal of Chla from LHC-I and LHC-II results in the disorganization of the complexes, degradation of Chlb and digestion of their polypeptides.

REFERENCES
1.Argyroudi-Akoyunoglou,J.H. and Akoyunoglou,G.(1979).The Chl-protein complexes of the thylakoids in greening plastids of Phaseolus vulgaris. FEBS Lett.104,78-84.
2.Anderson,J.M.,Waldron,J.C. and Thorne,S.W. (1978). Chl-protein complexes of spinach and barley thylakoids. FEBS Lett.99,227-233.
3.Argyroudi-Akoyunoglou,J.H. and Thomou,H.(1981).Separation of the pigment-protein complexes by SDS-sucrose density gradient centrifugation. FEBS Lett.135,177-181
4.Argyroudi-Akoyunoglou,J.H.(1984). The 77K fluorescence spectrum of the PSI complex CPIa. FEBS Lett.171,47-53.
5.Argyroudi-Akoyunoglou,J.H.(1980).Cation-induced transformation of pigment-protein complexes. Photobiochem. Photobiophys.1,279-287.
6.Argyroudi-Akoyunoglou,J.H. and Akoyunoglou,G.(1983).Su-

pramolecular structure of Chl-protein complexes in relation to the Chla fluorescence of chloroplasts at
R. or liquid N_2 temp.Arch.Biochem.Biophys.227,469-477.
7.Remy,R.,Tremolieres,A.,Duval,J.C.,Ambart-Breteville,F.
A. and Dubecq,J.R.(1982).Study of the supramolecular
organization of LHCP Chl-protein. FEBS Lett.137,271-275
8.Argyroudi-Akoyunoglou,J.H.,Castorinis,A.and Akoyunoglou,
G.(In press).Biogenesis and organization of the Chl-
protein complexes:Relation to the low temp.fluorescence
characteristics of developing thylakoids.Israel J.Bot.
9.Akoyunoglou,G.(1984).Thylakoid biogenesis in higher
plants:Assembly and reorganization.In:Advances in Photosynthesis Research,Vol IV, C.Sybesma (ed).Martinus
Nijhoff/Dr.W.Junk Publishers,The Hague,pp.595-602.
10.Ellis,R.J.(1981). Chl-proteins:synthesis transport and
assembly. Ann.Rev.Plant Physiol.32,111-137.
11.Argyroudi-Akoyunoglou,J.H.,Akoyunoglou,A.,Kalosakas,
K.and Akoyunoglou,G.(1982).Reorganization of the PSII
unit in developing thylakoids of higher plants after
transfer to darkness. Plant Physiol.70,1242-1248.
12.Akoyunoglou,G.(1982). Reorganization of thylakoid components during chloroplast development in higher
plants. Progr.Clin.Biol.Res.102B,171-188.
13.Akoyunoglou,A.and Akoyunoglou,G.(In press). Mechanism
of thylakoid reorganization during chloroplast development in higher plants. Israel J.Bot.
14.Akoyunoglou,G.,Argyroudi-Akoyunoglou,J.H.,Michel-
Wolwertz,M.R.and Sironval,C.(1966). Effect of intermittent and continuous light in Chl formation in
etiolated plants. Physiol.Plant.19,1101-1104.
15.De Greef,J.,Butler,W.L.and Roth,T.F.(1971). Greening
of etiolated bean leaves in far-red light. Plant
Physiol.47,457-464.
16.Argyroudi-Akoyunoglou,J.H.,Feleki,Z.and Akoyunoglou,
G.(1971). Formation of two Chl-protein complexes
during greening of etiolated bean leaves. Biochem.
Biophys.Res.Comm.45,606-614.
17.Viro,M.and Kloppstech,K.(1982). Expression of genes
for plastid membrane proteins in barley under intermittent light conditions. Planta 154,18-23.

BASIC RESEARCH ON THE MODE OF ACTION OF HERBICIDES: DIPHENYL ETHERS

PETER BÖGER
Lehrstuhl für Physiologie und Biochemie der Pflanzen,
Universität Konstanz, D-7750 Konstanz, Germany

INTRODUCTORY REMARK

In essence, the primary target of phytotoxic diphenyl ethers (DPEs) is the chloroplast with its membrane-embedded photosynthetic electron-transport and pigment system. As demonstrated in Fig.1, the following sites of diphenyl-ether attack have been found: [1] inhibition of photosynthetic electron transport, [2] peroxidative activity, [3] inhibition of carotenogenesis, and [4] inhibition of ATP-synthase. Induction of stress response has also been reported (1), as well as interference with (dark) mitochondrial respiration (2), but these effects apparently do not play a dominant role

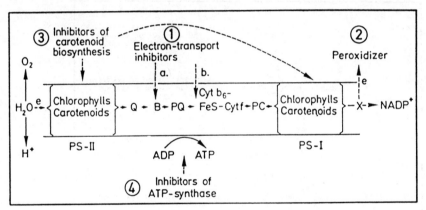

Fig.1: Targets of diphenyl ethers at the photosynthetic electron-transport and pigment system.
A part of a thylakoid is schematically drawn. PS II,I indicate the pigment apparatus; Q, primary electron acceptor of PS II; B, herbicide-binding protein (Q_B); PQ, plastoquinone pool; FeS, Rieske protein, presumably forming a complex with cyt(ochromes) b_6 and f; PC, plastocyanin

Proceedings of the 16th FEBS Congress
Part B, pp. 47–53

as far as the primary herbicidal activity of DPEs is
concerned. So, this report will briefly outline our
knowledge on the four plastidic targets. See reviews
(2,3) for more details; phenoxyphenoxy-type compounds
will not be considered.

In pesticide biochemistry, multiple modes of action
of one class of compounds are well known. As far as
herbicides are concerned, DPEs have to be regarded at
the moment as the most versatile ones. Fig.2 demonstrates some examples. It should be mentioned that no
detailed knowledge exists as yet on structure-activity
relationships to determine type and position of substituents which will shift the mode of action of DPEs
from one target to the other.

PHOTOSYNTHETIC ELECTRON TRANSPORT

Generally, the I_{50}-value for DPEs (oxyfluorfen, nitrofen, bifenox and the like) is $\geq 10^{-5}$ M, too high to
account for herbicidal activity (4). Complex substitu-

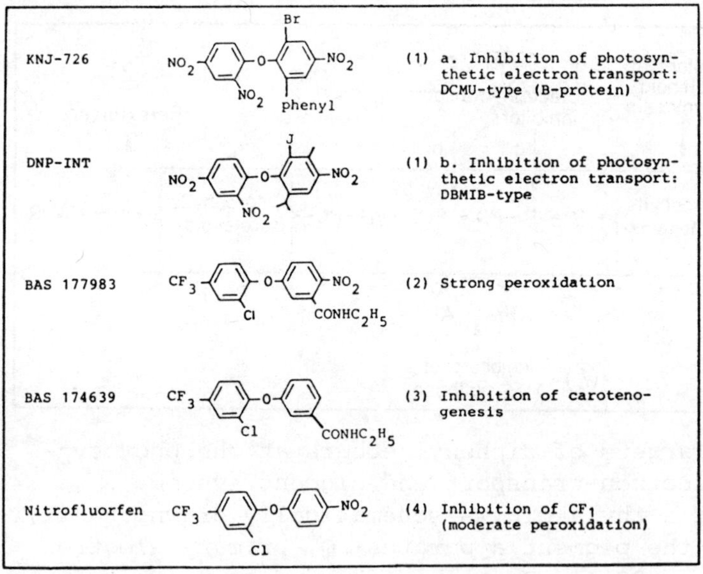

Fig.2: Structure and activity of some diphenyl ethers.
Position and type of substituents determine the activity
and mode of action. Numbers refer to Fig.1; comp. refs.
5,15,16,21.

tion may lead to efficient Hill-reaction inhibitors (5).
While most DPEs affect the reoxidation of plastoquinone
(cf. [2]), "DBMIB-type", like DNP-INT, case (b), see
Fig.2), some may also bind to the "herbicide-binding
protein" B (= Q_B), as does e.g. KNJ-726 (case a). Herbicides on the basis of direct electron-transport inhibition have not yet been developed. Efforts may be
worthwhile to synthesize and assay some more DPEs to
achieve high affinity to the Cyt b_6/f-complex in order
to circumvent resistance at B due to genetic alterations.

PEROXIDIZERS

In the light, certain p-nitrodiphenyl ethers at low
concentrations (like oxyfluorfen) induce breakdown of
polyunsaturated fatty acids (generally constituents of
membrane galactolipids). This peroxidation is accompanied by evolution of (saturated) short-chain hydro-
carbons of definite chain lengths (depending on the
type of fatty acid(s) present, see [6]). Peroxidation
is the essential basis for herbicidal activity using
DPEs like oxyfluorfen or bifenox.
   Using green tissue or algae, oxyfluorfen-induced
peroxidation proceeds best in red light and can be
"safened" by diuron (= DCMU), indicative of the photosynthetic electron transport being responsible for
"activating" the DPE. It is still unclear whether this
occurs by a (transient) 1-electron reduction of the
DPE itself or whether an (unknown) endogenous light-
induced radical reaction is enhanced in the presence
of a p-nitro-DPE. There is agreement that a primary
radical will subsequently start a peroxidative radi-
calic chain reaction (see 3,7 for details).
   Using cucumber cotyledons, carotenoids were proposed
as sensitizers for DPE activation (8, originally by
9). It appears, however, that this activation is not
substantial in photosynthetically competent cells.
   Ethoxyquin (10) or α-tocopherol acetate suppress
peroxidation in intact cells. In oxyfluorfen-treated
mustard seedlings, the level of endogenous antioxidant
vitamin C decreases inversely with increasing ethane
formation (11). By comparing different plant species,

it has been shown recently that a certain ratio of ascorbic acid/α-tocopherol in the cell determines tolerance against a peroxidizing DPE [12].

Peroxidation is exhibited not only by a p-nitro, but also by a p-Cl-DPE (comp.[2]) provided appropriate "enhancer" substituents are in the neighboring 3'-position (like -OCH3, -OC2H5, -CONH-alkyl, for details see [13, 14,15]).

CAROTENOID BIOSYNTHESIS

Diphenyl ethers of the m-phenoxybenzamide type interfere with carotenoid biosynthesis (16) leading to "bleaching" of the cell. Light is not necessary. This phytotoxic activity causes accumulation of phytoene (and little phytofluene) by preventing hydrogen abstraction from this carotene precursor. The phytoene-desaturase complex is non-competitively inhibited (17), as can be shown with a cell-free carotenogenic system (from Aphanocapsa, which converts labeled geranylgeranyl pyrophosphate into ß-carotene). As shown by this cell-free system, certain diphenyl ether-substituted diethylamines exert an influence on cyclase activity leading to accumulation of lycopene (this laboratory, unpubl. results).

As demonstrated in the table, presence of an active m-phenoxybenzamide yields a high ^{14}C-ratio of phytoene to ß-carotene (no.1), while the p-nitro analog (no.2) is inactive with respect to inhibition of phytoene desaturation (18). Oxadiazon, which also has bleaching activity, is included (no.3), demonstrating not to interfere with carotenoids (apparently it affects chlorophyll biosynthesis, see [19]).

ATP-SYNTHASE (CF1-COUPLING FACTOR)

At concentrations too low to block photosynthetic electron transport, certain chlorinated p-nitro-DPEs (nitrofen or nitrofluorfen, see Fig.2 and refs. 20,21) interfere with photophosphorylation ("energy-transfer inhibition") by competing with ADP at the plastidic CF1. Apparently, nucleotide exchange at the coupling factor

Inhibition of cell-free ß-carotene synthesis (ß-car). Aphanocapsa system with ^{14}C-geranylgeranyl pyrophosphate as substrate; after (18).

Compounds (10 µM)	Phytoene	Phytofluene	ß-Car	Phytoene / ß-car
Control	68	50	1004	0.07
(1) CF$_3$–◯–O–◯ 6' 5' 4', Cl, 2' CONHC$_2$H$_5$	1562	174	494	3.16
(2) CF$_3$–◯–O–◯–NO$_2$, Cl, CONHC$_2$H$_5$	137	53	1112	0.12
(3) (CH$_3$)$_3$C, N–N, OCH(CH$_3$)$_2$, Cl, Cl, O Oxadiazon	89	59	986	0.09

is affected (22). The action of these DPEs can be easily demonstrated by their interference with the "photosynthetic control" (cf.[2]) as well as by decrease of photophosphorylation, e.g. in a cyclic electron-transport system. For structural prerequisites see ref.[15].

ACKNOWLEDGMENT

Our studies on the mode of action of phytotoxic compounds were supported by grants from the Deutsche Forschungsgemeinschaft, Germany.

Chemical names of phytotoxic compounds used in the text, and of which no formula has been presented here: bifenox, methyl 5-(2,4-dichlorophenoxy)-2-nitrobenzoate; DCMU (diuron), 3-(3,4-dichlorophenyl)-1,1-dimethylurea; difunon, 5-(dimethylaminomethylene)-2-oxo-4-phenyl-2,5-dihydrofurane-carbonitrile-(3); nitrofen, 2,4-

dichlorophenyl-4'-nitrophenyl ether; norflurazon, 4-
chloro-5-methylamin-2-(3-trifluoromethylphenyl)pyri-
dazin-3(2H)one; oxyfluorfen, 2-chloro-4-(trifluoromethyl)-
phenyl-3'-ethoxy-4'-nitrophenyl ether.

REFERENCES

1. Gorske, S.F. and Hopen, H.J. (1978). Weed Sci.26,
   585-588; Kömives, T. and Casida, J.E. (1983). J.
   Agric. Food Chem. 31, 751-755.
2. Böger, P. (1984). Z. Naturforsch. 39c, 468-475.
3. Sandmann, G. and Böger P. (1982). Mode of action
   of herbicidal bleaching. In: Biochemical Responses
   Induced by Herbicides, D.E. Moreland, J.B. St.John,
   and F.D. Hess (Eds.) ACS Symp. Series no. 181,
   Amer. Chem. Society, Washington D.C., pp. 111-130.
4. Van den Berg, G. and Tipker, J. (1982). Pestic.
   Sci. 13, 29-38.
5. Draber, W., Knops, H.J., and Trebst, A. (1981).
   Z. Naturforsch. 36c, 848-852.
6. Sandmann, G. and Böger, P. (1982). Lipids 17, 35-41.
   Sandmann, G. and Böger, P. (1983). Lipids 18, 37-41.
7. Lambert, R., Kroneck, P.M.H., and Böger, P. (1984).
   Z. Naturforsch. 39c, 486.491.
8. Orr, G.L. and Hess, F.D. (1982), Proposed site(s)
   of action of new diphenyl ether herbicides. In:
   Biochemical Responses Induced by Herbicides, D.E.
   Moreland, J.B. St.John, and F.D. Hess (Eds.) ACS
   Symp. Series no. 181, Amer. Chem. Society,
   Washington D.C., pp. 131-152.
9. Masunaka, S. (1969). Residue Rev. 25, 45-58.
10. Kunert, K.J. and Böger, P. (1984). J. Agric. Food
    Chem. 32, 725-728.
11. Kunert, K.J. (1984). Herbicide-induced lipid per-
    oxidation in higher plants: The role of vitamin C.
    In: Oxygen Radicals in Chemistry and Biology,
    W. Bors et al. (Eds.). de Gruyter, Berlin-New York,
    pp. 383-386.
12. Finckh, B. and Kunert, K.J. (1985). J. Agric. Food
    Chem., submitted.

13. Lambert, R. and Böger, P. (1984). Adv. Photosynth. Res. (Proc. 6th Int. Congr. Photosynth.) Vol. IV, Nijhoff/Junk, The Hague-Boston-Lancaster, pp. 45-48.
14. Orr, G.K., Elliott, C.M., and Hogan, M.E. (1983). Plant Physiol. 73, 939-944.
15. Lambert, R., Sandmann, G., and Böger, P. (1983). Pest. Biochem. Physiol. 19, 309-320; Lambert, R., Sandmann, G., and Böger P. (1983). Mode of action of nitrodiphenylethers affecting pigments and membrane integrity. In: Pesticide Chemistry. Human Welfare and the Environment (IUPAC), Vol.3, J. Miyamoto and P.C. Kearney (Eds.). Pergamon Press, Oxford-New York-Toronto-Sydney-Paris-Frankfurt, pp. 97-102.
16. Lambert, R. and Böger, P. (1983). Pest. Biochem. Physiol. 20, 183-187.
17. Clarke, I.E., Sandmann, G., Bramley, P.M., and Böger, P. (1984). Pest. Biochem. Physiol., in press.
18. Sandmann, G., Clarke, I.E., Bramley, P.M., and Böger, P. (1984). Z. Naturforsch. 39c, 443-449.
19. Sandmann, G., Reck, H., and Böger, P. (1984). J. Agric. Food Chem. 32, 868-872.
20. Lambert, R., Kunert, K.-J., and Böger, P. (1979). Pest. Biochem. Physiol. 11, 267-274.
21. Ridley, S.M. (1983). Plant Physiol. 72, 461-468.
22. Huchzermeyer, B. and Loehr, A. (1983). Biochim. Biophys. Acta 724, 224-229.

MOLECULAR ORGANIZATION OF CHLOROPHYLL A IN THE LIGHT-HARVESTING COMPLEX (LHC$_{II}$) OF THYLAKOIDS

AGNES FALUDI-DÁNIEL, MUSTÁRDY L.A., KISS J.G.[‡],
GARAB Gy.I. and V.V. SHUBIN
Institute of Plant Physiology, Biological
Research Center Hungarian Academy of Sciences,
H-6701, Szeged, POB 521, Hungary and Bakh In-
stitute of Biochemistry Academy of Sciences
USSR, Moscow, USSR

INTRODUCTION

In higher plants and green algae approximately
half of the total chlorophyll is associated
with the light-harvesting complex (LHC$_{II}$)
which serves photosystem II (PS II). This pigment-protein complex ensures the balance in
excitation of the two photosystems a condition for optimum quantum efficiency of photosynthesis. LHC$_{II}$ also plays an important role in
controlling the distribution of absorbed excitation energy between the two photosystems in
response to physiological demands requiring an
excess of ATP or NADPH [1]. When PS II is over-
loaded surface exposed segments of LHC$_{II}$ polypeptides become phosphorylated. As a result,
the connectivity between PS II and LHC$_{II}$ decreases with a concomitant increase in the ab-
sorptive cross section of PS I. The structural
background to this process may be the existence
of "mobile antennae". These are phosphorylated
particles which separate off from PS II and
migrate from the granum into stroma membranes
[2]. Such a dynamic process implies a flexible
architecture sensitive to electrostatic interactions, which allows LHC$_{II}$ movements within
the photosynthetic membrane.

[‡]Clinic of ENT, Medical University, H-6701,
Szeged, POB 422, Hungary

Proceedings of the 16th FEBS Congress
Part B, pp. 55–60
© 1985 VNU Science Press

The chemical composition of LHC$_{\parallel}$ is reasonably well known. It can be purified, and in the presence of cations assembled to crystalline arrays which have been analysed by high resolution electron microscopy [3] and by X-ray diffraction spectroscopy [4]. However, the architecture of LHC$_{\parallel}$ in situ is not so well known because analytical procedures result in the decomposition of the macromolecular aggregate and the reconstituted complex may be somewhat different from the original. Therefore it is of interest to utilize non-destructive methods like polarization spectroscopy which can inform on LHC$_{\parallel}$ in situ in parallel with the reconstituted LHC$_{\parallel}$ aggregate.

This paper is a review of earlier investigations and discussion of more recent data on LHC$_{\parallel}$ obtained by circular dichroism (CD) measurements and fluorescence polarization spectroscopy.

RESULTS

The giant CD

It was reported earlier [5,6] that whole chloroplasts containing LHC$_{\parallel}$ exhibit a giant CD. This CD signal was different in wavelength from that of individual photosystems. Its amplitude expressed in terms of differential absorption (CD/Abs), was one order of a magnitude higher than the CD of whole chloroplasts not containing LHC. In greening chloroplasts the synthesis of LHC$_{\parallel}$ proceeded parallel with the increase of the characteristic LHC-CD, with peaks around 684 (+) and 672 nm (-) [7]. In purified LHC$_{\parallel}$ aggregated in vitro was a giant CD signal was measured spectrally the same as for LHC$_{\parallel}$ in vivo but of opposite sign [8]. The physical background of such giant CD-s may be rather complex [9]. Nevertheless,

they can be regularly encountered in chromo-
phores embedded in liquid crystals [10]. Thus,
the giant CD of LHC$_{II}$ aggregates might indicate
a liquid crystal-like structure but, as judged
from the CD of opposite sign, some parameters,
like pitch height and the tilt of pigment
molecules might be different [11].

Magnetic susceptibility

A characteristic feature of liquid crystals is
their magnetic susceptibility. It was reasonable to check the magnetic susceptibility of
chloroplasts with various LHC$_{II}$ content in comparison with the extracted and reaggregated
LHC$_{II}$. Measurement of the ratio of fluorescence
intensity emitted parallel and perpendicular
to the magnetic field (FP=$F_{II}/F_{\perp}$) as a function
of the magnetic field strength has shown that
magnetic susceptibility of the chloroplasts
was in close relationship with their LHC$_{II}$
content, and the artificial LHC$_{II}$ aggregate also
exhibited a high magnetic susceptibility. This
observation supports the idea on the liquid
crystal-like organization of LHC$_{II}$.

The dynamic behaviour of LHC$_{II}$ shown by the light-induced change in the CD signal

According to the "mobile antenna" hypothesis,
regulation of quantum distribution in thylakoids involves energetic and spatial separation of LHC$_{II}$ from PS II. This process was
found to be reflected in light-induced changes
of the characteristic CD signal of LHC$_{II}$ [12].
Chloroplasts of high photosynthetic activity
prepared from mesophyll cells of maize, spinach
or pea leaves were illuminated in a phosphoros-
cope which was placed in the sample compartment
of a JASCO AS 40 dichrograph equipped with a
data processor and side illumination. Illumination was high ($1.5.10^4$ erg cm^{-2}s^{-1}) white

light, and several light-minus-dark CD (ΔCD)
were accumulated. Upon illumination the CD
signal of chloroplasts decreased by approximately 5-15%. This change was reversible after
several minutes of darkness.

Spectral characteristics of the light-induced
changes of chloroplast CD were somewhat different from that of the dark signal: a/ ΔCD was
more conservative, b/ the peaks of ΔCD were
located at slightly shorter wavelengths, c/ the
half band width of ΔCD is narrower, d/ in the region of chlorophyll b absorption no appreciable
light-induced changes were observed.

Kinetics of light-induced CD reveals two
phases: an initial fast phase (rise time in the
range of seconds) and a slow phase lasting for
several minutes. Inhibition of the linear
electron transport by DCMU prevented ΔCD completely, while Antimycin A left the slow
phase of ΔCD unaffected.

It is not clear so far whether ΔCD originates
from a change in the molecular interaction
between chlorophyll-a molecules or from a
change of the circular differential scattering
[13], in any case it indicates structural
changes associated with operation of LHC$_{II}$.

CONCLUSIONS

CD studies have shown that: a/ both native and
artificial LHC$_{II}$ exhibit a liquid crystal-like
structure. Beside gross similarities they are
somewhat different in architecture as shown by
CD signals of opposite sign. b/ the liquid
crystal-like character of LHC$_{II}$ is supported
by the fact that LHC$_{II}$ aggregates are highly
susceptible to magnetic field, c/ in phosphorylating chloroplasts characteristic changes
of CD signal occur which might reflect structural changes of LHC$_{II}$ in vivo.

REFERENCES

[1] Haworth, P., Kyle, D.J., Horton, P., Arntzen, Ch.J. (1982). Chloroplast membrane protein phosphorylation. Photochem. Photobiol. 36, 743-748.
[2] Kyle, D.J., Ting-Yun Kuang, Watson, J.L., Arntzen, Ch.J. (1984). Movement of a sub--population of the light harvesting complex from grana to stroma lamellae as a consequence of its phosphorylation. Biochim. Biophys. Acta 765, 89-96.
[3] Kühlbrandt, W. (1984). Three-dimensional structure of the light-harvesting chlorophyll a/b-protein complex. Nature 307, 478-480.
[4] Li, J., Hollingshead, C. (1982). Formation of crystalline arrays of chlorophyll a/b-light-harvesting protein by membrane reconstitution. Biophys. J. 37, 363-370.
[5] Gregory, R.P.F., Raps, S., Thornber, J.P., Bertsch, J. (1972). Chlorophyll-protein--detergent complexes compared with thylakoids by means of circular dichroism. In Proc. of the 2nd Internatl. Congress of Photosynthesis (Forti, G., Avron, M., Melandri, A. eds.) W. Junk, The Hague 1503-1508.
[6] Faludi-Daniel, A., Demeter, S., Garay, A.S. (1973). Circular dichroism spectra of granal and agranal chloroplasts of maize. Plant Physiol. 52, 54-56.
[7] Faludi-Daniel, A., Mustárdy, L.A. (1983). Organization of chlorophyll a in the light harvesting chlorophyll a/b protein complex as shown by circular dichroism. Liquid crystal-like domains. Plant Physiol. 73, 16-19.
[8] Gregory, R.P.F., Demeter, S., Faludi-Daniel, A. (1980). Macromolecular organization of chlorophyll a in aggregated chlorophyll

a/b protein complex as shown by circular dichroism at room and cryogenic temperatures. Biochim. Biophys. Acta 591, 356--360.

[9] Pearlstein, R.M., Davis, R.C., Ditson, S.L. (1982). Giant circular dichroism of high molecular weight chlorophyllide-apomyoglobin complexes. Proc. Natl. Acad. Sci. USA 79, 400-402.

[10] Saeva, F.D. (1979). Cholesteric liquid crystal-induced circular dichroism. In Saeva F.D. ed. Liquid Crystals Marcek Dekker. Inc. New York, 249-273.

[11] Holzwarth, G., Holzwarth, N.A.W. (1973). Circular dichroism and rotatory dispersion near absorption bands of cholesteric liquid crystals. J. Opt. Soc. Am. 63, 324-331.

[12] Faludi-Dániel, A., Mustárdy, L.A., Shubin, V.V., Sobhi, M.A. (1983). Organization of the light-harvesting chlorophyll-protein complex (LHCP) as shown by differences circular dichroism (ΔCD) during greening, under light and stepwise degradation. Proc. 6th Internatl. Congress of Photosynthesis, Brussels, IV, 6, 733-736.

[13] Bustamante, C., Tinoco, I.Jr., Maestre, M.F. (1983). Circular differential scattering can be an important part of the circular dichroism of macromolecules. Proc. Natl. Acad. Sci. USA, 80, 3568-3572.

CHLOROPHYLL REARRANGEMENTS AT THE EARLY STEPS IN THE FORMATION OF THE PIGMENT SYSTEMS

A.A. SHLYK, L.I. FRADKIN, V.P. DOMANSKII, A.G. SAMOILENKO

Institute of Photobiology, BSSR Academy of Sciences, Minsk, USSR

Chlorophyll (Chl) is synthesized by multienzyme complexes of Chl-synthetase located in plastid membranes /1/. Even at the earliest stage of chloroplast development,the protochlorophyllide (Pchlde) and Chl molecules first-formed from Pchlde of etiolated leaves are assembled in groups with efficient intermolecular energy transfer. The proximity of the Chl biosynthetic apparatus to the pigment systems and the group-type organization of Chl biosynthesis may favor a rapid formation of the first units of the photosynthetic apparatus /1/. It is known that photosystem 1 (PS1) appears at the very start of greening while PS2 usually develops later and was recorded only after 1 h of illumination. The aim of the present work was to study the initial development of the pigment systems and the spatial aspects of their formation.

Following Pchlde photoreduction, the Shibata shift attributed to disaggregation of pigment molecules occurs. During this shift there takes place a rearrangement of chlorophyllide (Chlde) molecules, bringing them into contact with carotenoids (Car), so that energy transfer from Car to Chlde becomes feasible /2/. It is fully developed by the end of the shift.We found that in the case of partial photoconversion of the Pchlde pool the Shibata shift proceeds as well

Proceedings of the 16th FEBS Congress
Part B, pp. 61–66
© 1985 VNU Science Press

concomitantly with the appearance and evolution of energy transfer from Car to Chlde672 (data not shown). In this case, the initial energy transfer from Pchlde to Chlde is still present and only afterwards declines as in /3/. Thus, the appearance of energy transfer from Car to Chlde suggests the first rearrangement of Chlde molecules, while the disappearance of energy transfer from Pchlde results from the second rearrangement which displaces Chl(de) from Pchlde to a more distant position.

After the Shibata shift, further spectral changes produced by the accumulation of long-wave Chl are distinguishable. We observed /2/ a correlated growth of a new absorption band at 683nm and a fluorescence band at 720nm for 1 h of greening.Just after the Shibata shift (Fig1, 20-min light), the amount of longwave Chl is very small, the set of fluorescing centers is relatively homogeneous and the excitation spectra of the emission bands 682 and 720 are very similar up to 620nm. The excitation band of longwave fluorescence is at 672nm. After a 2-h illumination, the amount of longwave Chl slightly increases. The excitation spectrum for the increment in longwave emission was defined as the difference between the excitation spectra of 720nm fluorescence after 2 h and 20 min and had the maximum at 683nm. This spectrum has no real contribution of Chl672 which dominates at the moment in the fluorescence excitation spectrum as such. This implies the absence of energy transfer from the bulk Chl to its longwave form. Besides, spatial separation of these Chl pools follows from the distinctions in their closest environment which are revealed by the greater relative height and by the batochromic shift of the bands of energy transfer from Car to Chl683 in comparison with that to Chl672. The dark conversion of Chl672 into Chl683 indicates that Chl672 is a precur-

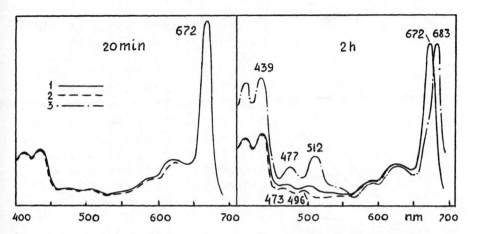

Fig.1 Excitation spectra of fluorescence at 720
(1) and 682nm (2) after 20-min and 2-h illumination of etiolated barley leaves; 3 - difference 1 for 2 h minus 1 for 20 min.

sor of Chl683 /4/. All this testifies that in
the course of Chl683 formation the next (third)
rearrangement of Chl molecules occurs.
That the Chl683 excitation band coincides
with the maximum in the action spectrum of PS1
known from /5/ permits to relate this translocation of Chl with the formation of PS1.It was
shown /2/ that already at this early stage of
greening, the PS1 pigment is built as an assembly of Chl forms with efficient energy transfer to the longwave Chl form emitting at 720nm.
Postetiolated leaves exhibit at room temperature delayed luminescence of PS2 with a short
retardation after the onset of illumination
/2/. Fig.2 presents the evolution of PS2 delayed luminescence in leaves given a flash and afterwards transferred to darkness or exposed to
white light of various intensities. Etiolated
leaves have no this luminescence at room tem-
perature.It appears a few minutes after a flash
even in darkness. The development of PS2 centers in the dark means that they are formed at

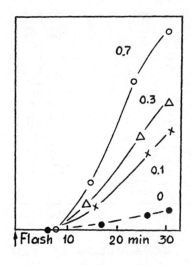

Fig.2 Delayed luminescence of 5-day-old etiolated barley leaves illuminated by a flash (2 ms) to convert Pchlde and subsequently either redarkened or transferred to continuous white light (0.1, 0.3, 0.7 mW/cm^2). Full circles indicate luminescence of leaves at the end of different dark periods (new leaves for each point).

the expense of the Chl672 pool, originating from the formerly present Pchlde, so that further Chl synthesis is not necessary. Flashed 6-day-old leaves display their delayed luminescence only after 10 min both in darkness and in light of any intensity. In other experiments, where not a flash but very weak continuous light was used to convert only 2% of Pchlde, delayed luminescence also arose after 10 min. This time is apparently needed for the synthesis of PS2 centers. Delayed luminescence grew faster at higher light intensity (Fig.2) even during the lag-phase in Chl accumulation. There exists, therefore, a particular light dependence of the development of PS2 emission, in addition to that well-known for the light-dependent Chl synthesis.

Excitation spectra of PS2 delayed luminescence have three components and do not differ for the samples with partial (about 50%) and complete Pchlde conversion (2 and 4 in Fig.3). It is of importance that after the partial conversion this spectrum has no band of energy transfer from the remaining Pchlde. Evidently sites of PS2 location are spatially separated

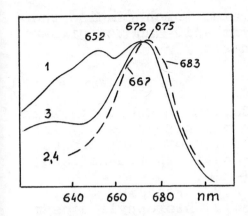

Fig.3 Absorption (1,3) and delayed luminescence excitation spectra(2,4) of 7-day-old etiolated barley leaves illuminated either by weak light of 650nm for partial conversion of Pchlde followed by light of 690nm for 1 h to stimulate luminescence development (1,2), or by white light (0.2mW/cm^2) for 1 h (3,4). Spectra are normalized on the main maxima.

from sites of Pchlde at this early step of development. Moreover, the excitation spectrum of delayed luminescence contains no band of energy transfer from the main pigment pool which determines the 672nm absorption and fluorescence excitation maxima of such leaves (Fig.3 and 1). Thus, PS2 formation involves a translocation of Chl not only from the site of synthesis but even further, from Chl672. It is the fourth rearrangement of Chl which occurs at the same time as the third one, so that PS1 and 2 grow in parallel from Chl672 serving as the supplying pool, the three entities being present simultaneously.

Further greening changes the conditions for Chl translocations and for energy transfer from Pchlde to Chl. The latter reappears after about 6 h of greening, then rapidly grows and by 24 h reaches the constant level of 50-60% /6/. It was proposed in /6/ that in the process of building of the pigment apparatus, when the assemblies of the both PSs expand, the distance between the Pchlde-forming sites and the accumulated Chl shortens and energy transfer is reestablished. These processes apparently take place in the supracomplexes which combine the machinery for Chl biosynthesis and the pigment apparatus of photosynthesis /7/.

REFERENCES

1. Shlyk, A.A.(1980). Current concept of organization of chlorophyll biosynthesis. In: Biogenesis and Function of Plant Lipids, P. Mazliak (ed). Elsevier/North-Holland, Amsterdam, pp. 311-320.
2. Shlyk, A.A., Rudoi, A.B., Fradkin, L.I., Averina, N.G. (1984). Chlorophyll biosynthesis in etiolated and greening leaves. In: Advances in Photosynthesis Research, v. IV, C. Sybesma (ed). M. Nijhoff/Dr. W. Junk Publ., The Hague, pp. 697-704.
3. Thorne, S.W. (1971). The greening of etiolated bean leaves. 1. The initial photoconversion process. Biochim. Biophys. Acta 226, 113-127.
4. Ogava, M., Konishi, M. (1980). Analysis of spectral properties after the Shibata shift by second derivative spectrophotometry. Plant Sci. Lett. 17, 169-173.
5. Hiller, R.G., Boardman, N.K. (1972). Action spectrum of cytochrome f photooxidation in greening bean leaves. Plant Physiol. 50, 183-185.
6. Shlyk, A.A., Fradkin, L.I., Domanskaya,I.N., Netkacheva, E.R. (1984). The energy migration in pigment assembly in relation to the chlorophyll biosynthesis. In: Protochlorophyllide Reduction and Greening, C. Sironval, M. Brouers (eds). M. Nijhoff/ Dr. W. Junk Publ., The Hague, pp. 297-306.
7. Fradkin, L.I., Chkanikova, R.A., Shlyk, A.A. (1981). Coupling of chlorophyll metabolism with submembrane particles, isolated with digitonin and gel-electrophoresis. Plant Physiol. 67, 555-559.

GENOME ORGANIZATION

THE MOSAIC GENOME OF WARM BLOODED VERTEBRATES

G. BERNARDI, B. OLOFSSON, J. FILIPSKI, M. ZERIAL,
J. SALINAS, G. CUNY, M. MEUNIER-ROTIVAL & F. RODIER

Laboratoire de Genetique Moleculaire, Institut
Jacques Monod, 2 Place Jussieu, 75005 Paris, France

INTRODUCTION

Density gradient centrifugation in the presence of
certain DNA ligands (Ag$^+$, BAMD; 1-3), allows the
separation of nuclear DNA from warm-blooded vertebrates
into four major components and several satellite and
minor components (4-9). The former comprise: (i) two
light components, L1 and L2, (5); and (ii) two heavy
components, H1 and H2; a third heavy component, H3, is
present at least in the human genome. The heavy
components represent about one-third of the genome and
account for the strong heterogeneity and marked
asymmetry of main-band DNAs from warm-blooded
vertebrates (4-8). In contrast, main-band DNAs from
most cold-blooded vertebrates show weak heterogeneities,
only slightly skewed CsCl peaks, and major components
having buoyant densities which are only or mainly in the
same range as the light components of warm-blooded
vertebrates (5, 10, 11, and paper in preparation). The
families of molecules forming the major components are
derived, by the unavoidable breakage which accompanies
DNA preparation, from much longer DNA segments, the
isochores (8), which have an average size well above 200
kb (6,7), and are fairly homogeneous in base composition
(6, 8, 12-15).
  Here we have studied: (i) the distribution of several
genes, of some families of interspersed repeats, and of
some integrated viral sequences in the major components
of genomes from warm-blooded vertebrates; and (ii) the
correlation between this distribution and the base
composition and codon usage of these sequences.

Proceedings of the 16th FEBS Congress
Part B, pp. 69–77
© 1985 VNU Science Press

RESULTS

Genomic distribution of genes, interspersed repeats and integrated viral sequences

Table 1 lists the sequences which were investigated and the major components in which they were found. The main findings can be summarized as follows: a) Single-copy genes are located in single major components. This indicates, in agreement with previous conclusions, (4-9, 13-15): (i) that the separation of major components corresponds to a real fractionation of the genome; and (ii) that large segments around the genes tested are compositionally fairly homogeneous. b) Clustered genes are located in the same major component, as expected if isochore size is large compared to gene cluster size (4-40 kb in the cases under consideration). c) In contrast, scattered genes belonging to the same family may be located in different major components. The α and β globin gene clusters are located in the H2 (or H3) and in the L2 components of mammalian DNAs, respectively. Other gene families, like the actin genes and pseudogenes, are scattered over all DNA components (16). d) Genes present in a given major component may be located on different chromosomes. In chicken, α^A and α^D globin genes are located on the largest chromosomes, the conalbumin gene is located on a chromosome of intermediate size, and the β and ρ globin genes are present on a small macro- or on a micro-chromosome (17); therefore, the major component in which all these genes are located, H2, is present on several chromosomes. e) Conversely, genes present in different major components may be located on the same chromosome. For example, the human Ha-ras 1 and β globin genes, which belong to components H3 and L2 respectively, are both located on chromosome 11. f) The distribution of genes and gene clusters within different major components is highly non-uniform. The data of Table 1 concern a total of 34 genes corresponding to 24 "loci" (defined here as isolated genes or gene clusters), and to 14 functionally unrelated proteins. About half of the loci examined for each genome are present in the heaviest components (H2 or H3), which only represent 8% or 4%,

70

respectively, of the DNA. g) <u>Families of interspersed
repeated sequences are concentrated in some major
components</u> (14). For instance, the BamHI family and the
CR-1 (Alu-like) family are almost only present in the
two light components of mouse (13) and in the heaviest
component of chicken (15), respectively. h) <u>Integrated
viral sequences are only or mainly located in a given
major component</u>. The integrated sequences of bovine
leukemia virus (BLV) and hepatitis B virus (HBV) from
the Alexander cell line were almost only found in
components H2 and H3, respectively; those of mouse
mammary tumor virus (MMTV) were only found in component
L2 of Balb-c mice (18, and paper in preparation). i)
<u>The distribution of genes and interspersed repeats in
the major components tends to be conserved in evolution</u>.
For instance, the α and β globin gene clusters, vimentin
and c-abl genes are located in components identical or
close in GC levels in different mammals. The same
applies to specific families of interspersed repeats
(13-15).

Gene composition and codon usage
a) <u>The GC contents of genes, exons and introns are
linearly related to those of the major components in
which they are located</u>. The slopes of the lines
representing these relationships are equal to 1.9 for
genes, to 3.0 for introns, and to 1.0 for exons. While
"light" genes are, on the average, only slightly higher
in GC than light components, "heavy" genes are
increasingly higher in GC than the corresponding heavy
components (Fig. 1). An increasing deviation from the
unit slope is also exhibited by introns and by 5' and 3'
untranslated sequences (not shown). In contrast, exons
have a unit slope, but are about 10% higher in GC, on
the average, than the components in which they are
located (not shown). Finally, integrated viral
sequences and long interspersed repeats seem to show a
closer match in composition with the major components in
which they are located, compared to genes (Fig. 1).
b) <u>The higher GC level of "heavy" relative to "light"
exons is due to a different codon usage</u> and not to the
amino acid composition of the corresponding proteins.

TABLE 1 : Localization of some sequences in the major
DNA components of warm blooded vertebrates (a).

Sequences	Major component	Sequences	Major component
Xenopus		Rabbit	
1. α globin	L1	21. α globin	H2*
2. β globin	L1	22. β globin	L2*
Chicken		Man	
3. α_D^A globin	H2	23. α_1 globin	H3*
4. α globin	"	24. α_2 globin	"
5. β globin	H2	25. β globin	L2
6. ρ globin	"	26. Aγ globin	"
7. conalbumin	H2	27. Gγ globin	"
8. ovalbumin	L2	28. δ globin	"
9. Y	"	29. ε globin	"
10. X	"	30. p-omc	H3*
11. vitellogenin	L2	31. vimentin	H1
		32. c-Ha ras 1	H3*
Mouse		33. c-myc	H1
		34. c-sis	H3*
12. α globin	H2	35. c-mos	H1*
13. β_M globin	L2	36. c-abl	H3*
14. β_m globin	"		
15. α_c actin	L2*	Viral & repeated seqs.	
16. α_s actin	H2*		
17. vimentin	L2	37. BLV	H2*
18. Ig_k const	L2	38. HBV	H3*
19. Ig^k var	L1	39. MMTV	L2*
20. c-abl	H2*	40. Mouse Bam H1	L1,L2

(a) Sequences were localized in separated major
components or, (asterisks), in preparative
BAMD-Cs_2SO_4 density gradients. References for
gene sequences will be given elsewhere. Non-
standard abbreviations: βM, β major; βm, β minor;
α_c, α cardiac ;α_s, α skeletal; p-omc, pre-pro-
opiomelanocortin. Inverted commas refer to
clustered genes.

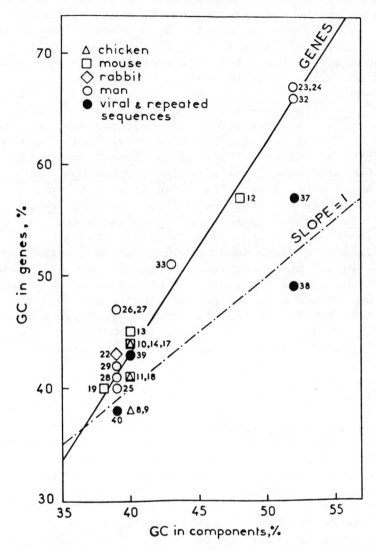

Figure 1. Plot of GC levels of genes and of viral and
long interspersed repeated sequences against the GC
levels and the buoyant densities of DNA components
in which they are located. Numbers indicate
sequences (see Table 1).

Indeed, if the codons used in "heavy" exons (53-67% GC) were replaced with the synonymous codons lowest in GC also used in the same exons, the GC levels of "heavy" exons would decrease to about 40%, a value as low as the lowest of "light" exons (40-55% GC), without any amino acid change. c) Since the vast majority of synonymous codons differ in third positions, one should expect that GC contents in codon third positions are different for "heavy" and "light" exons. This expectation is borne out, the GC level of codon third positions ranging from 43-69% to 61-90% for the "light" and the "heavy" genes, respectively. d) Genes located in "heavy" components exhibit a decreased discrimination against CpG doublets, (not shown) which tend to be avoided in vertebrate genomes. e) If the gene composition and codon usage "rules" (a-d, above) are generally valid, genes from any warm blooded vertebrate (i) should fall into compositional classes (such as those found for genes located in different components; Fig. 1); and (ii) these classes should, in turn, largely determine codon usage. Both the first and the second prediction are fulfilled (data not shown), proving the general validity of the "rules". Moreover, "light" genes predominate in the "light" genomes of cold-blooded vertebrates, as expected.

DISCUSSION

The mosaic genome organization discussed so far is typical of warm-blooded vertebrates. When the genomes of cold-blooded and warm-blooded vertebrates are compared with each other, it is clear that the main differences concern the presence of abundant, heavy components in the latter, as well as a predominance of "heavy" genes in warm-blooded vertebrates, and of "light" genes in cold-blooded vertebrates. These findings raise the question of the evolutionary origin of the heavy components present in the genome of warm-blooded vertebrates.
The evolutionary origin of the heavy components of the genome of warm-blooded vertebrates may be visualized as due to: (i) regional increases in GC levels of pre-existing "light" sequences; (ii) amplification of pre-existing "heavy" sequences. The first process is

predominates over other constraints, which may also be operational. b) <u>The heterogeneity in DNA composition is associated with chromosomal G or R banding</u>. The identification of isochores with the DNA segments present in G or R bands was previously suggested (8) on the basis of: (i) indications that G bands correspond to AT-rich, late-replicating DNA and R bands to GC-rich early replicating DNA; and (ii) the observation (8) that the increase in the heterogeneity of DNA composition when moving from cold-blooded to warm-blooded vertebrates (5) is paralleled by an increased G and R banding. This notion is now reinforced beyond reasonable doubt by: (i) the confirmation of the first two points mentioned above by recent results (paper in preparation); (ii) the fact that gene amplification leads to the appearance of homogeneous staining regions in chromosomes, as expected if the genome segments which are amplified are smaller than isochores; (iii) the presence in early replicating DNA, namely in R bands, of genes (human c-Ha ras 1 and α globin genes; mouse α globin gene) which are located in the heaviest component and the presence in late-replicating DNA, namely in G bands, of genes (human β globin gene) which are located in the lightest components (19).

CONCLUSIONS

The investigations reported here show that the <u>compositional compartmentalization</u> of the genome of warm-blooded vertebrates (i) largely dictates the base composition of genes and their codon usage; and (ii) plays a role in the timing of DNA replication and in the targeting of integration of mobile and viral sequences. From a more general viewpoint, it should be stressed that compositional compartmentalization (i) has an extremely wide evolutionary range, going as far as the mitochondrial genome (20); (ii) shows different patterns in different organisms, as exemplified here by cold-blooded and warm-blooded vertebrates; and (iii) plays a general role in genome structure and function; indeed, the different GC levels of isochores, their different CpG/GpC ratios, and the accompanying differences in potential methylation sites are bound to be associated with differences in DNA and chromatin structure, and possibly, with differences in the regulation of gene expression.

Preliminary reports on some parts of this work were published previously (21-24).

ACKNOWLEDGEMENTS

We thank the Fogarty International Center for Advanced Study in the Health Sciences, National Institutes of Health, Bethesda, Md. 20205, for a scholarship to G.B., the Institut National de la Sante et de la Recherche Medicale, Paris, France , the Associazione Italiana per la Ricerca sul Cancro, Milan, Italy, the Ministerio de Educacion y Ciencia, Madrid, Spain, for Fellowships to J.F., M.Z. and J.S., respectively, and the Association pour la Recherche Contre le Cancer, Villejuif, France, for financial support.

REFERENCES

1. G. Corneo, E. Ginelli, C. Soave and G. Bernardi, Biochemistry, 7, 4373 (1968).
2. J. Cortadas, G. Macaya and G. Bernardi, Eur. J. Biochem. 76, 13 (1977).
3. G. Macaya, J. Cortadas and G. Bernardi, Eur. J. Biochem. 84, 179 (1978).
4. J. Filipski, J.P. Thiery and G. Bernardi, J. Mol. Biol. 80, 177 (1973).
5. J.P. Thiery, G. Macaya and G. Bernardi, J. Mol. Biol. 108, 219 (1976).
6. G. Macaya, J.P. Thiery and G. Bernardi, J. Mol. Biol. 108, 237 (1976).
7. J. Cortadas, B. Olofsson, M. Meunier-Rotival, G. Macaya and G. Bernardi, Eur. J. Biochem. 99, 179 (1979).
8. G. Cuny, P. Soriano, G. Macaya and G. Bernardi, Eur. J. Biochem. 115, 227 (1981).
9. B. Olofsson and G. Bernardi, Eur. J. Biochem. 130, 241 (1983).

10. A.P. Hudson, G. Cuny, J. Cortadas, A.E.V. Haschemeyer and G. Bernardi, Eur. J. Biochem. 112, 203 (1980).
11. V. Pizon, G. Cuny and G. Bernardi, Eur. J. Biochem. 140, 25 (1984);
12. P. Soriano, G. Macaya and G. Bernardi, Eur. J. Biochem. 115, 235 (1981).
13. M. Meunier-Rotival, P. Soriano, G. Cuny, F. Strauss and G. Bernardi, Proc. Natl. Acad. Sci. U.S.A. 79, 355 (1982).
14. P. Soriano, M. Meunier-Rotival and G. Bernardi, Proc. Natl. Acad. Sci. U.S.A. 80, 1816 (1983).
15. B. Olofsson and G. Bernardi, Biochem. Biophys. Acta 740, 339 (1983).
16. P. Soriano, P. Szabo and G. Bernardi, EMBO J. 1, 579 (1982).
17. S.H. Hughes, E. Stubblefield, F. Payver, J.D. Engel, J.B. Dodgson, D. Spector, B. Cordell, R.T. Schimke and H. E. Varmus, Proc. Natl. Acad. Sci. U.S.A. 76, 1348 (1979).
18. R. Kettman, M.Meunier-Rotiva, J. Cortadas, G. Cuny, J. Ghysdael, M. Mammerickx, A. Burny and G. Bernardi, Proc. Natl. Acad. Sci. U.S.A. 76, 4822 (1979).
19. M.A. Goldman, G.P. Holmquist, M.C. Gray, L.A. Caston, A. Nag, Science 224, 686 (1984).
20. G. Bernardi, Folia Biologica 29, 82 (1983).
21. G. Bernardi in Mutations, Biology and Society, D. N. Walcher, N. Kretschmer, H. L. Barnett, Eds., (Masson, New York, 1978) p. 327.
22. C. Cuny, G. Macaya, M. Meunier-Rotival, P. Soriano and G. Bernardi, in Genetic Engineering, H.W. Boyer and S. Nicosia, Eds. (Elsevier-North Holland Biomedical Press, Amsterdam, 1978), p. 109.
23. G. Bernardi, in Recombinant DNA and Genetic Experimentation, J. Morgan and W. J. Whelan, Eds. (Pergamon Press, London, 1979), p. 15.
24. G. Bernardi, in Genetic Manipulation: Impact on Man and Society, W. Arber, et al., Eds. (Cambridge University Pres, Cambridge, 1984), p. 171.

THE MATRIX HYPOTHESIS OF DNA-DIRECTED MORPHOGENESIS, PROTODYNAMISM AND GROWTH CONTROL*

Klaus SCHERRER

Institut JACQUES MONOD, Université PARIS VII
2, Place Jussieu — 75251 PARIS Cedex 05 (FRANCE)

> "In this world, seeds of different kinds, sown
> at the proper time in the land, even in one
> field, come forth (each) according to its
> kind."
>
> MANUSMRITI (9:38)

INTRODUCTION

The objective of this essay is to try to correlate
rationally some enigmatic aspects of two domains of Cell
Biology which, in general, are treated separately. These
are cellular morphology and organisation on one hand, and
the organisation and function of genomic DNA on the
other. The hope is to show some perspectives of
understanding which may serve as a basis for future
experimental and theoretical investigation. As such this
essay, and particularly in its present short form, will
necessarily appear superficial to specialists in the
domains under consideration.

However, as demonstrated 15 years ago by the Cascade
Regulation Hypothesis (2, 3), an early attempt to draw

---

*The term MATRIX is used signifying the integrality of
the cells fibrous networks in nucleus and cytoplasm,
during interphase and metaphase. PROTODYNAMISM was
defined earlier (1) as meaning the integrality of the
organised mouvements of the cellular components,
excluding mere diffusion.

Proceedings of the 16th FEBS Congress
Part B, pp. 79–103
© 1985 VNU Science Press

attention to importance and complexity of post-transcriptional controls, it may be necessary sometimes to penetrate beyond the incomprehendable mass of details to the underlying general patterns, in spite of the initial oversimplification.

The present reflection originated from the experimental observation of the systematic punctuation of the eukaryotic DNA by AT-rich DNA segments (4) having precise locations in relation to genes (5) and acting essentially as spacers (review in (6); cf. this volume, preceeding article). This led us to explore possible theoretical explanations of this phenomenon of long range DNA organisation. Some of these ideas evolving independently, were found to converge partially with those exposed in a theoretical analysis by T. CAVALIER-SMITH (7) about the C-value paradox (8). Without the ambition to complete nor to comment his extensive and erudite analysis, the present discussion develops some ideas which possibly extend that anterior work, but are developped from a more mechanistic viewpoint of Molecular Biology.

Morphogenesis of organism and organ is necessarily based on properties of the individual cell, essentially the number and direction in space of consecutive cell divisions in a clone, modulated by cell to cell interaction. In some cases at least it is evident that this process must be based on the morphology of the individual cell and its functional organisation. How these properties arise is, however, a complete mystery at present. Some think that genes are not necessary for morphogenesis (9), but others consider that morphogenesis is essentially based on the self- assembly of proteins and their enzymatic derivatives. Examples are some of the matrix networks, in particular the tubulin fibers which self- assemble, indeed, even in vitro . Although co-polymerisation of several different components may allow for some modulation in the assembly of structures, the complexity and specificity of the individual phenotype of cell and organ, however, seems to set a limit to the application of this kind of process. That matrix fibers are involved in cellular and extra-cellular structure is unquestionable (cf. recent review volume of

J. Cell. Biol., and in particular (10); however what
directs their assembly, their overall organisation and
specificity ? The enigma seems still complete.

A quite different enigma relates to the genomic DNA in
eukaryotes. To put it simply, there is too much of it and
of the wrong kind! Calculations show that no more than a
few percent of typical eukaryotic DNA can be accounted
for by structural genes. To make matters worse, animals
and plants of comparable morphology may contain vastly
different amounts of DNA (the so-called C-value paradox,
8) or, apparently, different kinds of DNA. Recent studies
show that plant cells may contain anywhere from 0.6 pg to
35 pg of DNA (RANJEKAR pers. comm.; cf. 11), amphibians 3
- 8 pg (12) and Necturus 100 pg (13). Crabs have up to
90%, mice about 6% of AT-rich satellite DNA, whereas rats
are apparently devoid of this kind of DNA. The comparison
of the DNA of Triturus and Xenopus shows that the about
seven fold difference in DNA content does not concern
unique frequency DNA transcribed into pre-mRNA and mRNA
but repetitive DNA of all frequency classes (13). In
plants the difference concerns neither simple sequence
(highly repetitive), nor unique (coding?) DNA but the
intermediate frequency class and, in particular, its
AT-rich fraction (RANJEKAR, pers. comm.; cf. 11).

We have found recently that eukaryotic DNA is
systematically punctuated by AT-rich DNA segments (4)
which frame units of genome organisation (5), and
transcription, and eventually genes and gene fragments
(exons) in pre-mRNA (6). Integrating the known facts
about these AT-rich elements in eukaryotic DNA discussed
in the preceeding article (this volume; 6), we are again
faced by the old dilemmma concerning eukaryotic DNA, that
of "too much" (uneconomical !) and "of the wrong kind"
(no reading frames), a dilemma exposed most concisely by
the C-value paradox mentioned above (8; and review in 7).
So why does nature insist on piling up "unnecessary" DNA
when scientists feel that the cell does not need it? It
must be "junk" DNA (14) or, worse, a kind of perversion
of the "selfish" DNA (15)! The attempt to overcome this
intellectual deadlock must obviously consider the
proposition that other possible functions may be ascribed

to the surplus DNA; this is the main objective of the Matrix Hypothesis developed here.

If we begin by rejecting the a priori notion that all of this "junk" DNA is useless, and take more seriously what would otherwise be considered as spurious coincidence (and this choice is possibly rather a "philosophical" question or attitude) then a dual pattern of possible significance of this DNA seems to emerge. It relates to the architecture of cell and chromosomes and their "mechanics" on the one hand, and to cellular topology and "protodynamism" in the widest sense on the other. In other words: within the Matrix Hypothesis the "extra" DNA is postulated to relate to the structural and dynamic organisation of the cell, and to morphogenesis.

The incredible speed and flexibility of mouvement of the cellular components often opposes the concepts of a static internal architecture. Furthermore, the concept of high mobility of cellular macromolecular components has spread over to the genome itself. We are witness to a literal "dissolution" of the rigid genome organisation, brought about by natural or experimental gene mobility, DNA transposition and translocation. However, although genes seem to be able to mouve most rapidly from place to place, and although it is possible to achieve experimentally the expression of almost any gene in any host, the fact is that within a species the genome organisation is remarkably conserved.

In living matter the seemingly static architecture is thus just a temporary facett of its dynamic organisation. And the variability and mobility of genes and DNA sequences at the level of the genome may be considered as a prerequisite for the generation of the more stable variants of organisation specific to a species, and to its somatic genotype and phenotype. And the question arises to what extent these two aspects of the cells physiology might relate and condition each other.

The central proposition of the Matrix Hypothesis to be developped here is the consideration that the not-protein coding part of the cells genomic DNA might govern largely and directly the cells architecture and dynamic organisation. The concept that the role of DNA is to

82

produce enzymes and proteins and their derivatives, which might eventually self-assemble in a para-cristalline manner, is extended to include the idea that the non-coding part of the DNA may directly dictate the assembly of cellular components into a matrix network which then becomes the core of the cells static and dynamic architecture. This idea differs from the proposition of CAVALIER-SMITH (7) to the extent that the DNA is not considered to be _itself_ a nuclear skeleton but acts as a template to build the matrix network, constituted of protein and possibly RNA, which eventually becomes independant of the DNA. This proposition does not exclude but complements the mechanism of protein self-assembly, which is all-evident in some precise cases. Finally, the Matrix Hypothesis has the potentiality to account logically for the excessive amounts and variations in DNA content in different species, and to project some intrinsic logic into some seemingly absurd features of eukaryotic DNA, such as the fragmentation of the gene and the necessity for its post-transcriptional reconstitution.

In the following we will formulate the several propositions included in this scheme and discuss their experimental and theoretical background.

THE BASIC POSTULATES OF THE MATRIX HYPOTHESIS

1) The extra-genic, non protein-coding part of genomic DNA governs organisation and assembly of the cellular matrix: the topology of specific sites in the DNA involved in matrix-protein interaction determines _directly_ the extent and topological organisation of the matrix network into which, in turn, the DNA is suspended. The topology of these sites and hence mere DNA length in between individual sites amounts to a novel type of genetic information.

2) To allow for a predefined three-dimensional structure in which specific proximal or distal segments in the DNA are joined at specific points of the matrix, the DNA : matrix-protein interaction is governed by a

83

specific <u>code</u> involving combinations of <u>pleiotropic</u>
<u>signals</u> ; as a consequence, such DNA sequences tend
hence to be repetitive, and matrix proteins will be
only partially specific to a gene domain, to a
cellular sector or a tissue.

3) The DNA not only determines cellular and nuclear
volume (cf. 7) but also cell morphology, and organizes
the skeletal structures in early stages of lineage
determination, when the nuclei of stem cells virtually
fill the cellular lumen.

4) In crucial steps of differentiation, the decondensed
DNA of specific gene domains, genes or gene fragments
condition the build-up of local matrix networks, which
integrated, define overall somatic cell morphology and
volume. Genes are thus placed in specific topological
sectors of the matrix, of the cell and nucleus; the
necessity to keep this topology genetically stable
leads to a relatively stable localisation of genes in
the chromosomal DNA, conditioning the "chromosome
field" (cf. 16).

5) Extra-genic and intra-genic transcribed DNA spacers
interact in a gene-specific manner with specific
matrix "channels" and condition and support sector-
specific processing and transport of pre-mRNA; in turn
the pre-mRNA contains signals conditioning build-up
and dynamism of gene specific matrix channels on which
its processing occurs (cf. 17). The organisational
principle of a specific cells dynamic architecture and
RNA processing and transport system ("PROTODYNAMISM")
is hence thought to be conditioned directly by DNA and
pre-mRNA itself.

6) Chromosomes are held in specific positions relative to
each other during inter- and metaphase by direct DNA
and protein mediated interaction, ectopic pairing and
matrix elements.

7) A pattern of point to point alignment of the sister
chromatids during meiotic and mitotic recombination
and sister chromatid exchange, allows for crossing-
over at specific topologically fixed sites of the DNA;
this topology - relating to the cells genome and
morphological organisation (cf. postulate 4) - is

characteristic for a given species and constitutes a
barrier to inter-species synaptonemal alignment and,
hence, to the fertility of hybrids.
8) Topology of growth, i.e. direction in space and number
of sequential cellular divisions are directly or
indirectly based on the quantitative and qualitative
specificity of the DNA : matrix-protein interaction; a
cellular clone of a definitive line will thus have the
potentiality to fill a given morphologically defined
volume; these mechanisms are modulated by cell to cell
interaction involving extra-cellular matrix elements.
9) Available sites on the DNA must be satisfied by a
corresponding number of specific matrix components;
the programmed unbalance of this relation leads to DNA
replication and cell division.
10) Any unprogrammed and unbalanced perturbation of the
DNA-matrix or RNA-matrix interactions leads to the
disruption of programms of temporal and spatial gene
expression, of growth control and morphogenesis.

THE BASIC MECHANISMS

The basic postulate of the matrix hypothesis is that
the "extra-genic", non protein-coding DNA has a directing
function in the organisation of the static and dynamic
architecture of the cell, which partially conditions its
phenotypic function (postulates 1 to 3). At each step of
differentiation partially different fractions of the DNA
will be involved. The DNA carrying genes for specific
cell function would hence also influence spatial
organisation and morphology; quite obviously, the latter
must be adapted to cell function. There is thus a logic
in an arrangement which will link genetically
cell-specific gene expression with the blueprint of the
infrastructure necessary to support both the mechanism
and control of that genes expression and the execution of
its phenotypic function.

The postulate of a direct action of the nuclear DNA in
the cells architecture meets a quite obvious and trivial
difficulty in the compartmentalisation of the eukaryotic

cell: we see the cell basically as a dual architectural
entity, composed of nucleus and cytoplasm. But typically,
stem cells or cells arrested in differentiation as
resting lymphocytes, have minimal cytoplasm. Furthermore,
in most cells the nucleus is, in fact, an ephemeral
structure. Disrupted during cell division, it can not be
part nor condition of the permanency of the cells
architecture and organisation, which must constitute a
continuum throughout interphase and metaphase. Since the
structures conditioning this architecture must be
maintained throughout cell division, at least some of the
matrix networks must be faithfully duplicated in every
cell division. Indeed, e.g. centriole duplication often
occurs at the onset of the S phase, and the daughter
centrioles separate only later on, moving to opposite
poles prior to morphological segregation and
redistribution of the inactivated chromosomes; then only
the new nuclei are formed.

The filamental networks of the cell are hence likely to
represent the only permanent structures throughout the
cell cycle which, in conjunction with the plasma-
membrane skeleton, represent the permanent organisation
of the cell. This and other facts led some to consider
that: "DNA, gene and chromosomes are not thus important"
(9), and that the continuity of the cell is largely given
by some non-genic mechanisms based on the self assembling
potential of living matter. What then is the basis of the
opposite idea: that DNA may govern directly , and not
only through gene expression and the assembly of its
products, matrix organisation?

We may consider the cell as a unit space to be filled
by a three dimensional network. The question arises how,
within this network, positions and inter-connections are
defined according to the function of specific cellular
sectors or transport channels.

Data arising over the past ten years demonstrate with
increasing strength that the cell is highly sectorized,
not only morphologically but also in respect to
localisation of DNA and (pre-)mRNA. The old observation
that in normally differentiating cells nucleoli occupy
specific positions is being complemented by the recent

finding that satellite DNA occupies specific topological
positions (18) forming a finite number of "pseudo-
micronucleoli". Even more to the point are the
experiments showing by _in situ_ hybridization of specific
repetitive sequence probes that specific DNA may be
located in topologically defined sectors of the nucleus,
as are some specific transcripts (19). Such data are
complemented by the fact that newly induced, and/or cell-
specific proteins appear in delimited sectors of the
cytoplasm and hence are not synthesized randomly all over
the cell (20, 21). All these data tend to show that the
(unmanipulated!) cell has a highly specific static and
dynamic architecture and functional organisation. Our
challenge is hence to try to understand the molecular
basis of such an organisation in which, almost
inevitably, the filamenteous networks will play a crucial
role. Indeed, the DNA, pre-mRNA and mRNA, as well as the
polyribosomes, are long known to be attached to nuclear
and cytoplasmic matrix or skeleton (cf. discussion in
17).

From a theoretical standpoint, the cells basic structure is hence to be understood as a three- dimensional
network or lattice in which every position is defined.
Since this model concerns a living cell, and not the
steel skeleton of a building, this lattice has to be
dynamic and not merely static: lines of defined positions
have to form vectors of functional interconnection and of
dynamic change. In a regular lattice involving straight
lines at right angles, every point in space is defined by
three coordinates, e.g. X10, Y10, Z10, or in the general
case by three types of "redundant signals": Xn, Yn, Zn.
In turn, such a lattice can be reconstituted by
assembling multiple straight segment of given length e.g.
Xa-Xb, Ya-Yb, Za-Zb, Xb-Xc, etc... Clearly however, as in
geometry the triangle is defined by its sides length, any
kind of irregular three-dimensional network can also be
built on this basis, provided the existance of a
combinatory of redundant signals placed at specific
distance which define unequivocally the points of contact
of the variably shaped fibres constituting the network.
Applied to biology, the problem is thus to propose

mechanisms which allow construction of a three-
dimensional matrix, by which the cell could be sectorized
and in which given genes could occupy specific positions,
and where, furthermore, the gene products, RNA and
protein, would be generated and transported along
specific vector channels.

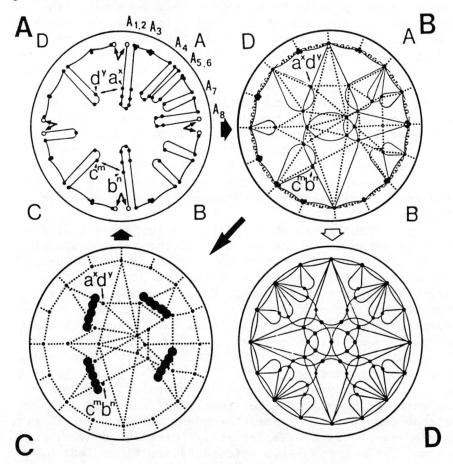

Figure 1: Schematic representation of the basic
propositions of the Matrix Hypothesis   (A) The linear
organisation of 4 chromosomes is shown with the sites of
potential specific interaction (black dots) having
specific positions a(n), b(n), c(n) or d(n) in the DNA,
each one loaded with specific pleiotropic factors. Some

of them (e.g. A1) are in decondensed chromatin, forming the classical LAEMMLI loops (44), others remain in heterochromatic state (e.g. A3). (B) Interaction takes place in site-specific manner (e.g. in between sites ax and dy, cm and bn,etc..) under the control of the signals and factors bound to each site and to telomeres (rings): a three dimensional network is created in which every position is determined by the pleiotropic signals and factors common to interacting sites. From the sites of interaction, constituting "roots" of polymerisation, the matrix network is formed corresponding, thus, to the fraction of DNA in decondensed chromatin loops; the basis of these are at the nuclear lamina and hence envelope. In course of further differentiation this envelope retracts from the periphery leaving behind some matrix elements. (C) The cell has gone through mitosis and the interconnected mitotic chromosomes will start to decondense according to "A" into chromatin, to be reinserted at specific sites into the matrix network (not shown in "A"). However in differentiation, additional loops may form conditioning new sectors of matrix, and the chromatin of other domains may have become heterochromatic, leading to the loss of the corresponding matrix sectors; such events might correspond to those of "Quantal Mitosis" (45). (D) Shows the fully decondensed state of chromatin conditioning the (theoretical?) maximal expansion of the network.

At this point of our discussion intervenes the central proposition of the Matrix Hypothesis: that it is the DNA itself which directs the overall organisation of the three-dimensional network of cellular filaments, and that the transcripts i.e. the primary and secondary pre-mRNA recognize and extend in a dynamic fashion this kind of organisation. Accordingly, the fraction of the transcribed and untranscribed DNA, interspersed with genes but taking part neither directly nor indirectly in protein synthesis, is thought to contain an inventory of pleiotropic signals which, in given specific combinations, can be recognized by specific proteins. By interacting with specific DNA sequences and in between themselves, these define specific points of the matrix. From such "roots", the further assembly of the filamentous network could be completed, possibly by self-assembly of fiber proteins.

In other words : DNA, and possibly pre-mRNA, would directly constitute building templates for the organised assembly of the static and dynamic parts of networks which, once constituted, would in turn provide static and dynamic recognition points for specific segments of the nucleic acids. Since the DNA signals directing this assembly are thought to be of pleiotropic nature, a three-dimensional lattice would result in which segments of specific DNA from the same or different chromosomes would interact directly or indirectly. As a result, any segment of the DNA taking part in this system would find itself in precise positions in the lattice and hence in specific sectors of nucleus and cell. Fig. 1 and its legend formulate and illustrate this basic proposition in more detail. Secondarily, the combinatory of proteins interacting with thus defined positions of the DNA would assemble automatically into an organised filamentous network of its own which, once constituted, might become temporarily independant of its nucleic acid building templates. This is the case in mitosis when the metaphase chromosomes condense; the reconstitution of the daughter cell nuclei would consist in part in the re-insertion of the DNA segments into their assigned positions within the matrix. In every cell division, according to the fraction of DNA involved (i.e. the decondensed part of chromatin) the decision to maintain or alter this organisation might constitute a basic event of cell differentiation. In this fashion might be comforted the seemingly conflicting postulates of the apparent non-genic permanancy of the cells architecture and its dependancy on the genetic apparatus of cell and species, as well as its modification in course of differentiation.

Some of the basic implications of this model seem to correlate reasonably well with present knowledge about nucleic acids and cellular matrix. Being pleiotropic, the putative signals at the contact points would have to correspond to repetitive DNA sequences, and the matrix structures would have to include a quite extensive but defined population of proteins (cf. 10). In fact, as in the case of the non-histone proteins and of the pre-mRNA and mRNP "recognition" proteins (22), thought to control gene expression, we are confronted here again with the properties of a multikey system of pleiotropic signals discussed e.g. within the Cascade Regulation Scheme (3). These are of fundamental theoretical necessity in any kind of biological (and other) system of control of information. In the case discussed here, the system would have the additional potential capacity to organise the DNA into an architecture in which given genes would reside in specific localisations, where different and in the DNA unlinked genes could be temporarily linked constituting centers of cooperative action. From there gene products could be delivered to specific transport and expression channels, leading to specific sectors of the cytoplasm, thus conditioning the phenotype. This architecture would also define the overall morphology and size of the cell, and secondarily that of supra- cellular compounds and organs.

EXPERIMENTAL CORRELATIONS AND THEORETICAL EXTRAPOLATIONS

The postulate that DNA content conditions the size of a cell - its main architectural feature - was proposed years ago by CAVALIER-SMITH (7); the matrix hypothesis, among other propositions, adds an inter-dependant protein matrix to this DNA network. The haploid DNA content shows a linear correlation when plotted versu the volume of specific cells (23). We have to keep in mind that selection in evolution acts on the phenotype exclusively, and that the DNA as the archive of the cells blueprints has to provide simultaneously for the emergence of modification as well as for the capacity to integrate new solutions without changing the basic patterns of the plan; this is the case for instance when cells grow bigger adapting to a given ecological niche.

The matrix hypothesis (postulates 1 to 3) allows for a

91

straightforward interpretation of the correlation of cell volume and DNA content. If the DNA conditions and is part of a specific three-dimensional network as a building template for e.g. an erythroblast, and if such a cell and its nucleus grow bigger in some species, to maintain this network spanning the nucleus and integrating the specific genes expressed in this cell, the DNA must expand itself. The only solution is to intercalate more and more spacer DNA in between genes and, possibly, gene domains (exons). If this DNA is in addition directly involved in the DNA: specific matrix-protein intraction then, due to the pleiotropy of these signals, this DNA will be repetitive in sequence. Cellular and DNA mass will grow in concertation, but the blueprint of organisation, the genes and, in first approximation, the DNA complexity will remain stable.

Proceeding to more specific architectural features: we have already mentioned that the inter-connection of specific DNA segments has the potentiality to assign every gene to a specific sector of cell and nucleus. The phenomenon of ectopic pairing in polytene chromosomes of Drosophila (cf. e.g. 24), linking specific interbands in between and within chromosomes and with nucleoli, gives a quite precise "macroscopical" image of the existance of specific linkage of genomic domains. Ectopic pairing is also visible in between metaphase chromosomes (25), and it is known that the latter, obeying specific rules, occupy precise positions relative to each other in the metaphase plates (26). Furthermore, paternal and maternal chromosome sets remain linked at least through the first 3 cell divisions after fertilisation (27).

There is hence ample evidence for specific inter-connection of chromosomes in interphase and metaphase. The contribution of the matrix hypothesis (postulate 6) is to propose that this kind of mechanisms goes straight down to the individual unit of chromosome architecture and function in interphase and metaphase: to the equivalents of the polytene chromosome bands and of the units of transcription and replication, which are thought interconnected in between themselves and with the matrix. Furthermore, chromosome translocations and gene transposition may reveal the existance of such types of linkage. The intragenic chromosome translocation in leukemic cells (28) may be the result of a pathology in which dynamically linked gene fragments escape the controls that keep them separate and which permeates by DNA recombination a temporary, functionally conditioned association. Indeed, such translocations suggest that the genes involved are temporarily in close molecular contact with each other. Such events may thus not occur by chance but may be conditioned by organisation and function of cell and genome.

Another postulate which divided and still divides Molecular and Classical Biologists is that of the "chromosome field" (cf. remarks of F. CRICK in LIMA DE FARIA, 16b). It is based on the observation that within a species, and also between related species, some specific genes reside in specific relative positions of the individual chromosome arms in relation to centromeres and telomeres and to each other. When multiple chromosome arms carrying e.g. ribosomal genes, are arranged in parallel on a X/Y system of coordinates, with their centromeres on the ordinate and the telomeres on a line at a 45° angle (16), then the specific genes are found in the same relative position on the specific chromosome arms defining a "chromosome field". This has been interpreted as the result of an internal structural "message" originating from the centromere and organizing the sequential insertion of specific genes; an explanation hardly acceptable to the molecule-minded biologist. If however the cell is functionally sectorized and this sectorisation depends genetically on the DNA (postulates 3 and 4), then classical evolutionary pressure will keep specific genes at their specific localisation in relation to each other, and in their sequential order on the chromosomes. Furthermore, for this kind of mechanism it will not matter into how many chromosomes the DNA will be divided, only the relative order of genes and other structural DNA segments will be important, and not the chromosome number per se . (The 46 chromosomes of Muntjak muntjak or the 6 of Muntjak Reevesi will be able to condition an allmost identical

93

phenotype, 29). Indeed, according to the matrix hypothesis, the basic mechanism of sectorisation and organisation implies simply permanent and dynamic matrix attachment points, placed at given distances and in a given sequential order along the DNA, conditioning the organisation of structure and expression of genome and phenotype. If this sequential order of genes is punctuated by centromeres, telomeres or simply by constitutive heterochromatin, and if spindle fiber attachment points along the chromosome are centromeric or dispersed (30) are details of chromosome mechanics, superimposed on the basic features of long range DNA organisation.

It is however important to notice that, within the framework of such an organisation, topological positions of signals and mere distance in the DNA start to matter. <u>Nucleotide numbers alone</u> (never mind their sequence!) between two signals <u>will amount to specific genetic information</u> . Two novel and related types of genetic information must thus be postulated (postulate 2), in addition to the genetic code of protein assembly: 1) a code of pleiotropic signals defining the specificity of DNA-matrix protein interaction, and 2) the topology of sites of DNA-matrix interaction given by the distance in the DNA of the corresponding signals and their sequential arrangement.

It is evident that the type of DNA assigned to these functions will obey completely different rules in regard to effects of mutation, deletion and evolution, compared to the protein-coding parts of the genome. Furthermore, the chromosome morphology, in as far as it reveals gross features of this latent organisation, will partially reflect a latent image related to the phenotype. This organisation might be reflected in the banding pattern of chromosomes which characterize a species, but also relate different species to each other (31). Indeed, the telomeric fusion of the 40 chromosomes of <u>Mus Musculus</u> into fewer metacentric chromosomes in <u>Mus Posciavino</u> (32) will still produce a mouse, incidentally of different size. The turning around of a chromosome arm correlates, however, with the physiological difference between man and Chimpanzee, which differ in their morphology and the building plan of their nervous system, although they share the same primary sequences in their hemoglobin. Structural genes and gross chromosome patterns are thus maintained but details of overall organisation changes.

Once established this scheme of defined long range DNA organisation and topology, several further implications become apparent. We may mention in particular those concerning the mechanisms of meiotic crossing over and somatic sister chromatid exchange (postulate 7). Legitimate and/or illegitimate recombination implies that the sister chromatids align and have the possibility to interact at precise positions, which may be localised in extragenic, or possibly intragenic (introns) spacers . The units of meiotic complementation correspond grossly to the polytene chromosome bands (33), and although intra- band and intra-coding sequence recombination occurs (e.g. in genic conversion), apparently it occurs at lower frequency (per cell division) compared to meiotic recombination. As the examples of aberrant crossing over show, intra-genically in the cases of e.g. the hemoglobin LEPORE deletion (34), or the chromosome translocation associated with Burkitts Lymphoma (28, 35) or extra-genically in the cases of the yeast "Petite" mutation (36), aberrant recombination may lead to disaster for cell and organism. The point to point alignment of the chromatids in the synaptonemal complex implies, however, that the genes and gene fragments to be exchanged are in precise positions when recombination occurs: again topology i.e. relative DNA distance matters, to fix and maintain the pattern of signals conditioning this alignment.

We may touch here at the rules of the molecular basis of speciation. Indeed, the mule or hinny living happily with the genes of two different species can not reproduce since horse and donkey sister chromatids can not align properly: they are lysed instead of forming a healthy synaptonemal complex (37).

The evolutionary pressure driving a phenotype to adopt to its ecological niche will hence lead to genetic separation of the successful variant if, by the mechanisms of the matrix hypothesis proposed, morphological phenotype and genotype are <u>directly</u> interdependant (and not only through the bias of peptides which can be shared by widely different species) and if the pattern of chromosomal signals thus created matters in the mechanisms of sexual reproduction.

Proceeding to other implications we may recall that, within the Matrix Hypothesis, the ultimate justification for a rather rigid structural organisation of the genomic DNA is thought to relate to the specific phenotype, and thus to the mechanisms of gene expression which condition phenotypic expression. In other words: genes have to cooperate (e.g. the alpha and beta (Hemo-)globin chains encoded on different chromosomes), and their pre-mRNA, mRNA and protein products have to reach specific sectors of the cell by specific transfer channels as e.g. in the case of Myelin (20). The basic overall organisation of cell and nucleus by the genomic DNA is hence thought to be complemented by a more dynamic DNA-Matrix interaction in which the transcribed DNA would give over the primary transcripts at specific positions to the matrix, on which RNA processing takes place (17). Indeed several components of pre-mRNP complexes are shared by the matrix structures such as the SnRNA (17, 37) and the poly(A) binding protein (17).

Since the very specificity of pre-mRNA processing is thought to be influenced by differential attachment of the transcribed DNA at specific points of the matrix (such DNA signals might operationally have the properties of "transcription" enhancers, 39), the primary mono- or polycistronic pre-mRNA could be differentially selected and yield different mRNA, according to the diffe-rentiation state of cell and its stage-specific matrix. DNA modifications such as methylation, and DNA-protein interactions within chromatin could thus lead to post-transcriptional effects at the level of the controls of processing.

If the DNA has the potential ability to organise the static and dynamic matrix network in relation to gene expression, and in particular, if some proteins could be transfered from DNA to RNA (e.g. SV40 T-antigen attached to both ? 40), then the further possibility is given that it is the primary transcripts and successive processing intermediates that carry out, during processing and transport, an organizing function (postulate 5). Pre-mRNA might hence at the same time be template and substrate to the processing and transport machinery, extending and supplementing the architectural and organising function of the DNA, which could be modulated by successive processing steps. It has been obvious for a long time that the mRNA in its final form cannot carry all the information necessary for all the collateral mechanisms involved in its transport and expression; the pre-mRNA however has no limits in this respect, and was proposed to carry in its structure the chronology of mechanistic and regulative interventions necessary for the delivery of its genetic message (cf. Fig. 19 in the "Cascade Regulation"; 3).

The topology of the DNA: matrix-protein interaction may thus differentially influence the processing of pre-mRNA. The latter might serve as a template for the organisation of processing and transport channels on the matrix leading to the cytoplasm. Finally, proteins of DNA: matrix interaction may be transferred to the RNA and prolong this interaction at pre-mRNA level.

A last implication of the matrix hypothesis (postulates 8 and 9) to be discussed relates to morphogenesis of supra-cellular structures, of cellular clones and eventually organs. Some components of the matrix networks are known not to be limited to the individual cell but transcend its limits. By defining supra-cellular compounds in conjunction with sequential vectorial control of cell division, they have the potential to fill in a specific volume of pre-defined shape. Before touching at these matters we will first have to come back to the putative mechanisms of sectorisation in the individual cell.

If the cell is sectorized in respect to the matrix networks, i.e. the contact points of interaction involving specific activated DNA segments, conditioned by differential (allelic !) activity of the chromatid sets, then the line of subdivision of the cell resp. the directionality of division starts to matter. Quite obviously, it can divide the cell and the matrix networks strictly symetrically, or asymetrically to various degree. Some observations show indeed a clearcut correlation between plane of cell division (conditioned by spindle orientation) and events of differentiation occuring after a specific number of divisions (e.g. in moss protonema formation, 41). Thus, a programmation of the number and direction of consecutive cellular divisions must be postulated in line with programms of differentiation.

On the other hand, simple logic tells us that the number of cell divisions in a clone must be programmed since the final volume of a cell compartment or an organ is predetermined. Combining the number of divisions and their directionality in space within a program, any morphological shape can be predetermined; of course such programs have to be modulated by cell to cell interaction within and between cellular clones. The example of the six compartments of the Drosophila wing, separated by virtual lines partially unrelated to anatomical features (42) demonstrates the necessity for the existance of such programs. Since somatic mutagenesis by X-rays leads to the local breackdown of such virtual lines (43), DNA must be involved directly or indirectly in their establishment and maintenance.

The precise molecular mechanisms conditioning these programs are totally unknown at present. Postulates 8 and 9 of the Matrix Hypothesis propose one possibility to imagine a solution by molecular mechanism implicating the DNA-matrix interaction. Conditioning cellular sectorisation, they have obviously also the potential to control directionality of division. Together with a count-down mechanism determining numbers of division, the DNA- matrix interaction might be both rigid and flexible enough to determine numbers and direction of sequential cell division.

The further implication arises then, if such systems exist, that the pathology of overall growth control, i.e. uncontrolled division and invasiveness of cells, might originate in the breakdown of the molecular mechanisms conditioning these programs of differentiation of specific growth control and morphogenesis (postulate 10). It can not escape the reader that the cellular oncogenes, the products of which are located everywhere in the cell where there are matrix elements, from the DNA to the plasma membrane, might represent good candidates to participate in the molecular mechanism conditioning these programs.

IN CONCLUSION

The attempt was made here to introduce some new ideas concerning the enigmatic molecular basis of morphogenesis and the static and dynamic organisation of the eukaryotic cell, and to propose mechanisms of its possible inter-dependance on still equally enigmatic characteristics of genome and DNA organisation and function. Some ramifications of these ideas were discussed but more remain untold. There was no space to evaluate and detail here basic knowledge on matrix and DNA structure; the author apologizes to the eminent collegues working in these fields for not having discussed their work which, of course, served as a basis of reflection.
To the engaged and lucid scientist it is unacceptable to cover up our ignorance by postulating absurdity in nature; we have the obligation to try to push further the limits of the mechanistic comprehension of the phenomenon of life. This idea is at the basis of this essay and is the source of its imperfections. Sometimes we have to put to test seed and soil, beeing nothing more than the humble instruments of the evolution of nature and of its human comprehension.

ACKNOWLEDGEMENTS

The author thanks all friends and collegues who participated by discussion in the intelletual elaboration of this essay, and in particular the most critical and stimulating collegues in India, who challenged the ideas

outlined here during a lecture tour. Warm personal thanks
go to Sheldon PENMAN who taught me much on matrix and new
ways of looking at it, to François JACOB who critically
evaluated the basic ideas of the scheme, to François
ZAJDELA, Cecile LEUCHTENBERGER, Jacques MOREAU and Sohan
MODAK with whom I discussed specific aspects, and in
particular to Kinsey MAUNDRELL who helped me to bring
ideas and language into a comprehendable form. This work
was supported by the French CNRS, INSERM, the Ministère
de la Recherche et de la Technologie, the Fondation pour
la Recherche Médicale Française and the Association pour
la Recherche sur le Cancer (ARC).

BIBLIOGRAPHY

(1) SCHERRER, K. (1966) A. Soc. Helv. Nat. $\underline{146}$, 75–92
(2) SCHERRER, K. and MARCAUD, L. (1968) J. Cell.
     Physiol. $\underline{172}$, 181–212
(3) SCHERRER, K. (1980) in "Eukaryotic Gene Regulation",
     Kolodny ed., Vol.I, CRC Press, pp. 57–129
(4) MOREAU, J., MATYASH-SMIRNIAGUINA, L. and SCHERRER,
     K. (1981) Proc. Natl. Acad. Sci. USA $\underline{78}$, 1341–1345
(5) MOREAU, J., MARCAUD, J., MASCHAT, F.,
     KEJZLAROVA-LEPESANT, J., LEPESANT, J–A and SCHERRER,
     K. (1982) Nature $\underline{295}$, 260–262
(6) SCHERRER, K. and MOREAU, J. (1985) Proceedings of
     the 16th FEBS Congress, Moscow 1984, VNU Science
     Press (Utrecht 1985); in press; cf. this volume
(7) CAVALIER-SMITH, T. (1978) J. Cell Sci. $\underline{34}$, 247–278
(8) THOMAS, C.A. (1971) A. Rev. Genet. $\underline{5}$, 237–256
(9) LIMA DE FARIA, A. (1983) in "Molecular evolution and
     organization of the chromosome", (Elsevier, ed.,
     Amsterdam), page 3 ff
(10) FEY, E.G., CAPCO, D.G., KROCHMALNIC, G. and PENMAN,
     S. (1984) J. Cell Biol. $\underline{99}$, 203s–208s
(11) RANJEKAR, P.K., PALLOTA, D. and LAFONTAINE, J.G.
     (1978) Biochem. Gen. $\underline{16}$, 957–970
     RANJEKAR, P.K. (1983) pers. comm.
(12) SOMMERVILLE, J. (1977) in "Biochem. of Cell
     Differentiation", J. Paul Ed., Int. Rev. Biochem. $\underline{15}$

,79-156

(13) ROSBASH, M., FORD, P.J. and J. BISHOP (1974) Proc. Natl. Acad. Sci. USA 71 , 3746-3750

(14) OHNO, S. (1972) J. Hum. Evol. 1 , 651-662

(15) DOOLITTLE, W.F. (1982) in "Genome Evolution", G.A. Dower and R.B. Flavell ed. (Academic Press); page 3; and therein

(16) LIMA DE FARIA, A. (1980) Hereditas 93 , 1-46

(-b) LIMA DE FARIA, A. (1979) in "Specific Eukaryotic Genes", Alfred Benzon Symposium 13 (Munksgaard, 1979), page 25

(17) MAUNDRELL, K., MAXWELL, S., PUVION, E. and SCHERRER, K. (1981) Exptl. Cell Res. 136 , 435-445

(-b) MARIMAN, E.C., VAN EEKELEN, C.A., REINDERS, R.J., BERNS, A.J. and VAN VENROOIJ, W.J. (1982) J. Mol. Biol. 154 , 103-119

(18) MANUELIDES, L. (1982) in "Genome Evolution", G.A. Dower and R.B. Flavell ed. (Academic Press); page 263

(19) LIFSCHYTZ, E., HAREVEN, D., AZRIEL, A. and HAYWARD, W.S. (1983) Cell 32 , 191-199

(20) COLMAN, D.R., KREIBICH, G., FREY, A.B. and SABATINI, D.D. (1982) J. of Cell Biol. 95 , 598-608

(21) KUHLMANN, W.D., BOUTEILLE, M. and AVRAMEAS, S. (1975) Exptl Cell Res. 96 , 335-343

(22) VINCENT, A., AKHAYAT, O., GOLDENBERG, S. and SCHERRER, K. (1983) EMBO J. 2 , 1869-1876

(23) PRICE, H.J. (1973) Experientia 29 , 1028-1029

(-b) COMMONER, B. (1964) Nature 202 , 960-968

(24) KAUFMANN, B.P., McDONALD, M.R., GAY, H., WILSON, K., WYMAN, R., OKUDA, N. (1948) Carnegie Inst. Year Book 47 , 144-155

(25) DU PRAW, E.J. (1970) "DNA and Chromosomes" (Holt, Rinehart and Winston, Inc.), page 186 (cf. Fig. 11.3)

(-b) LIMA DE FARIA, A. (1983) in "Molecular evolution and organization of the chromosomes", (Elsevier, ed., Amsterdam), page 641 ff

(26) BENNETT, M.D. (1982) in "Genome Evolution" G.A. Dower and R.B. Flavell ed. (Academic Press, Amsterdam); page 239

(27) ODARTCHENκυ, N. and KENEKLIS, T.(1973) Nature 241 ,528-529

(28) MANOLOVA, Y., MANOLOV, G., KIELER, J., LEVAN, A. and KLEIN, G. (1979) Hereditas 90 , 5-10

(29) LIMA DE FARIA, A. (1980) Hereditas 93 , 47-73

(30) LAGOWSKI, J.M., YU, M.Y., FORREST, H.S. and LAIRD, C.D. (1973) Chromosoma 43 , 349-373

(31) SETH, P.K., DE BOER, L.E.M., SAXENA, M.B. and SETH, S. (1976) in "Chromosomes Today" 5 (Pearson and Lewis ed. (Wiley, New York) page 315-322

(-b) CASPERSON, T., DE LA CHAPELLE, A. SCHRODER, J. and ZECH, L. (1972a) Exp. Cell Res. 72 , 56-59

(32) CAPANNA, E., GROPP, A., WINKING, H., NOACK, G. and CIVITELLI, M-V. (1976) Chromosoma 58 , 341-353

(33) JUDD, B.H., SHEN, M.W. and KAUFMAN, T.C. (1972) Genetics 71 , 139-156

(-b) SHANON, M.P., KAUFMAN, T.C., SHEN, M.W. and JUDD, B.H. (1972) Genetics 72 , 615-638

(34) CHEBLOUNE, Y. and VERDIER, Y.(1983) Acta Haem. 69 ,294-302

(35) KLEIN, G. (1981) Nature 294 , 313-318

(36) BERNARDI, G. (1979) Trends Biochem. Sci. 4 , 197-201

(37) MAXWELL, S., MAUNDRELL, K., PUVION-DUTILLEUL, F. and SCHERRER, K. (1981) Eur. J. Biochem. 113 , 233-247

(38) CHANDLEY, A.C., JONES, R.C., DOTT, H.M., ALLEN, W.R. and SHORT, R.V. (1974) Cytogenet. Cell. Genet. 13 , 330-341

(39) YANIV, N. (1984) Biol. Cell 50 , 203-216

(40) RIO, D.C. and TJIAN, R. (1983) Cell 32 , 1227-1240

(-b) KHANDJIAN, W., LOCHE, M., DARLIX, J-L, CRAMER, R., TURLER, H. and WEIL, R. (1982) Proc. Natl. Acad. Sci. USA 79 , 1139-1143

(41) JOHRI M.M. (1978) in "Fontiers of Plant Tissue Culture", T.A. Thorpe ed. (Univ. Calgary Bookstore, 1978; page 27

(42) CRICK, F.H.C. and LAWRENCE, P.A.(1975) Science 189 ,340-347

(43) LAWRENCE, P.A. and STRUHL, G. (1982) The EMBO J. 7 , 827-833

(44) PAULSON, J.R. and LAEMMLI, U.K. (1977) Cell 12 , 817-828

(45) HOLTZER, H., WEINTRAUB, H., MAYNE, R. and MOCHAN, B.
     (1972) in Currents Topics in Developmental Biology,
     vol. 7, A.A. Moscona and A. Monroy ed. (Academic
     Press); page 228
(-b) WEINTRAUB, H., CAMPBELL, G.L. and HOLTZER, H. (1972)
     J. Mol. Biol. 70 , 337-350

ABOUT THE SIGNIFICANCE OF AT-RICH DNA SEGMENTS IN EUKARYOTIC GENOME ORGANISATION AND FUNCTION

Klaus SCHERRER and Jacques MOREAU

Institut JACQUES MONOD, Université Paris VII
2 Place Jussieu, 75251 PARIS Cedex 05

> "Es war einmal ein Lattenzaun,
> mit Zwischenraum, hindurchzuschaun.
> Ein Architekt, der dieses sah,
> stand eines Abends plötzlich da-
> und nahm den Zwischenraum heraus
> und baute draus ein grosses Haus".
> "There used to be a picket fence
> with space to gaze from hence to thence.
> An architect who saw this sight
> approached it suddenly one night,
> remouved the spaces from the fence,
> and built of them a residence".
>
> Christian MORGENSTERN (1)

1) INTRODUCTION

Although detailed sequence knowledge of eukaryotic DNA is rapidly accumulating, relatively little is known concerning long range DNA sequence organisation that could be related to known features of chromosome architecture and function in replication, transcription, meiotic and somatic recombination, differentiation and, possibly, oncogenic transformation.
A particular enigma relates to the fact that an estimated 90 % of the eukaryotic DNA apparently contains no structural genes, and might not contribute to gene expression; furthermore closely related species may have vastly different DNA contents (C-value paradox) although having (by order of magnitude) similar sequence

Proceedings of the 16th FEBS Congress
Part B, pp. 105–122
© 1985 VNU Science Press

complexities. Indeed, the DNA of species differs by the
frequency of representation of given sequences in the
various classes of repetitiveness, rather than by total
sequence complexity. This is particularly evident
comparing plant genomes e.g., which have DNA contents of
0.6-35 pg/ cell (2) or those of amphibians which have
3.1-78 pg/cell (3). Hence such differences bear on total
DNA content and possibly gross genome organisation rather
than on the number and differences of the structural
genes present.

General features of eukaryotic DNA, starting with the
"2nd rule of CHARGAFF" pointing out that eukaryotic DNA
has always an excess of A+T (about 60 % A+T), have been
widely explored (cf. e.g. review in 4). In particular, in
a great number of species was studied the phenomenon of
the existence of DNA satellites which eventually
subdivide the genomic DNA into about a dozen (induced)
density fractions containing in some cases specific genes
(5). Until very recently however the only evidence
concerning a possibly specific function of satellite DNA
(excluding repetitive genes as e.g. rDNA) was the
knowledge about the localisation of light AT-rich
satellites at centromeric regions (6).

Cytogenetic data, particularly in the cases of polytene
and lampbrush chromosomes, indicate strongly that
elements in the DNA must exist to devide the genome into
functional units of middle size-range, varying in number
and size from species to species. The number of such
units defined by chromosome architecture and function,
and by genetics, may vary from 10.000 in Diptera to
100.000 in vertebrates. This crude calculation underlines
the major problem in searching for the existence of DNA
features which serve as a basis for this type of
organisation. Placed at minimal distances of 10-100 Kbp,
such putative repetitious elements are too scarce to be
easily detected by nucleotide sequence analysis, by even
the most rapid techniques; on the other hand, they are
too frequent to be analysed by the very crude methods
mentioned above.

In a deliberate attempt to search for features relating
to intermediate and long range DNA organisation, we

therefore resorted to another experimental approach. It was based on a working hypothesis developed over many years since we observed by chance that eukaryotic DNA contain numerous AT-rich segments (7, 8). Our model postulated that DNA is systematically punctuated by AT-rich sequences of various size, placed inside and outside the transcriptional units (9, 10). Technically, our new approach is based on electron microscopy of partially denatured DNA, spread in defined conditions to reveal specific patterns of denaturation. This has enabled us to establish maps of AT-rich segments which can then be placed in relation to the corresponding restriction maps ("AT-mapping"). For this purpose electron microscopy has a resolution of 50-100 nucleotides and is capable of scanning molecules of 100-1000 Kbp, i.e. the length range appropriate for this ananlysis.

The first experiments confirmed the basic supposition: a systematic punctuation of eukaryotic DNA by AT-rich segments at distances correlating with those of the spacing of the chromosomal units of structure and function (10-40 Kbp) (11). Furthermore, other results were obtained correlating these sequence elements with the localisation of specific genes analysed in cloned genomic DNA (12).

The AT-rich segments were termed "AT-rich linkers" ("ATRLs") since they seem to assume essentially an architectural function in the DNA as spacers "linking" the basic units of genome function and expression involved in transcription and protein synthesis. Thus, they correspond to "inter-space" ; however, as so nicely said in Christian MORGENSTERN's poem, inter-space may have a function per se and, furthermore, may be used to accomodate other superimposed functions eliminated from "within" the basic units. Indeed, such "spacers" may hide many signals relating to chromosome architecture and function, as e.g. the potentialisation for transcription of a chromatin segment, and also for two other fundamentally different functions which may be termed "chromosome mechanics" on the one hand and morphogenesis on the other. As such they are thought to relate to long term organisation and variation of the genome, to its expressional patterns and, possibly, to the static and dynamic architectural organisation of cell and organism.

The latter idea is detailed in an accompanying theoretical paper "The Matrix Hypothesis of DNA-Directed Morphogenesis, Protodynamism and Growth Control" (13; this volume). We will try here to trace the steps of experimental observation that led to the proposition of such a model, summarizing the results of AT-mapping, and then explore the ramifications which relate the phenomenon observed to other known features of genome architecture and function.

2) EXPERIMENTAL DEFINITION OF AT-RICH DNA SEGMENTS

DNA is partially denatured in 75-85 % formamide at 60 mM Na+ and 24.5°C (+/- 0.1°C). No fixation is applied, in order to allow for the establishment of an equilibrium of de- and renaturation which depends on the AT-content of a segment and on the GC-content of the framing sequences. The DNA is then spread for electron microscopy by the classical Kleinschmidt technique and the position of the denaturation bubbles relative to the ends of the molecules is determined (cf. 12). The general AT-content of DNA segments observed by denaturation varies in between species with different, but also with an identical general AT/GC ratio of the genomic DNA ; within a species it may vary between different genomic domains. In consequence, the experimental conditions must be adjusted to allow for 80-100 % denaturation of the segments with the highest AT content.

This method thus allows us to establish a map of differential DNA melting ("AT-MAP") which can be superimposed on the map of restriction sites, which is of diagnostic value : in contrast to the latter, the AT-map has direct significance in relation to DNA organisation and function. Basically three types of characteristic AT-rich elements can be observed :
a) <u>SINGLE AT-RICH LINKERS</u> (ATRLs) are about 800 (+/- 300 bp) long (11) and contain 70-95 % AT (<u>Pro</u> <u>memoria</u> : the genetic code allows for 48% A+T in a random sequence of

all codons) ; 80-100 % of spread ATRLs are denatured. On
average, they are spaced by 10 to 40 Kbp of DNA (11).
b) CLUSTERS OF AT-RICH LINKERS ("AT-clusters") are up to
10 Kbp long and include more than two ATRLs. Within the
cluster, ATRLs are spaced by 0.5 to 3 Kbp only, and may
fuse into longer "bubbles" upon denaturation ; their
length histogram shows the same modal peak of 800 (+/-
300 bp) but extends up to 3.5 Kbp. AT-clusters are found
spaced by 20 to 100 Kbp (11).
c) AT-RICH BREAKS ("AT-breaks") are, by definition,
placed within transcribed domains. In the globin domains
they are on average shorter and less AT-rich than the
ATRLs ; a 25-75 % denaturation allows us to estimate an
AT content of 60-70 %. In introns of highly dispersed
genes they may be as AT-rich as the ATRLs (cf. 3.3).

3) THE EXPERIMENTAL FACTS

3.1) AT-rich linkers and their clusters frame
     organisational domains of genomic DNA

    The analysis of total eukaryotic DNA showed immediately
that the punctuation by ATRLs represents a general
feature of middle to long range DNA organisation (11),
and allowed us to propose the basic model shown in Fig.
1.This model is based on the analysis of various cloned
genomic DNA segments, including the domains of the
chicken and duck alpha and beta globin genes (about 30
Kbp of each analysed), all Xenopus globin genes, the
human beta globin genes (30 Kbp ; partial), of the
Drosophila P1 (80 Kbp) and P6 genes (55 Kbp), the LSP-1
alpha, beta, gamma and LSP-2 genes, and finally the
cellular oncogenes c-erb (45 Kbp), c-mil (60 Kbp), c-sis,
c-myb and c-myc.
    In each case a gene or group of genes was found to be
framed by ATRLs present singly or in clusters (12). These
elements hence frame organisational domains which are
relatively G-C rich and contain the genes and the
transcribed extragenic and intragenic spacers. In cloned
gene- specific DNA, as in total DNA, the individual

AT-rich segments themselves are relatively short (800 +/-
300 bp if occuring as single units) however their
clusters may spread over DNA segments of up to 10 Kbp.
This is particularly striking in Drosophila DNA
(Fig.2), where AT-clusters of up to 10 Kbp, interspaced
every 10-15 bp,results in a repetitive pattern of 23 Kbp.
This spacing approximates to the cytologically and cyto-
genetically defined pattern of polytene chromosome band/
interband length, and to the average transcription units
(14,15). In vertebrates, DNA clusters seem to be more
widely spaced, and placed 50-100 Kbp apart.

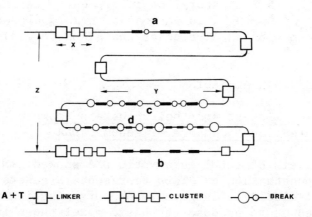

Figure 1 : Model of the distribution of the AT-rich
segments in eukaryotic DNA : (▬▬) genes or gene
fragments; (—□—) ATRLs; (—○—) AT-rich breaks; (X)
AT-rich clusters dispersed over 3-10 Kbp on average; (Y)
distance in between ATRLs (on average 10-40 Kbp); (Z)
distance in between clusters (20-100 Kbp).
Examples: chick alpha (a) and beta (b) globin gene
domains; (c) Xenopus globin genes and Drosophila LSP
genes; (d) highly dispersed genes as c-erb or ovalbumin.

The domains thus formed are further subdivided by
ATRL's or "AT-rich breaks". Interestingly, in Drosophila
(cf."Fig.2" and 15) and Xenopus (MOREAU et al, unpubl.)

110

individual genes seem to be framed at their 5'- and 3'-
messenger-termini by such elements, sometimes
encompassing the TATA boxes (e.g. in case of the
Drosophila P1 gene) and the 3' downstream (pre)-mRNA
terminal "boxes". This recalls the situation of the
Dictostelium actin genes, where the coding sequence is
placed into a practically pure AT background (16), but
also that of the sea urchin histone gene domain where
every gene is separated by an AT-rich segment (17, 18).
In duck and chick, however, the globin gene domains are
interrupted by a single break in between the embryonic
and adult genes (see below and Fig. 3); in this case the
"TATA"- and "ATA"(AAUAAA)- boxes, that frame in birds
also every gene, are placed in a very GC-rich background.
Finally, in highly dispersed genes (see below chapter
3.3) introns may contain very AT-rich "breaks".

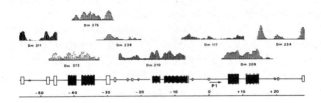

Figure 2 : AT-map of the P1 gene domain of Drosophila
melanogaster . This domain includes three polytene
chromosome bands and interbands; the average spacing of
the AT-cluster is 23 Kbp. The height of the boxes
indicates the frequency of denaturation of every segment
indicated on the axis; hatched areas represent AT-rich
clusters where the precise positions of individual ATRLs
was not further detailed (taken from 15).

Thus, AT-clusters seem to delimit large genomic domains
in the 20-100 Kbp range which, in the case of Drosophila
may correlate with the band/interband units. ATRLs, as
seen e.g. in the case of the avian globin genes, frame

the organisational domains of groups of genes (Fig. 3).
AT-breaks subdivide the domains in between ATRLs and/or
clusters and isolate individual genes as well illustrated
by the Dictostelium Actin genes, the sea urchin
histone, and the amphibian and mammalian globin genes.
The distribution of AT-rich elements correlates thus with
domains of genome organisation; they represent
essentially spacers, from the scale of chromosome
architecture down to that of genes and the peptide
domains (exons) within a gene.

3.2) The example of the avian alpha globin gene domain

   There is no space here to develop all the above
propositions, and to discuss extensively the results
concerning the role of the AT-rich DNA segments. We have
therefore chosen to discuss as an example the results
concerning a specific gene domain, that of the alpha
globin genes in the chick and duck, which are
traditionally the main object of our investigations (19,
20). As shown in Fig. 3, this 25 Kbp domain contains
(from the 5' side): a cluster of ATRLs, the embryonic PI
gene, an AT-break, the adult ALPHA D (minor) and ALPHA A
(major) globin genes, and another ATRL closing the
domain.
   First observation: the ATRLs frame the organisational
domain of this family of genes; this hold true also for
the BETA globin gene domain (12). Comparing chick and
duck shows that this basic organisation is maintained in
evolution, although with some variations (12 and
KRETSOVALI et al, unpubl. res.). Second: the map of
repetitive DNA elements present in the domain coincides
largely with that of the ATRLs (21, 22): the same
observation also holds true for the cluster of ATRLs
placed on the 3' side of the beta globin gene domain of
the chick (23). Similar observations were made for the
Xenopus globin genes (MOREAU et al, unpubl. obs.). We
may therefore conclude that ATRLs often include or are
close to repetitive DNA elements.
   Comparing the AT-map with that of other features of DNA
mapped within the same domain, more correlations become

apparent. The ATRL placed on the 3' side of the chicken globin genes is also close to a DNA segment which includes multiple sites of DNAse hypersensitivity and differential methylation (24). The same holds true for another ATRL (not shown in Fig. 3) placed 8 Kbp further downstream (cf.12).

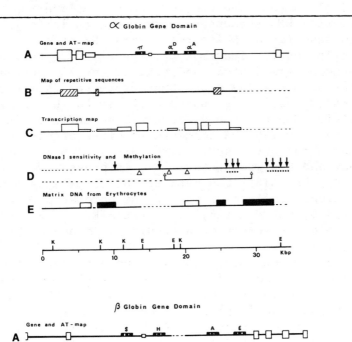

Figure 3 : AT-map of the globin gene domains of the chick and correlations (A) AT and gene map (12); (B) map of repetitive sequences (21);(C) domain transcribed in adult erythroblasts: height of boxes = nuclear RNA hybridisation (21); (D) Hyper-(....) and normal (⌐⌐) DNAse sensitivity, (filled arrows) differential methylation (24).(E) segments enriched in erythrocyte matrix DNA: (▬) strong, (⌐⌐) weak signals (41).

All these observations tend to indicate that ATRLs
might relate to chromatin structure and organisation. A
more direct indication of the same kind results from the
mapping within the ALPHA globin domain of sites of
permanent matrix attachment. The framing segments, both
5' and 3' to the gene cluster, which include repetitive
and AT-rich DNA sequences, were found enriched in the
matrix associated (DNAse resistant) DNA of the
transcriptionally inactive chicken erythrocytes. A unique
DNA segment immediately adjacent to the 5' located
cluster of ATRLs was also found protected, demonstrating
that these results are not simply due to the presence of
repetitive DNA sequences, known to be enriched in matrix
DNA (25). AT-rich DNA segments as sites of matrix
attachment of other genes were lately also identified by
LAEMMLI and his group (Cell 38 , in press). We may
conclude that ATRLs may mark the sites of attachment to
the nuclear scaffold of one of the chromatin loops
proposed by LAEMMLI (26), and that ATRLs in general are
close to sites involved in stable and dynamic chromatin
organisation.

The last facet to be discussed here concerns the
possible involvment of ATRLs in transcription. Indeed,
the data of WEINTRAUB et al (24) indicate the existence
of a strong transcription termination site 1.5 Kbp
downstream from the chicken ALPHA A globin gene, and of a
weaker one at about 2.5 Kbp downstream. The latter would
place transcription termination of the domain within the
3' ATRL. Our own data confirm this latter observation
(21, and BRODERS unpubl. res.), and show that the domain
of about 20 Kbp in between the ATRLs is indeed
transcribed throughout. The transcription product of this
domain thus corresponds to the giant globin pre-mRNA
observed previously (27, 28). The first and last strong
transcription signals were obtained within the segments
around the ATRLs, containing repetitive and unique DNA,
which frame the domain on the 5' and 3' side. The DNA
segments containing the ATRLs may thus also include
signals for transcription initiation and termination of
the 20 Kbp domain, but might also be transcribed

114

independantly.

3.3) AT-rich breaks are eliminated by RNA processing

The AT-rich breaks situated within the ALPHA globin gene domain are most conspicuously placed in segments eliminated by RNA processing from the putatitve primary transcripts including the full domain (cf. 21, 28). AT-rich segments may therefore represent spacers inside transcribed domains as well as between them. This principle became apparent by the AT-mapping of highly dispersed genes in which exons are distributed over 10-30 Kbp, as per example in the case of the cellular proto-oncogenes (c-onc).

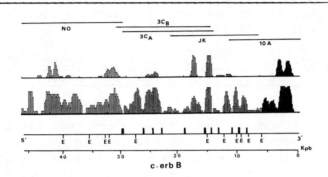

Figure 4 : AT-map of the c-erb B gene (33)

The upper lines show five recombinant DNA clones studied (with their overlaps). Two histograms of denaturation are shown. The upper one represents molecules denatured at 75% formamide, and the lower one at 80% formamide. Below the histogram, the exon localisation is indicated by black boxes; (E) Eco RI restriction sites (clone recombinant by J.COLL and D.STEHELIN).

Fig. 4 shows as an example the AT-map of the c-erb B gene from the chick. Clearly, in addition to a cluster of ATRLs on the 5' side of the gene, every intervening sequence contains an AT-rich segments which allows us to "map" the GC-rich exons. Since these AT-rich breaks may in some cases be shorter than the ATRLs, the resolution of the mapping procedure (of the order of 100 bp) often does not allow very precise mapping of the introns and furthermore, short exons may be engulfed by very AT-rich introns. The principle of the AT-richness of introns is, however, clearly demonstrated; it is confirmed by the available sequence data on dispersed genes, as e.g. in the case of the ovalbumin gene (29). But also the cytochrome oxidase gene of yeast mitochondria shows the same principle in some of its introns (30); interestingly in the first intron 600 bp are GC-rich and 400 AT-rich; all lethal processing mutations are located in the GC-rich highly structured part (31) whereas the AT-rich part seems genetically neutral (30).

3.4) The observation of a systematic integration of proviral DNA into AT-rich host DNA segments

There were indications that AT-rich DNA might play a role in gene transposition. Not only are some prokaryotic sites of transposition AT-rich (32) but in eukaryotic chromosomes telomeric and centromeric domains known to contain AT-rich type satellite DNA are preferential sites of ectopic attachment and chromosome translocation. Hence, we started a survey of cloned recombinant DNA including transposed elements, domains of DNA amplification, and oncogenic provirus integration sites. The former two investigations are not yet conclusive; however, the latter one yielded clearcut results.

At the present state of analysis we can report that in 8 cases out of 8 studied the proviral DNA of transforming RNA- and DNA- tumor viruses was found integrated within or in the immediate neighbourhood of AT-rich DNA segments (33, and unpubl. res.). Fig. 5 gives as an example the AT-map of the integration site of the provirus E-26; other cases studied were B77-ASV (Li1), MH-2, 4 variants

of MSPV, and SV40. This observation tends to indicate a
tropism of proviral DNA elements (at least of the stable
integration sites effective in transformation) for
AT-rich host DNA segments. This result contradicts the
currently accepted notion that proviral DNA may integrate
at random into the host genome (34).
   The nature of the AT-rich segments involved is of
course unknown at present, however some cases of proviral
DNA integration into introns are known (35). Chromosome
translocations are also known to occur within introns
such as in the case of the DNA of the Burkitt's lymphoma
cells, where the IVS containing the (AT-rich!) switching

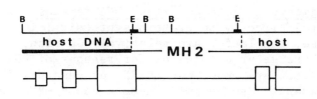

Figure 5 : AT-map of the site of integration into the
host genome of the provirus MH-2 Denaturation map (80%
formamide) of genomic DNA integrated in phage lambda
containing the MH-2 retrovirus.The upper line shows the
restriction map, (E) Eco RI (B) Bam HI and the LTR
localisation (black boxes), the lower line indicates the
localisation of AT-rich sequences (the height of the
boxes indicates the relative frequency of denaturation
relating to the local AT- content) (clone recombinant by
J.COLL and D.STEHELIN).

segment of the immunoglobulin gene on chromosome 14 is
linked to the first IVS of the c-myc proto-oncogene on
chromosome 8. Furthermore, the activation of the c-erb B
proto-oncogene in ALV transformed cells correlates with
the translocation of an LTR just before the first intron
of the c-erb B gene (36).
Although these observations are poorly understood, the

117

systematic nature of the integration of the proviral DNA into AT-rich host DNA segments, confirmed recently by another punctual observation (37) is a further indication of the potential importance of these elements for chromosome organisation and function.

4) THE SIGNIFICANCE OF AT-RICH SEGMENTS IN EUKARYOTIC DNA

Summarizing the conclusions that can be reached by combining the currently available data, and by theoretical deduction, some basic postulates are proposed here that might be useful in guiding the further discussion of experimental data.

AT-rich segments in general "link" DNA domains involved directly or indirectly in protein synthesis ; in the general case, the latter are relatively GC rich, as imposed by the genetic code, or for reasons of RNA secondary structure important in RNA processing. Thus, AT-rich segments also delimit in some cases mRNA domains (exons) corresponding to individual polypeptide functions.

AT-rich LINKERS, CLUSTERS and BREAKS are basically SPACERS separating domains at various levels of genome organisation and function ; they are likely to contain shorter signal sequences which are not necessarily AT-rich.

AT-rich clusters are likely to be involved in chromosome mechanics and dynamics; they may amplify into longer domains forming constitutive heterochromatin, telomeres, into kinetochores and centromeres of specific function in chromosome "mechanics", all of which are known to include AT-rich "satellite" DNA.

AT-rich linkers frame transcriptional units. They may contain promotor and terminator sites for the RNA polymerase.

AT-rich clusters and linkers may define , in addition to transcriptional units, units of replication, of meiotic recombination and chromosome architecture.

AT-rich breaks interrupt transcription units and are placed in between genes or gene fragments (exons); they define units of RNA processing and, possibly, of polypeptide function.

AT-rich segments may coincide with or are in the close vicinity of sites of repetitive DNA, of DNAse hypersensitivity, of sites of matrix attachment, and in some cases of enhancers of transcription.

AT-rich DNA segments are preferential sites of oncogenic provirus integration , they may generally be involved in phenomena of DNA rearrangment, of gene transposition or switching.

The hypothetical rationale of the existance, frequency, extent and topology of AT-rich DNA as inter- and intra-genic spacers, is proposed, in addition to their function in chromatin structure and transcription and processing of RNA, to be the consequence of a direct organisational function of DNA and pre-mRNA in cellular architecture and dynamism. DNA is thought to direct by site-specific interaction with specific proteins the assembly of the matrix networks which are the basis of the cells architecture, and hence to direct cellular morphogenesis. Accordingly, spacers are not only thought to provide (possibly AT-rich) signals in the DNA for attachment of the proteins involved in this assembly, but they provide specific distance per se . This allows the maintenance of DNA signals and specific genes in specific topological positions in relation to each other, primarily in the DNA and, in consequence, indirectly in specific sectors of the nucleus and cell.

Indeed, it has become evident in recent years that the genome is highly organised in relation to the cellular structures, that specific DNA occupies specific topological positions in the nucleus (38) and that specific types of mRNA are channelled to specific domains of the cytoplasm (39, 40). These novel functions of DNA would be based on a novel type of genetic information, controlling topology and relative distance of specific sites in the DNA. The AT-rich DNA segments, their quality, length and distribution would hence reflect this type of organisation in respect to both aspects: 1) the materialisation of the matrix assembly, and 2) the spacer-distance function. We develop these ideas further

119

in a paper on "The "Matrix Hypothesis of DNA Directed Morphogenesis, Protodynamism and Growth Control" (13; this volume).

We may conclude by stating that a systematic punctuation of the eukaryotic DNA by AT-rich segments exists and that these segments occupy specific positions in relation to gene organisation and function, and to other structural features of the DNA and the chromosomes. That these ATRLs are the preferred targets of transforming proviral DNA tends to indicate that they may contain essential signals relating to the cells and viral gene expression. As other basic elements of the genome (e.g. introns, repetitive sequences, sites of methylation, of DNAse hypersensitivity, etc...), it can not be expected that single and simple functions are involved. The experimental exploitation and theoretical interpretation of the phenomenon of the AT-rich DNA segments is thus liable to be long and complex. On the other hand the establishment of AT-maps is easy, and adds another feature characterizing a specific DNA domain in relation to its restriction map; in contrast to the latter, and as possibly also the map of repetitive DNA elements, it is liable to relate directly to genome organisation and function.

ACKNOWLEDGEMENTS

The authors thank all collaborators and colleagues who contributed to the work discussed in particular F.BRODERS, S.RAZIN and J.RZESZOWSKA-WOLNY. The technical assistance of C.MICHON is gratefully acknowledged. We are very grateful to Dr Kinsey MAUNDRELL who critically read and edited the manuscript, and to Chantal CUISINIER who typed this paper. This work was supported by the French CNRS, INSERM, Association pour la Recherche sur le Cancer (ARC) and the Fondation pour la Recherche Médicale Française.

BIBLIOGRAPHY
(1) MORGENSTERN, CH. (1963) The Gallow Songs, ed. by
     University of California Press
(2) RANJEKAR, P.K., PALLOTA, D. and LAFONTAINE, J.G.
     (1978) Biochem. Genet. 16 , 957-970; and pers. comm.
(3) SOMMERVILLE, J. (1977) Int. Rev. Biochem. 15 , 79-156
(4) ILYIN, Y.V. and GEORGIEV, G.P. (1982) Crit. Rev. in
     Biochem. 12 , CRC Press pp. 237-287
(5) SORIANO, P., SZABO, P. and BERNARDI, G. (1982) The
     EMBO J. 1 , 579-583
(6) PARDUE, M.L. and GALL, J.G. (1970) Science 168 ,
     1356-1358
(7) SCHERRER, K. MARCAUD, L. ZAJDELA, F., LONDON, I.M.
     and GROS, F. (1966) Proc. Natl. Acad. Sci. USA 56 ,
     1571-1578
(8) SCHERRER, K. (1971) FEBS Letters 17 , 68-72
(9) SCHERRER, K. (1973) Karolinska Symposia on Research
     Methods in productive Endocrinology 6th. Symposium,
     95-129
(10) SCHERRER, K. (1980) Kolodny Ed. in "Eukaryotic Gene
     Regulation", Vol.I CRC Press
(11) MOREAU, J., MATYASH-SMIRNIAGUINA, L. and SCHERRER, K.
     (1981), Proc. Natl. Acad. Sci USA 78 , 1341-1345
(12) MOREAU, J., MARCAUD, L., MASCHAT, F.,
     KEJZLAROVA-LEPESANT, J., LEPESANT, J-A. and SCHERRER,
     K. (1982) Nature 295 , 260-262
(13) SCHERRER, K. (1985) Proc. 16th FEBS Congress Moscou
     1984 VNU Science Press (Utrecht 1985); this volume
(14) BEYER. A (1983) Mol. Biol. Rep. 9 , 49-58
(15) MOREAU et al, 1985 (submitted to MGG)
(16) FIRTEL, R.A., TIMM, R., KIMMEL, A.R. and Mc KEOW
     (1979) Proc. Natl. Acad. Sci. USA 76 , 6206-6210
(17) PORTMAN, R., SCHAFFNER, W. and BIRNSTIEL, M. (1976)
     Nature 264 , 31-34
(18) SCHAFFNER, W., KUNZ, G., DAETWYLER, H., TELFORD, J.,
     SMITH, H.O. and BIRNSTIEL, M.L. (1978) Cell 14 ,
     655-671
(19) SCHERRER, K., IMAIZUMI-SCHERRER, M-T., REYNAUD, C-A.
     and THERWATH, A. (1979) Mol. Biol. Rep. 5 , 5-28
(20) VINCENT, A., GOLDENBERG, S., STANDART, N, CIVELLI,
     O., IMAIZUMI-SCHERRER, M-T., MAUNDRELL, K. and
     SCHERRER, K. (1981) Mol. Biol. Rep. 7 , 71-81

(21) BRODERS, F. 1984, Thèse de Doctorat, Université PARIS VII
(22) BRODERS, F. et al (1985) (manuscript in prep.)
(23) VILLAPONTEAU, B., LANDES, G.M., PANKRATZ, M.J. and MARTINSON, G. (1982) The Journal of Biol. Chem. 257 , 11015-11023
(24) WEINTRAUB, M., LARSEN, A. and GROUDINE, M. (1981) Cell 24 , 333-344
(25) GOLDBERG, G.I., COLLIER, I. and CASSEL, A. (1983) Proc. Natl. Acad. Sci. USA 80 , 6887-6891
(26) PAULSON, J.R. and LAEMMLI, U.K. (1977) Cell 12 , 817-828
(27) SPOHR, G., IMAIZUMI, M-T. and SCHERRER, K. (1974) Proc. Natl. Acad. Sci. USA 71 , 5009-5013
(28) REYNAUD, C-A, IMAIZUMI-SCHERRER, M-T. and SCHERRER, K. (1980) J. Mol. Biol. 140 , 481-504
(29) HEILIG, R., MURASKOWSKY, R., KLOEPFER, C. and MANDEL, J-L. (1982) Nucl. Acids Res. 10 , 4363-4382
(30) LAZOWSKA, J., JACQ, C. and SLONIMSKY, P.P. (1980) Cell 22 , 333-348
(31) MICHEL, F. and DUJON, B. (1983) The EMBO Journal 2 , 33-38
WARING, R.B. and DAVIES, R.W. (1984) Gen 28 , 277-291
(32) MEYER, J., LIDA, S. and ARBER, W. (1980) M.G.G. 178 , 471-473
(33) MOREAU et al, 1984 (submitted to Nature)
(34) SHIMOTOHNO, K. and TEMIN, H.M. (1980) Proc. Natl. Acad. Sci. USA 77 , 7357-7361
(35) SCHNIEKE, A., HARBERS, K. and JAENISCH, R. (1983) Nature 304 , 315-320
(36) FUNG, Y.K.T., WYNNE, G.L., CRITTENDEN, L.B. and KUNG, M.J. (1983) Cell 33 , 357-368
(37) SHIH, C.K., LINIAL, M., GOODENOW, M.M. and HAYWARD, W.S. (1984) Proc. Natl. Acad. Sci. USA 81 , 4697-4701
(38) LIFSCHYTZ, E., HAREVEN, D., AZRIEL, A. and BRODSLY, H. (1983) Cell 32 , 191-199
(39) KUHLMANN, W.D., BOUTEILLE, M. and AVRAMEAS, S. (1975) Exptl Cell Research 96 , 335-343
(40) COLMAN, D.R., KREIBICH, G., FREY, A.B. and SABATINI, D.D. (1982) The Journal of Cell Biology 95 , 598-608
(41) RAZIN, S, RZESZOWSKA- WOLNY, J., MOREAU, J. and SCHERRER, K. (1984) submitted to the EMBO J.

ATTENUATION IN SV40 FUNCTIONS AT LATE TIME AFTER INFECTION AND IT IS AUGMENTED BY AGNOPROTEIN

NISSIM HAY[+] AND YOSEF ALONI[+*]

[+]Department of Genetics, Weizmann Institute of Science, Rehovot 76100, Israel and [+*]Department of Molecular Biology, Princeton University, Princeton, NJ 08544

INTRODUCTION

The structural similarity between the major leader of 16S mRNA of SV40 and the leader of amino acid operons in bacteria is striking (1-3). This similarity raised the possibility that the major leader of 16S mRNA participates in an attenuation mechanism that regulates the expression of the downstream structural gene, VP1 (2,4). Like the leaders of amino acid operons in bacteria, the major leader of 16S mRNA can be folded into two alternative secondary structures. One of them consists of two stem-and-loop structures (1 and 2; 3 and 4) and was termed the attenuation conformation (see Fig 1A) (2). The alternative secondary structure contains one stem-and-loop structure (2 and 3) which overlaps with that of the attenuation conformation. It was termed the readthrough conformation (see Fig 1B) (2). The 3 and 4 stem-and-loop, in the attenuation conformation, is followed by a string of U's. This structure acts as a transcription termination signal which prevents transcription from continuing into the structural gene (5,6). Analogous to the leaders of the mRNAs of amino acid operons in bacteria the major leader of 16S mRNA

Proceedings of the 16th FEBS Congress
Part B, pp. 123–140
© 1985 VNU Science Press

A. Attenuation

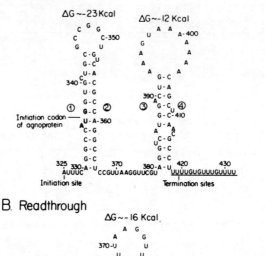

B. Readthrough

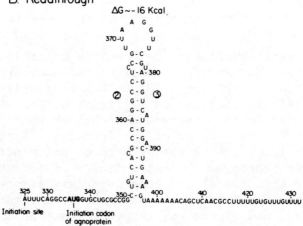

Fig 1   Schema of alternative conformation in the attenuator RNA

A.   Attenuation conformation showing typical pausing (1 + 2) (17) and termination signals (3 + 4) (2,5).

B.   Readthrough conformation.   For details see Hay _et al_ (2).   The ΔG were calculated as described by Tinoco _et al_ (33).   The residue number is from Tooze (34).

of SV40 codes for a small protein known as agnoprotein (7,8).

In bacteria, where transcription and translation are coupled, the translation process of the leader peptide regulates the attenuation of transcription (3). We have suggested that in SV40, where transcription and translation are uncoupled, the final product of translation of the leader's codons, i.e. the agnoprotein regulates the attenuation of transcription (1,2,4). According to this suggestion the agnoprotein is transported from the cytoplasm to the nucleus and it has dual functions. In the nucleus it enhances attenuation of transcription by stabilizing the attenuation conformation in the nascent RNA (see Fig 1A). In the cytoplasm by stabilizing the same conformation at the 5' end of the 16S mRNA it enhances translation of VP1. In this conformation the AUG start codon of the agnoprotein is sequestered in the 1;2 stem-and-loop structure (see Fig. 1A) and the scanning ribosome bypasses it (9-15) and initiates translation from the downstream AUG of VP1. A similar mechanism has been suggested to regulate the synthesis of VP2 and VP3 (1,4). It has been postulated that attenuation during SV40 late transcription regulates the synthesis of the relative amounts of the capsid proteins one to each other and to the copy number of the viral DNA (1,2,4). By that, the efficiency of capsid formation and the process of encapsidation are controlled.

As an approach to verify the physiological significance of attenuation in the life cycle of SV40 and for testing our hypothesis for the role of agnoprotein in enhancing attenuation, we have developed a system of isolated nuclei in which efficient transcription - termination at the attenuation site of SV40 occurs. This is evident by the production of a 94 nt attenuator RNA as revealed by gel-electrophoresis (5).

In the following studies we have used the isolated nuclei system, under conditions that lead to attenuation. The results indicate that attenuation is temporally regulated i.e. it is predominant towards the end of the infection cycle and they further suggest that agnoprotein enhances attenuation.

RESULTS

I Increased Attenuation is Directly Correlated with the Progress of Infection

In order to verify the physiological significance of attenuation in the life cycle of SV40 we have first determined when, during the SV40 infection cycle, attenuation is predominant. For this, at various times during the late phase of the SV40 life cycle, nuclei were isolated from the infected cells and incubated in vitro under the standard conditions (100 mM NaCl, 10 μM (α-^{32}P) UTP) that lead to the production of the 94 nt attenuator RNA (5). ^{32}P-RNA was extracted and viral RNA was purified by hybridization to and elution from SV40 DNA immobilized on nitrocellulose filters. The ^{32}P-viral RNA was then analyzed by gel-electrophresis under denaturing conditions. Fig 2 shows that only minor quantities of the attenuator RNA are synthesized at the beginning of the late phase of the SV40 infection cycle. While, long viral transcripts accumulate (A and B in Fig 2). The long RNA represents transcripts of the viral DNA fragments that are remote from the major transcription initiation site. This is evident from their hybridization, after elution from the gel, with the late fragments b (0.76-0.0 mu) and d (0.0-0.17 mu) as well as with the early fragments a (0.67-0.37 mu) and c (0.37-0.17 mu) (see Fig 2) (2). The hybridization with the early fragments could represent either early or late transcripts. Almost no hybridization occurs with the promoter proximal fragment e. In contrast, the viral RNA synthesized at a later time in the infection cycle produces a major 94 nt RNA (C in Fig 2). This RNA was previously characterized and was termed attenuator RNA (2,16,17). It hybridizes to fragment e (0.67-0.76 mu) and it maps between the major initiation site of late transcription at residue 325 and residue 419. Almost no long viral RNA is synthesized at this time post-infection. The RNA of about 125 nt is most likely of cellular origin. Thus, the system of isolated nuclei reveals that while readthrough is occurring at the beginning of the late phase, attenuation is predominant towards the end of the infection cycle. These results imply that regulation at the attenuation site has a physiological significance.

II Time Course of Synthesis of Agnoprotein

In our original model we postulated that agnoprotein has a trans-acting negative effect on late transcription (1,2,4,7). In order to test this hypothesis we have first studied when, during the infection cycle, agnoprotein is synthesized. For this, at various times after infection cells were labeled for 3 h with ^{14}C-arginine and the synthesized proteins analyzed by gel-electrophoresis. We chose to label the cells for 3 h because this has previously been shown to be the half-life of agnoprotein (7,8). The gel was exposed to X-ray film for 6 h for quantitating the major capsid proteins, VP1, VP2 and VP3 and for 24 h for quantitating the agnoprotein. As can be seen in Fig 3A the synthesis of the capsid proteins is increased up to 42 h p.i. At 50 h p.i. there is no further increase in their synthesis but there even is some decrease. In contrast, the agnoprotein is synthesized primarily at the latest

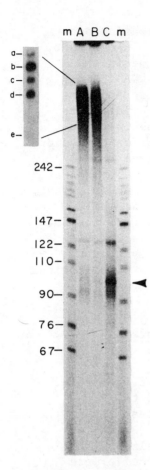

Fig 2 Size analyses of viral RNAs produced in nuclei isolated from SV40 infected cells at various times after infection

At various times after infection nuclei were isolated from SV40 infected cells and incubated in a standard transcription reaction mixture (5). The labeled viral RNA produced were purified and analyzed by gel-electrophoresis. Each lane was loaded with equal amounts of viral RNA. A-nuclei isolated at 24 h p.i. B-nuclei isolated at 36 h p.i. C-nuclei isolated at 48 h p.i. m-labeled DNA fragments used as size markers. Labeled RNA was eluted from lane A, as indicated and hybridized to a blot of SV40 DNA restriction fragments obtained by cleavage of SV40 DNA with EcoRI, BglI and HpaI restriction enzymes (2). The arrow points to the position of the 94 nt attenuator RNA.

time after infection (Fig 3B). These results together with the observation that attenuation is predominant towards the end of the late phase (see Fig 2) demonstrate a direct correlation between the amount of agnoprotein in the cell and the level of attenuation.

III There is Reduced Synthesis of Attenuator RNA in Nuclei Isolated from Cells Infected with SV40 Mutants that do not Produce Agnoprotein

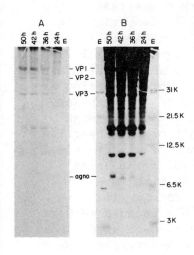

Fig 3 Time course of synthesis of agnoprotein

At various times after infection 0.5 x 10^6 cells were labeled for 3 h with ^{14}C-arginine, collected in 0.1 ml sample buffer (10 mM sodium phosphate, pH 7.2, 7 M urea, 1% SDS, 1% β-mercaptoethanol and 0.01% bromophenol blue) lysed and analyzed on a 15% polyacrylamide gel containing 0.1% SDS in 6 M urea. The gel was fluorographed and dried. The autoradiogram was obtained by exposing the dried gel to Kodak XR-2 film at -80°C. A-6 h exposure B-24 h exposure m-molecular weight markers.

For examining directly whether agnoprotein enhances the synthesis of the attenuator RNA in isolated nuclei, cells were infected with several mutants of SV40 that lack the coding frame of agnoprotein. Nuclei were isolated and the production of the attenuator RNA was analyzed in comparison to that produced in nuclei isolated from WT infected cells. The mutants used were: (1) dl 1616 in which the entire coding region of agnoprotein is deleted (18). (ii) dl 1811 in which nt 305-345 are deleted. This deletion removes the AUG start codon of agnoprotein, the major initiation site at residue 325 and the first stem-and-loop structure (1;2) of the attenuation conformation of the WT attenuator RNA (see Fig 1). In this mutant the major initiation site of late transcription is shifted upstream to residue 290 (19). As a result of the deletion an alternative more stable RNA secondary structure can be formed upstream of the termination signal ($\Delta G=-24$ Kcal). In comparison to WT, the readthrough conformation is unchanged (see Fig 4, dl 1811 and for comparison see Fig 1). (iii) The mutant $\Delta 79$ is an insertion mutant in which 2 nt C and G were inserted at the HpaII site. This insertion has almost no effect on the stabilities of the secondary structures of both the attenuation and readthrough conformations. However, as a result of the insertion there is a shift in the coding frame of agnoprotein. The new coding frame encodes for a 31 amino acids protein. The new stop codon UAG is at residues 432-434 (see Fig 4 WT/$\Delta 79$). This protein, if translated, is probably very unstable because we were unable to detect it in infected cells even after short pulse-labeling and exposures of the X-ray films for long durations (7; and Hay and Aloni; unpublished results).

Nuclei were prepared from the various infected cells and incubated <u>in vitro</u> in the presence of (α-^{32}P) UTP for 15 min in a standard transcription reaction mixture which lead to premature termination and to the production of the 94 nt attenuator RNA (5). ^{32}P-RNA was extracted and viral RNA selected by hybridization to and elution from filters bearing SV40 DNA. The ^{32}P-labeled viral RNA was then analyzed by gel-electrophoresis under denaturing conditions. Fig 5 shows a significant reduction in the amount of the attenuator RNA and an increase of long RNA transcripts in all the mutants used. With dl 1626 there is a complete disappearance of the attenuator RNA, because in this virus the entire coding region of the attenuator RNA is deleted (18). With dl 1811 there is a faint band of about 90 nt which could result from

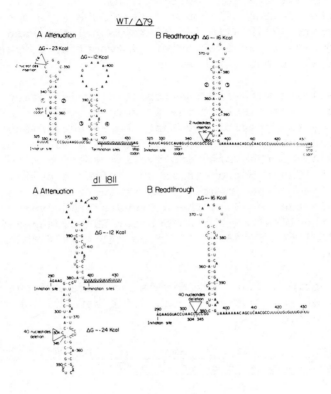

Fig 4 Schemes of alternative conformations of the attenuator RNA region in mutants of SV40

dl 1811 was obtained from Prof. W. Fiers and Δ79 from Prof. G. Khoury. Note that the alternative conformations can exist both in the attenuator RNA and at the 5' end of the major 16S mRNA. A-attenuation conformation showing stem-and-loop structure in which the 3; 4 structure (ΔG = -12 K cal) signals transcription termination (2). B-readthrough conformation. For details see Hay et al (2). The ΔG were calculated as described by Tinoco et al (32). The residue number is from Tooze (33).

partial termination at the termination signal (residue 419 in the attenuation conformation). In a short pulse with limited UTP concentration there is a pause at this site (2). With Δ79 there is a faint band corresponding to an RNA longer by two nt as compared with the WT attenuator RNA.

The experiment with Δ79 was repeated by isolating the nuclei at later times of the infection cycle in order to exclude the possibility that the reduced amount of the attenuator RNA is a consequence of a slower progression of the infection cycle rather than to the absence of the agnoprotein in the infected cells. In none of these experiments, even at later times than 56 h p.i. has the level of the attenuator RNA ever reached the level of the attenuator RNA produced in nuclei isolated at 48 h p.i. from cells infected with WT virus.

These experiments provide direct evidence for the function of agnoprotein in enhancing attenuation in isolated nuclei.

IV There is an Increased Amount of Viral RNA in the Cytoplasm of Cells Infected with Δ79

In our original model we have postulated that in the cytoplasm, during translation, agnoprotein can reduce its own synthesis by stabilizing the RNA conformation, at the 5' end of the 16S mRNA, by sequestering its own AUG start codon (see A in Fig 1). Consequently, the downstream AUG start codon of VP1 becomes functional and VP1 is synthesized (2). In Δ79 infected cells this regulation cannot operate because of the lack of functional agnoprotein in the infected cells and still VP1 is synthesized at high levels (7). We argue that the synthesis of high levels of VP1, in Δ79 infected cells, can be accomplished because of reduced attenuation of SV40 late transcription (see Fig 5) and

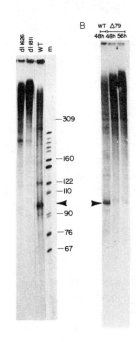

Fig 5 Size analyses of viral RNAs produced in nuclei isolated from cells infected with various mutants of SV40.

At 48 h p.i. nuclei were isolated from cells infected with the various mutants of SV40, as indicated. Nuclei were isolated from Δ79 infected cells also at 56 h p.i. The nuclei were incubated for 15 min at 30°C in a standard transcription reaction mixture. The labeled viral RNA produced were purified and analyzed by gel-electrophoresis. Each lane was loaded with equal amounts of viral RNA. m-labeled DNA fragments used as size markers. The arrow points to the position of the 94 nt attenuator RNA.

a resultant increase in the synthesis of viral RNA and its accumulation in the cytoplasm of infected cells. The increased amount of viral mRNA should be able to compensate for the less efficient translation of VP1 in Δ79 infected cells.

In order to test this argument we compared the levels of viral RNAs in the cytoplasms of cells infected with WT and Δ79. At 48 h p.i. nuclear and cytoplasmic fractions were prepared, RNAs were extracted from the cytoplasm and DNAs extracted, by the Hirt procedure (20) from the nuclear fractions. Two fold dilutions of RNAs and DNAs were dot blotted onto nitrocellulose paper and hybridized with a probe of SV40 labeled DNA. Fig 6 shows that for an equal amount of viral DNA, the

cytoplasm of cells infected with the Δ79 mutant
contains approximately twice the amount of viral RNA
present in the cytoplasms of WT infected cells.

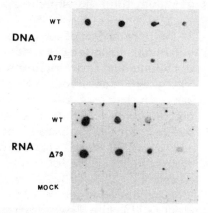

DNA WT Δ79

RNA WT Δ79

MOCK

Fig 6   Quantitation by dot-blot hybridization of viral
RNA present in the cytoplasms of WT and Δ79 infected
cells

At 48 h p.i. cells were infected with WT SV40, Δ79 or
mock-infected. Cytoplasmic and nuclear fractions were
prepared by lysing the cells with 0.5% NP$_{40}$. RNAs
were extracted from the cytoplasmic fractions and
viral DNAs were extracted, by the Hirt procedure (20)
from the pelleted nuclei. The RNA fractions were
treated with DNase and the DNA fractions were treated
with RNase. Two-fold dilutions of DNA and RNA were
dot-blotted on nitrocellulose paper and hybridized
with nick-translated SV40 DNA. The paper was dried
and exposed to an X-ray film.

DISCUSSION

The present studies have shown that attenuation is
temporally regulated i.e. with the progress of SV40
infection there is increased attenuation. At 24 h and

36 h p.i. most of the transcribed viral RNA chains are long. At 50 h p.i. there is a sharp decrease of long viral transcripts and in parallel there is synthesis of a 94 nt attenuator RNA. These results imply that regulation at the attenuation site has a physiological significance. At the latest time in infection the encapsidation process is extensive. Attenuation probably controls the efficiency of encapsidation by adjusting the relative amounts of the capsid proteins one to each other and also to the copy number of the viral DNA. In this respect it is worth noting that although mutants with deletions in the leader region are viable, they are all somewhat defective in the rate of production of infectious virions in established cell lines. This is indicated by both (i) the delayed appearance and smaller sizes of the plaques they produce and (ii) the lower rates of production of p.f.u. during a single growth cycle (21,22).

Protein analysis during the growth cycle of SV40 showed an increased synthesis of agnoprotein as the infection cycle progressed (see Fig 3). Similar observations were reported previously (23). This result together with the observation that attenuation is also increased with the progress of infection, demonstrates a direct correlation between the amount of agnoprotein in the cell and the level of attenuation in isolated nuclei, suggesting a possible involvement of agnoprotein in attenuation. The observation that SV40 mutants, that do not produce agnoprotein failed to synthesize the 94 nt attenuator RNA, especially with the two nucleotide insertion mutant Δ79, in which the stability of the secondary structure of nascent RNA is unchanged, provide direct evidence for the function of agnoprotein in enhancing attenuation. It should be mentioned that it has recently been suggested that agnoprotein interacts in a specific way with VP1 and that agnoprotein plays a role in virion assembly. This suggestion was based on

135

an observation that a VP1 defective mutant could be suppressed by a point mutation in the agnoprotein (24). We believe that a direct involvement in virion assembly, as a major role for agnoprotein is unlikely, because the assembly process occurs in the nucleus and the agnoprotein is found predominantly in the cytoplasm (1,23). In any case, interaction between VP1 and agnoprotein would not exclude the regulatory role of agnoprotein as suggested in our original model (1,2,4). Moreover, because VP1 is known to be transported from the cytoplasm to the nucleus, interaction between VP1 and agnoprotein can facilitate the transport of the agnoprotein to the nucleus where it can function in enhancing attenuation.

In our original model we have also suggested the existence of an anti-attenuation factor that either competes with the agnoprotein by stabilizing the readthrough conformation in the nascent RNA or by interacting with the RNA polymerase allowing it to transcribe through the attenuation site (1,2,4). We now have some evidence for the existence of a cellular anti-attenuator factor (King and Aloni, manuscript in preparation). If there is an additional viral anti-attenuator factor we believe that it should be one of the viral early gene products (Hay and Aloni, unpublished results). The results with the mutant dl 1811, that does not synthesize agnoprotein, tend to support the existence of an anti-attenuator factor, because in this virus even though the attenuation conformatin of the nascent RNA is more stable than in WT, there is almost no synthesis of attenuator RNA. This may indicate the importance of the readthrough conformation. For the same reason we suggest that there is almost no attenuation at early times in the infection when the low amount of agnoprotein in the cell cannot compete with the anti-attenuator factor and readthrough conformation.

In the present experiments attenuation was analyzed in isolated nuclei. That agnoprotein may enhance attenuation also in vivo is suggested by the experiments showing higher levels of viral cytoplasmic RNA in cells infected with Δ79, a mutant that does not synthesize agnoprotein, as compared to infection with WT virus (Fig 6).

Furthermore, we have previously shown that in vivo the RNA polymerase pauses at sites close to the 1;2 stem-and-loop structure (see Fig. 1 and 17). It is assumed that the formation of the 1;2 stem-and-loop structure prevents the formation of the competing 2;3 readthrough conformation and consequently the transcription-termination signal, 3;4 is formed (1,2,4). We further suggest that at the latest time after infection the agnoprotein enhances the formation of the 1;2 stem-and-loop structure leading to increased number of polymerase molecules at the pause sites (17). During in vitro elongation in isolated nuclei the termination signal 3;4 is formed and the attenuator RNA is synthesized (1,2,4,5,6,16,17). In Δ79 infected cells because of the absence of functional agnoprotein (7), the stability of the 1;2 stem-and-loop structure is reduced and the proportion of newly synthesized molecules haveing the competing 2;3 readthrough conformation is increased. Consequently, during in vitro elongation the synthesis of the attenuator RNA is reduced and there is an increased synthesis of long RNA molecules.

As concerned with the generality of the attenuation mechanism in animal viruses and cells the following is worth mentioning. It has recently been shown that attenuation of transcription exists in the autonomous parvovirus, minute virus of mice (MVM) (25) and it has been suggested to exist in polyoma virus (26) VSV (27) and retroviruses (28). In Ad-2 and Ad-5 premature-termination at specific sites were found to be temporally regulated being predominant, as in SV40,

at the late period of the infection cycle (29;
Seiberg, M., Levine, A.J. and Aloni, Y. manuscript in
preparation). Attenuation in specific eukaryotic
genes has also been documented (30-31). We believe
that more experimental systems in which attenuation is
functioning will soon be found.

ACKNOWLEDGEMENTS

We thank Ruchama Leiserowitz for technical assistance,
Dr. E.B. Jakobovitz for comments on the manuscript and
Noël Mann for preparing the manuscript. Y.A. thanks
Dr. A.J. Levine for his kind hospitality in his
laboratory where this work was completed. A major
part of this work is in press in Mol. Cell. Biol.
1985.

This research was supported by U.S. Public Health
Service research grant CA 14995 and in part by the
Norman V. Vechsler Endowment Fund. A part of the work
reported in this paper was undertaken during the
tenure of an American Cancer Society - Eleanor
Roosevelt - International Cancer Fellowship awarded to
Y.A. by the International Union against cancer.

REFERENCES

1. Aloni, Y., N. Hay, H. Skolnik-David, P.
   Pfeiffer, R. Abulafia, R. Pruzan, E.
   Ben-Asher, E.B. Jakobovits, O. Laub and A.
   Ben-Zeev. 1983. In: Developments in
   Molecular Virology IV (Kohn A. and Fuchs eds.
   Martinus Nijhoff Publishers, Boston).
2. Hay, N. H. Skolnik-David and Y. Aloni. 1982.
   Cell 29:183-193.
3. Yanofsky, C. 1981. Nature 289:751-758.

4. Aloni, Y. and N. Hay. 1983. Molec. Biol. Rep. 9:91-100.
5. Hay, N. and Y. Aloni. 1984. Nucleic Acids Res. 12:1401-1414.
6. Pfeiffer, P., N. Hay, R. Pruzan, E.B. Jakobivits and Y. Aloni. 1983. EMBO J. 2:185-191.
7. Hay, N., M. Kessler and Y. Aloni. 1984. Virology 137:160-170.
8. Jay, G., S. Nomura, C.W. Anderson and G. Khoury. 1981. Nature 291:346-349.
9. Kozak, M. 1978. Cell 15:1109-1123.
10. Kozak, M. 1980. Cell 22:7-8.
11. Kozak, M. 1981. Curr. Top. Microbiol. Immunol. 93:81-123.
12. Kozak, M. 1981. Nucleic Acids Res. 9:5233-5252.
13. Kozak, M. 1982. Biochem. Soc. Symp. 47:113-128.
14. Kozak, M. 1982. Microbiol. Rev. 47:1-45.
15. Kozak, M. 1983. Cell 34:971-978.
16. Skolnik-David, H., N. Hay and Y. Aloni. 1982. Proc. Natl. Acad. Sci. USA 79:2743-2747.
17. Skolnik-David, H. and Y. Aloni. 1983. EMBO J. 2:179-184.
18. Subramanian, K.N. 1979. Proc. Natl. Acad. Sci. USA 76:2556-7560.
19. Haegeman, G., D. Iserentant, D. Gheysen and W. Fiers. 1979. Nucleic Acids Res. 7:1799-1814.
20. Hirt, B. 1967. J. Mol. Biol. 26:365-369.
21. Barkan, A. and J.E. Metz. 1981. J. Virol. 37:730-737.
22. Mertz, J.E., A. Murphy and A. Barkan. 1983. J. Virol. 45:36-46.
23. Nomura, S., G. Khoury and G. Jay. 1983. J. Virol. 45:428-433.
24. Margolskee, R.F. and D. Nathans. 1983. J. Virol. 48:405-409.
25. Ben-Asher, E. and Y. Aloni. 1984. J. Virol.

52:266-276.

26. Montandon, P.E. and N.H. Acheson. 1982. J. Gen. Virol. 59:367-376.

27. Testa, D., P.K. Chanda and A.K. Banerjee. 1980. Unique mode of transcription in vitro by vesicular stomatitis virus. Cell 21:267-275.

28. Benz, E.W., R.M. Wydro, B. Nadal-Ginard and D. Dina. 1980. Nature 288:665-669.

29. Mok, M., A. Maderious and S. Chen-kiang. 1984. Mol. Cell. Biol. 4:2031-2040.

30. Andreadis, A. V,-P. Hsu, G.B. Kohlhaw and P. Schimmel. 1983. Cell 31:319-325.

31. Gariglio, P., M. Bellard and P. Chambon. 1981. Nucleic Acids Res. 9:2589-2598.

32. Tweeten, K.A. and G.R. Molloy. 1981. Nucleic Acids Res. 9:3307-3319.

33. Tinoco, I., P.N. Borer, B. Dengler, M.D. Levine, O. Uhlenbeck, D. Crothers and J. Gralla. 1973. Nature (London) New Biol. 246:40-41.

34. Tooze, J. 1981. Appendix A The SV40 nucleotide sequence p. 799-841. In J. Tooze (ed.) DNA tumor viruses, 2nd ed. Cold Spring Harbor Laboratory, Cold Spring Harbor, N.Y.

DYNAMIC STRUCTURAL CHANGES IN CHROMATIN UPON TRANSCRIPTION

A.D.MIRZABEKOV, V.L.KARPOV, O.V.PREOBRAZHENSKAYA, S.G.BAVYKIN, S.I.USACHENKO[x], A.I.LYSHANSKAYA[+], I.M.UNDRITSOV, V.V.SHICK, A.V.BELYAVSKY
Institute of Molecular Biology, The USSR Academy of Sciences, Moscow V-334
x Institute of Cytology, Leningrad 194064
+ Institute of Nuclear Physics, Leningrad 188350

INTRODUCTION

The basic unit of chromatin structure is a nucleosome core particle. It contains about 145 bp of DNA and the histone octamer consisting of two molecules of each histone H2A, H2B, H3, and H4. Together with histone H1 and spacer DNA of variable length, the core particle makes up a nucleosome. In the course of transcription, chromatin undergoes some structural transitions which can lead to either complete unraveling and linearization of DNA with attached histones or to removal of histones. In either case, certain changes in the DNA-histones contacts must be observed.

In the present report, we summarize our studies on the effect of chromatin activation on DNA-histone interactions. In these studies we used a number of new approaches developed in our laboratory.

If the nucleosome could unravel in transcribed chromatin, this would cause some rearrangement of histones on DNA. However, we have not found any essential differences in the primary organization (i.e. sequential arrangement of histones along DNA) of nucleosomal core particles between repressed and active nuclei. On the other hand, such unraveling could be caused by non-histone proteins associated with active chromatin, for example HMG 14 and HMG 17. We have not observed, however,

Proceedings of the 16th FEBS Congress
Part B, pp. 141–147
© 1985 VNU Science Press

any effect of these proteins on the primary organization of the cores. Finally, our study of the histone content in regulatory and coding regions of active genes has demonstrated removal of histones from chromatin upon its transcription and allowed us to suggest a mechanism regulating gene activity.

Primary organization of nucleosomal cores in active and repressed nuclei

To determine the arrangement of histones along DNA in nucleosomes and that of RNA polymerase subunits along promoter, we used our new method for sequencing the arrangement of proteins along DNA, which includes crosslinking proteins to DNA partly depurinated under mild conditions (1). Using this method, we have compared the primary organization of nucleosomal core particles in active in transcription and replication nuclei from yeast, Drosophila embryos and rat liver and in completely repressed nuclei from sea urchin sperm and chicken erythrocytes (2). To our surprise, no essential structural difference shows up between these particles. Fig. 1 presents a high resolution map for the arrangement of histone contacts on DNA in these core particles. It is worth mentioning here that isolation of the cores causes the appearance of a new contact for histone H2A, located at a distance of 75 nucleotides from the 5' core DNA ends. There is also an additional binding site for sea urchin sperm histone H2B at 58 nucleotides from the 5' DNA ends which is probably formed by an unusually extended N-terminal part of these H2B molecules.

Yeast cells are actively involved in replication and more than 40 percent of their DNA participate in transcription. Hence, yeast core particles should contain an essential portion of nucleosomes from transcribed chromatin regions. As we found no difference in the primary organization of the cores from active and repressed

nuclei, we have concluded that the overall inactivation of chromatin does not affect the arrangement of histones along DNA in the cores. These
data also show that the core structure is highly
conserved in evolution.

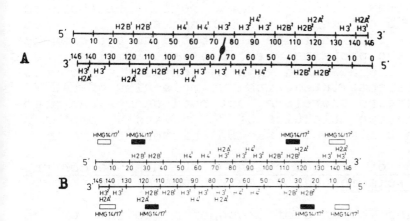

Fig. 1. Arrangement of histones on DNA: (A) in
the nucleosome core particles isolated from active nuclei of rat liver, Drosophila embryos,
yeast or from repressed nuclei of sea urchin
sperm and chicken erythrocytes; (B) in the particles containing two molecules of HMG 14 and
HMG 17 proteins from chicken erythrocytes.
Distances along both DNA strands are given in
nucleotides from the 5'-ends. Superscripts 1 and
2 denote two copies of each protein molecule.
Black and white rectangles mark, correspondingly,
strong and weak binding sites for HMG proteins.

Primary organization of nucleosomes containing HMG 14 and HMG 17 proteins

In order to study the effect of HMG 14 and 17
proteins (which seem to be associated with active
chromatin) on the nucleosome structure, we reconstituted cores and H1-containing nucleosomes

with HMG 14 and 17 proteins and crosslinked the proteins to DNA. Particles containing two molecules of HMG 14/17 were isolated by gel electrophoresis, and the arrangement of proteins on DNA was determined. The data for the cores are summarized in Fig. 1B. Two HMG molecules occupy two sites in both terminal regions of the core DNA. No changes in the arrangement of histones on DNA that could be attributed to the presence of these proteins were observed. Similar results were also obtained with H1-containing nucleosomes reconstituted with two molecules of HMG 14/17. It appears therefore that nucleosomes can accomodate two molecules of HMG 14 and 17 proteins without disturbing the DNA-histone contacts.

Effect of transcription on the histone content in chromatin

The hsp 70 genes of Drosophila, coding for the major heat-shock proteins, provide an excellent system for studying the structural changes occurring in chromatin upon activation. These potentially active genes can be easily transferred within a few minutes from inactive to active state by elevating temperature of Drosophila cells from normal 24°C to above 30°C. To test chromatin structure in different regions of the genes, we used two plasmid probes. One contained the 5'-terminal gene regions with gene regulatory sequences within plasmid pUR222. The other included an internal part of the coding region recloned in plasmid pBR322. Another pBR322 plasmid with a non-transcribed insertion within Drosophila ribosomal gene was used as a probe for repressed chromatin. The presence of histones on these regions of genes in different states of activation was estimated by the "protein image" hybridization procedure developed in our laboratory (3). First, histones were crosslinked to DNA directly in nuclei, then free DNA and DNA attached in the initial material to core histo-

nes or to histone H1 were separated into three
diagonals by two-dimensional gel electrophoresis.
transferred from the diagonals and immobilized
onto DBM-paper and, finally, DNA was successively hybridized with various ^{32}P-labeled probes.
Fig. 2 shows the hybridization patterns obtained
with the material from control cells and cells
subjected to heat shock. Hybridization with probes for non-transcribed ribosomal gene insertion
showed no difference between the two kinds of
cells (Figs. 2Ac and Bc) and evidenced the presence of both core histones and histone H1 in
the repressed chromatin. In control cells, the
coding region of hsp 70 genes showed the same
histone content as the repressed chromatin (Fig.
2Ab). On the other hand, the disappearance of H1
and core histones image diagonals upon hybridization of crosslinked material from the shocked
cells with the coding region probe (Fig. 2Bb)
indicates the absence of histones on DNA in fully activated and efficiently transcribed genes.
No histones are observed on the regulatory hsp
70 gene regions in both control and induced cells
(Figs. 2Aa and 2Ba). In moderately induced hsp
70 genes, this approach showed the disappearance
of histone H1 and partial depletion of core
histones (3).

CONCLUSIONS

On the basis of the experimental data presented
above (3), we suggest a model for dynamic structural transitions in chromatin induced by transcription and a transcription regulation mechanism acting on the level of chromatin structure.
   The lack of histones in the gene promoter region makes this region exposed and available for
RNA polymerase molecules which can enter and be
accumulated there, waiting for a signal to start
transcription. When transcription begins, the
RNA polymerase molecules remove histone H1 coo-
peratively from all transcribed area, thus

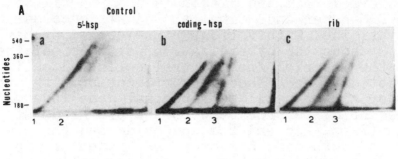

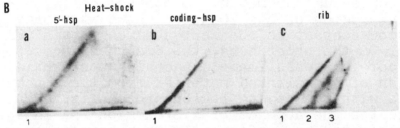

Fig. 2. Presence of histones in different chromatin regions of control (A) and heat-shocked (B) Drosophila tissue-culture cells. Crosslinked within nuclei, DNA-histone complexes were electrophoresed in the first direction (from right to left), then the proteins were digested in the gel by Pronase, and the single-stranded DNA fragments obtained were electrophoresed in the second direction (from top to bottom) into three diagonals, namely: (1) uncrosslinked DNA; (2) DNA crosslinked to core histones; (3) DNA crosslinked to histone H1. DNA from the gel was transferred onto DBM-paper and successively hybridized with ^{32}P-labeled probes for the 5'-terminal region (a) and coding region (b) of hsp 70 genes and for the repressed ribosomal gene insertion (c).

unfolding the silent chromatin 30 nm fiber into 10 nm fiber, and also displace directly the his-

146

tone octamer from the transcription sites. Upon
intensive transcription, RNA polymerases expell
all histones by occupying DNA and thus unfold the
10 nm fiber into completely linearized DNA. The
displacement of core octamers by polymerases
seems to proceed in a reversible way, so that the
core particles reassociate when the DNA becomes
available to the histone octamer. We suggest that
the primary organization of the initial and reas-
sociated core is very similar and therefore both
particles possess the folded configuration. The
displaced histone octamers can be temporary accomodated by some acceptors. It appears that histone modification, in particular their acetylation, and the presence of non-histone proteins facilitate reversible displacement of histones
rather than unfold nucleosomes in transcribed
chromatin. Thus, according to this model, the
removal of histones from promoters constitutes a
switching mechanism of gene activation whereas
histone modification and the presence of non-
histone proteins associated with active chromatin
play a role in quantative regulation of transcription.

References

1. Mirzabekov, A.D., Shick, V.V., Belyavsky, A.V.
   and Bavykin, S.G. (1978). Primary organization
   of nucleosomal core particles of chromatin: sequence of histone arrangement along DNA. Proc.
   Nat. Acad. Sci. USA 75, 4184–4188.
2. Bavykin, S.G., Usachenko, S.I., Shick, V.V.,
   Belyavsky, A.V., Lyshanskaya, A.I., Undritsov,
   I.M., Zalenskaya, I.A. and Mirzabekov, A.D.
   (in press). Primary organization of nucleosome
   core particles from active and repressed nuclei.
   Molekularnaya biologia (USSR).
3. Karpov, V.L., Preobrazhenskaya, O.V. and Mirzabekov, A.D. (1984). Chromatin structure of hsp
   70 genes, activated by heat shock: selective re
   moval of histones from the coding region and
   their absence from the 5'-region. Cell 36,423–431.

DIFFERENTIAL EXPRESSION OF THE XENOPUS VITELLOGENIN MULTIGENE FAMILY

J.R. TATA, W.C. NG, A.P. WOLFFE and J.L. WILLIAMS
National Institute for Medical Research, The Ridgeway,
Mill Hill, London NW7 1AA, U.K.

ABSTRACT

Although many multigene families are coordinately regulated, it is also becoming increasingly clear that individual genes within some families are unequally or differentially expressed in the same or in different tissues. This report describes how the hormone estrogen differentially activates the four expressed vitellogenin genes (gene A1, B1, A2 and B2) in the liver of male and female Xenopus. In both whole animals and a primary cell culture system developed in our laboratory, we find that the vitellogenin genes are activated de novo in male hepatocytes in the order B1 > A1 > A2 ≥ B2 genes. This pattern is also observed during late metamorphosis when the genes first acquire competence to respond to the hormone. There is however some flexibility in this pattern of differential expression, since by raising or lowering the dose of the hormone added to primary cell cultures or during secondary induction, one observes a more or less accentuated difference in the kinetics of accumulation of the four mRNAs. These effects on transcription and accumulation of the different mRNAs are also reflected in the relative overall DNase I sensitivity of the A and B groups of vitellogenin genes. However, the parallelism between transcription and conformation of the genes does not hold during hormone withdrawal when transcription rates drop back to control levels but the DNase I sensitivity remains elevated. This dissociation may be explained by the possibility that transcription requires continuous presence of the hormone or hormone-receptor complex in the nucleus, whereas the hormonally induced DNase I sensitivity may only return to the control levels upon cell division.

Proceedings of the 16th FEBS Congress
Part B, pp. 149–160
© 1985 VNU Science Press

INTRODUCTION

Many inducible and constitutively expressed genes are present as small multigene families. Examples of developmentally and irreversibly regulated multigene families include those encoding globin, actin and myosin. Other gene families are reversibly inducible in differentiated cells and include those encoding ovalbumin, vitellogenin and α_{2u}-globulin. Expression of the latter genes is regulated by hormones, such as sex steroids, thyroid hormones and glucocorticoids. An important question arises as to whether or not the individual gene members of such families are coordinately and equally expressed during development or hormonal induction. Also, it is not known whether or not a fixed pattern of coordinate or differential regulation of expression is maintained throughout development and in adult life. This review addresses these questions by considering a reversible, hormonally regulated multigene family which has been extensively studied in the authors' laboratory.

HORMONALLY REGULATED MULTIGENE FAMILIES

Hormones have proved to be useful tools as inducers or regulators in unravelling the relationship between structure and function of animal genes (1). The advent of gene cloning and recombinant DNA techniques has enabled us to understand some important features of hormonal regulation of gene expression. Among these are the high degree of species, tissue and hormone specificity of the genes regulated and the reversibility of the process, which in turn emphasize the importance of the interaction between the hormone-receptor complex and the genome. The recent findings on the interaction between steroid hormones and genes encoding chicken egg white proteins, vitellogenin and mammary tumor virus, illustrate this point well (see ref. 2 for several reviews).

Steroid hormones regulate transcription of specific genes, which is manifested either as a de novo activation or a modulation of the rate of transcription. In both cases, the hormone has to be continuously present so that the effect is rapidly reversed upon its withdrawal. This reversibility is an important feature since it allows one to study both the induction and de-induction processes in the context of gene structure, and which has been advantageously exploited in the regulation by estrogen of chicken egg white protein genes (1,3). In studies on the three contiguously located genes of the chicken ovalbumin family (termed ovalbumin, X and Y), it was found that upon estrogenic induction their transcription in oviduct nuclei was found to vary by a factor of 100-fold (4). It is important to note that the relative differential nuclease sensitivities of these genes did not correspond to the differences in their rates of transcription (5), a factor of some importance in considering receptor-gene interaction. In our laboratory, we have devoted considerable attention recently to how estrogen influences the conformation and expression of the Xenopus vitellogenin multigene family.

XENOPUS VITELLOGENIN GENES

Among the important advantages of studying Xenopus vitellogenin genes over other model systems used for analyzing hormonal regulation of gene expression are: 1) the dormant genes can be activated de novo by estrogen in cells from male animals; 2) the full physiological process can be reproduced in primary cell cultures, thus allowing accurate determination of the reversible changes in conformation and transcription of genes; 3) the virtual absence of DNA synthesis or cell proliferation during the early phase of hormonal stimulation.

The Xenopus vitellogenin gene family
In Xenopus laevis, four genes encoding vitellogenin are actively expressed (6), although pseudogenes or additional genes expressed at a very low level cannot be ruled out. The four expressed genes, termed A1, A2, B1, B2, exhibit a 95% sequence homology between the two genes within the A and B groups and an 80% homology between the two groups. The A1 and B1 vitellogenin genes are linked with a 15 kb DNA segment, but it is not known if the other two genes are (7).

Regulation of vitellogenin genes by estrogen

In all oviparous vertebrates the formation of egg yolk
proteins is directly regulated in the liver by estrogen
(8).   Several studies have shown that a single administration of the hormone causes a massive increase in the
accumulation of vitellogenin mRNA in the liver of both
males and females.   A characteristic feature in all
species studied is the 'memory effect', i.e. the response
to a secondary hormonal stimulation is more rapid and of a
higher magnitude.   A few studies have determined the
effect of estrogen on both the rate of transcription
per se and the stability of Xenopus vitellogenin mRNA
(9,10-12).   The rapid and massive accumulation of the
mRNA is largely due to a stabilization of the message in
the presence of the hormone relative to the rate of
induced transcription.   The hormone is continually
required not only to maintain transcription of the mRNA
but also the stability, which explains the rapid loss upon
hormone withdrawal of induced mRNA already accumulated
(8,13).

UNEQUAL EXPRESSION OF XENOPUS VITELLOGENIN GENES

Transcription and organization of groups A and B vitellogenin genes

In our earlier studies on differential regulation of
vitellogenin genes, we observed that the transcription of
A and B groups of genes and the accumulation of their
mRNAs did not occur at the same rate or to the same
extent.   In one study, we performed run-off transcription
assays on liver nuclei isolated from male and female adult
Xenopus treated with estrogen in vivo (10).   During
primary induction in males, the B group genes were found
to be significantly, but not greatly, more sensitive to
hormonal activation than the A group genes. However,
these differences disappeared or were greatly attenuated
in females or following secondary induction in males.
During the hormone withdrawal phase, the run-off transcription rates rapidly declined to nearly 'zero' levels
as in naive male liver nuclei. The differential hormonal
activation of transcription of A and B group genes was
paralleled by an increased general DNase I sensitivity

152

measured in the same batch of nuclei. However, upon
hormonal withdrawal the elevated DNase I sensitivity of
all vitellogenin genes was maintained for several weeks
even though their transcription had virtually ceased. A
similar dissociation between transcription and overall
DNase I sensitivity has been described for chicken
ovalbumin genes (3). By allowing for a longer time
interval to elapse (4-6 months), the elevated estrogen-
induced DNase I sensitivity of Xenopus vitellogenin genes
did eventually return to the basal levels found in naive
male Xenopus liver (10). The exact cause for this slow
return to the inactive gene conformation is not known but
may be related to the slow turnover of parenchymal cells
in Xenopus liver. These results are schematically
presented in Fig. 1.

Since cell cultures would allow a more accurate analysis
of the early phase of response to the hormonal stimulus,
as well as of the reversal of hormonal effects, in another
approach we studied the activation of vitellogenin A and B
group genes by estrogen directly in primary cultures of
hepatocytes (13). Again, the B group mRNAs accumulated
more rapidly than did the A group messengers upon addition
of estradiol to cell cultures. Also, if the hormone
concentration was not maintained but allowed to drop by
metabolism (14), then the accumulated mRNA decayed
rapidly with a $t_{1/2}$ of about 3-4 hr, indicating directly
that the hormone is required not only for transcription
but also for maintaining the mRNA in a stable state.

Transcription and accumulation of transcripts of
individual vitellogenin genes
Because of the 95% coding sequence homology of the two
genes constituting the A and B groups, it was difficult to
quantitatively measure the concentration of messenger RNA
encoded by each of the four Xenopus vitellogenin genes.
However, by devising a disc assay based on very stringent
hybridization and washing conditions, it was possible to
determine the steady state level of each individual mRNA
as well as the absolute rate of transcription of each
gene (15). The results obtained by this assay showed

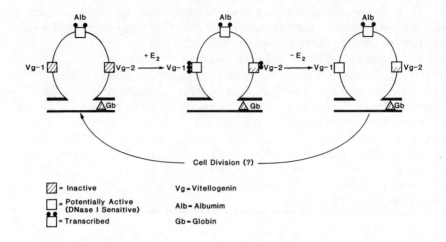

Fig. 1. Scheme depicting the enhanced overall DNase I sensitivity coupled to transcription of two Xenopus laevis vitellogenin genes induced by estradiol-17β administration (+E$_2$), and the dissociation between gene conformation and transcription upon hormone withdrawal (-E$_2$). Genes Vg-1 and Vg-2 are two vitellogenin genes initially transcribed unequally in male Xenopus liver. The involvement of cell division in the DNase I sensitivity returning to control male levels is hypothetical. Scheme based on data from Williams and Tata (10).

that the four genes were not coordinately or equally expressed under most conditions of early stages of hormonal induction.

The rate of accumulation of mRNAs corresponding to the four genes in livers of immediately post-metamorphic froglets of both sexes following their continuous immersion in a solution of estradiol (at this stage no vitellogenin transcription would be expected to occur in female animals) or in primary cultures of adult male hepatocytes, increased in the order of B1 > A1 > A2 ≥ B2. Since other experiments have shown that vitellogenin mRNA is extremely stable in the presence of estradiol (11,12), it was concluded that the pattern of initial increase in steady-state levels of each mRNA reflected the individual rate of transcription and RNA processing in the nucleus. This was confirmed by direct measurement of the absolute rate of transcription of the four genes. In the experiment shown in Table 1, cultures of female hepatocytes were hormonally stimulated in vitro in order to obtain the highest possible rate of transcription.

Table 1

Absolute rate of transcription of individual vitellogenin genes upon estrogen activation of cultured hepatocytes from adult female Xenopus (15).

Gene	Absolute rate of transcription (molecules cell^{-1} hr^{-1})
A1	265
A2	182
B1	670
B2	117

Experiments in which the time-course and dose of hormone were varied showed that the pattern of accumulation of B1 > A1 > A2 ≥ B2 mRNA can be flexible. Thus, the results summarized in Fig. 2 show that at 10^{-6}M estradiol added to the hepatocyte cultures the A1 - B1 pair of genes was the first to be activated (within 60 min) but the A2 - B2 pair of mRNAs began to accumulate at later times. The difference in the concentration of mRNA between the two pairs was gradually reduced with time of exposure to the hormone, which may explain why such differences in accumulation of individual mRNAs were not observed by

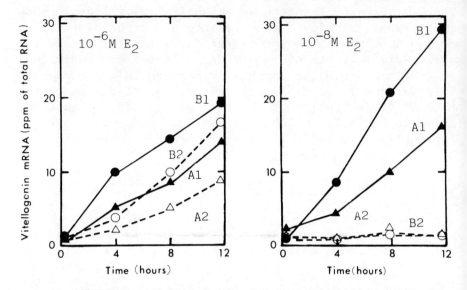

Fig. 2. Kinetics of accumulation of mRNA specified by the four Xenopus vitellogenin genes in male Xenopus hepatocyte cultures after primary induction by two different concentrations of estradiol (E_2). Note the different absicca scale in the two panels. Data adapted from Ng et al. (15).

other workers following long-term stimulation with estrogen in vivo (16). If the dose of the hormone were lowered 100-fold and the overall transcription rate reduced, then during the first 12 hr only the A1 - B1 pair of gene transcripts could be detected. Although we do not know the exact reason for the flexibility of response that we observe, it is quite likely a reflection of the different promoter strengths, and/or intensity of interaction between the estrogen-receptor complex and the regulatory sequences of the two pairs of genes. An examination of the sequences upstream of the 5' end of each of the four Xenopus vitellogenin genes (17) may reveal some interesting differences in the elements thought to be involved in steroid hormone receptor interaction with specific genes (2).

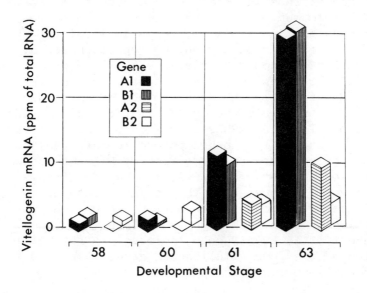

Fig. 3. Accumulation of the four Xenopus vitellogenins
         mRNAs in the liver of Xenopus larvae at different
stages of development after immersion for three days in
water containing 10^{-6}M estradiol.   Data of Ng et al.(15).

Unequal expression of individual genes during development
When during development is the above unequal expression
pattern established? Is such a pattern maintained
throughout development as well as in the adult tissue?
Answers to these questions are relevant to our eventual
understanding of the relationship between the organization
of the individual vitellogenin genes and their interaction
with estrogen receptor.

The pattern of expression in the order B1 > A1 > A2 ≌ B2
vitellogenin genes found in adult Xenopus liver is already
established in stage 66 froglets (15).   When the
accumulation of the four mRNAs was measured in livers of
tadpoles before and during metamorphosis, after exposure
to estrogen for three days, a similar unequal pattern of
expression was observed in earlier developmental stages

(Fig. 3). Little or no transcription of any of the vitellogenin genes was visible in tissue from embryos before developmental stage 58, which is about mid-metamorphosis. At stage 60, very low levels of transcripts were first detected but no reproducible pattern of individual mRNAs could be discerned. However, at stages 61 and 63 the genes were significantly responsive, exhibiting virtually the same pattern of expression as that seen in froglets and in adults (Fig. 2). (The equal amounts of Al and Bl mRNAs in stages 61 and 63 livers in Fig. 3 was due to the long exposure to estrogen, but shorter periods were characterized by Bl mRNA concentration exceeding that of Al mRNA, as seen for froglet and adult liver). Thus, once the hepatocytes acquire competence to respond to the hormone an unequal pattern of expression is established which is then maintained throughout life, even though the absolute rate of transcription of the four vitellogenin genes increases considerably during development.

DISCUSSION

The unequal pattern of expression of the individual genes of the Xenopus vitellogenin gene family and its developmental establishment raise some interesting questions. For example, the acquisition of competence for these genes to be activated in response to estrogen most likely reflects the first appearance of hormone receptor in the developing liver (18). It may also reflect some change in the conformation of genes making them more accessible to the receptor. Recently, we have detected a hypomethylation at three sites at the 3' end of the Bl gene which is developmentally regulated in female but not male Xenopus (19). However, the hypo-methylation was not hormonally regulated and was independent of whether or not the gene was transcribed. The significance of these three CpG residues remains unclear, but it would be of some interest to verify if such a developmentally regulated and sex specific process is also applicable to the same 3' region of the other three vitellogenin genes.

158

The coordinate, though unequal, regulation of transcription of the A1 and B1 vitellogenin genes is compatible with the fact that these two genes are linked (7). Differences in the intensity of interaction between estrogen-receptor complex and regulatory sequences determining promoter function of these genes may explain why the A1 - B1 pair is more sensitive to the hormone than the A2 and B2 vitellogenin genes. There is now good evidence for certain conserved sequences upstream from the promoters of chicken steroid hormone regulated genes, including vitellogenin gene, that are recognized by and interact with the relevant receptor (2,20). It would therefore be interesting to compare the sequences in the 5' flanking region of the four Xenopus vitellogenin genes. Indeed, a recent study shows that two symmetrical GGTCANNNTGACC elements are present at about -310 to -370 b.p. upstream from the transcription initiation site in all four Xenopus vitellogenin genes (17). However, another such element is present at -550 to -650 position only in the A1 - B1 gene pair but is absent in the A2 and B2 genes. Could this difference explain the unequal expression of the individual members of the vitellogenin multigene family? Whatever the answers to these questions will turn out to be, it is clear that the regulation of their expression by estrogen has already served as a valuable model in analyzing the organization and activity of multigene families as well as for understanding hormonal regulation of gene expression.

ACKNOWLEDGEMENTS

We are grateful to Professor W. Wahli for the cloned cDNAs specifying the four Xenopus vitellogenin genes and to Mrs. E. Heather for expert preparation of the manuscript.

REFERENCES

1. Tata, J.R. (1984). The action of growth and developmental hormones. In: Biological Regulation and Development, Vol. 3B, R.F. Goldberger and K.R. Yamamoto (Eds). Plenum Publishing, New York, pp.1-58.

2. Eriksson, H. and Gustafsson, J.-A. (Eds). (1983). Steroid Hormone Receptors: Structure and Function. Elsevier, Amsterdam.

3. Palmiter, R.D., Mulvihill, E.R., McKnight, G.S. and Senear, A.W. (1977). Cold Spring Harbor Symp. Quant. Biol. 42, 639-647.

4. LeMeur, M., Glanville, N., Mandel, J.L., Gerlinger, P., Palmiter, R. and Chambon, P. (1981). Cell 23, 561-571.

5. Lawson, G.M., Knoll, B.J., March, C.J., Woo, S.L.C., Tsai, M.-J. and O'Malley, B.W. (1982). J. Biol. Chem. 257, 1501-1507.

6. Wahli, W., Dawid, I.B., Wyler, T., Jaggi, R.B., Weber, R. and Ryffel, G.U. (1979). Cell 16, 535-549.

7. Wahli, W., Germond, J.-E., Heggeler, B.T. and May, F.E.B. (1982). Proc. Natl. Acad. Sci. USA 79,6832-6836.

8. Tata, J.R. and Smith, D.F. (1979). Recent Prog. Horm. Res. 35, 47-95.

9. Brock, M.L. and Shapiro, D.J. (1983). J. Biol. Chem. 258, 5449-5455.

10. Williams, J.L. and Tata, J.R. (1983). Nucl. Acids Res. 11, 1151-1166.

11. Brock, M.L. and Shapiro, D.J. (1983). Cell 34, 207-214.

12. Wolffe, A.P., Perlman, A.J. and Tata, J.R. (1984). The EMBO J. (in press).

13. Wolffe, A.P. and Tata, J.R. (1983) Eur. J. Biochem. 130, 365-372.

14. Tenniswood, M.P.R., Searle, P.F., Wolffe, A.P. and Tata, J.R. (1983). Mol. Cell. Endocrinol.30, 329-345.

15. Ng, W.C., Wolffe, A.P. and Tata, J.R. (1984). Develop. Biol. 102, 238-247.

16. Felber, B.K., Maurhofer, S., Jaggi, R.B., Wyler, T., Wahli, W., Ryffel, G.U. and Weber, R. (1980). Eur. J. Biochem. 105, 17-24.

17. Walker, P., Germond, J.-E., Brown-Luedi, M., Givel, F. and Wahli, W. (1985). Nucl. Acids Res. 12, 8611-8626.

18. May, F.E.B. and Knowland, J. (1981). Nature 292, 853-855.

19. Ng, W.C., Baker, B.S. and Tata, J.R. (1985) FEBS Lett. (in press).

20. Jost, J.-P., Seldran, M. and Geiser, M. (1984) Proc. Natl. Acad. Sci. USA 81, 429-433.

STRUCTURAL ASPECTS OF CHROMATIN REPLICATION

R.TSANEV
Inst.Molecular Biology,Bulg.Acad.Sci.,1113 Sofia,Bulgaria

The existence of specific DNA-protein complexes makes the reproduction of the genetic apparatus considerably more complicated than the replication of DNA itself. In eukaryotic cells the interaction of DNA with histones re- sults in two levels of DNA folding - nucleosomal (cf.1) and higher order structures (2). The interaction of the resulting chromatin fibers with some nonhistone struc- tures leads to a third level revealed as chromatin loops attached to a nuclear skeleton (3-5).

This complex structure is presumably either truely re- produced in a proliferative cell cycle,or altered in a differentiating cell cycle. Thus,it is of utmost import- ance to reveal the behavior of the chromosomal proteins and their complexes with DNA during replication.

The metabolic stability of histones (6) and the hete- rogeneity of the nucleosomes due to the existence of histone variants raise the problem of how the nucleoso- mal pattern,which shows some tissue variations (7),is transmitted to the progeny. To solve this problem the first question to be answered is how do old and new his- tones interact with the parental and the newly synthe- sized DNA strands.

We have studied this point by differential labelling of DNA and histones and following the association of the latter with the new and the old DNA strands (8,9). In one of our approaches (9) we have covalently linked the his- tones to DNA,dissociated the unbound protein and followed in a density gradient the distribution of old and new histones with respect to old and new DNA strands,one of which was made heavy by BUdR incorporation. These experi- ments have shown that the old histones remain associated with the parental DNA strands,while the new are bound to the newly synthesized DNA strands. This conclusion was confirmed in similar experiments where DNA has been sub- stituted with BUdR for two generations (10).

These data suggest but do not prove that the site of

Proceedings of the 16th FEBS Congress
Part B, pp. 161–170
© 1985 VNU Science Press

histone deposition is the replicating chromatin. The experiments designed to check this point have led to controversial results. The first data led to the unexpected conclusion that new histones were distributed at random while parental histones associated with new DNA (11-13). To account for these results it was proposed that new histones joined the old chromatin ahead of the replication fork,while parental histones associated with the replicating DNA by sliding.

Other experiments,however,have demonstrated that new histones in fact join nascent DNA (14,15). It seems that data showing a random distribution of histones are due to their redistribution induced by shearing and fixation with formaldehyde (16,17). The H2a-H2b pair seems to be especially sensitive and was found randomly distributed even under milder conditions,in contrast to the arginine rich histones found preferentially associated with new chromatin (18).

Bearing in mind the variagated chromatin structures,another important question is how old and new histone cores segregate between the two daughter DNA molecules. Evidence for a unilateral trans-segregation has been reported (19,20),but these results may have a different interpretation (cf.21). In our experiments (22) chromatin replicated during cycloheximide-inhibited histone synthesis was digested with Bsp I restriction nuclease. The fragments obtained and the corresponding DNA were fractionated in different density gradients. In agreement with other data the results have shown that such chromatin contains half the normal content of histones,but that it has no long stretches of naked DNA - the fragments have a buoyant density intermediate between that of DNA and that of normal chromatin. When chromatin with inhibited histone synthesis was digested with micrococcal nuclease the DNA fragments showed no multimers higher than pentamers with a large amount of dimers and monomers.These results led to the conclusion that old and new histones segregated in groups of no more than 5-6 nucleosomes which were distributed bilaterally between the two daughter DNA molecules. Such a distribution was confirmed by experiments using histones labelled with heavy amino acids /23,cf.also 24).

In other experiments with crosslinked histones (25) it was found that new histone octamers had a preference to be aligned together,but the size of the segregation group was not determined. It is not excluded that the size of these groups may be different in different cases.It also seems possible that at the start of replication the first segregation groups of old histone octamers remain associated with the old DNA in a trans position and then the alternating pattern of old and new clusters is produced.

An interesting problem is the mechanism which may determine a stronger binding of the histone cores to one of the DNA strands. This seems difficult to explain bearing in mind the dyad symmetry of the nucleosome. However,interaction between isolated core particles was shown to introduce an asymmetry in the relative arrangement of the two H2a-H2b dimers (26). Thus,it appears possible that in chromatin there might be also such factors which could induce even a higher degree of asymmetry. This may permit the preferential interaction of one of the two DNA strands with some strong binding sites,such as the arginine residues,which could fix the histone core to one of the unwinding strands of the double helix.

We have tried to check experimentally whether such an asymmetric interaction could be detected in the DNase I digestion pattern of the nucleosomes (27). Such an approach is justified by data indicating that reduced cleavage rates may arise from a reduction of DNA flexibility due to tight binding by histones (26). The two DNA strands of EAT cells were differentially labelled with 14C-TdR in vivo and with 3H-TdR in vitro in the presence of cycloheximide to eliminate symmetry due to the presence of new histone cores interacting preferentially with the new 3H-labelled strand which presumably will interact less strongly with the old histones.

The results obtained show that in control experiments carried out in the absence of cycloheximide,the digestion patterns of the two strands coincide,while in chromatin from cycloheximide-treated cells the newly synthesized strand is attacked more strongly and shows a profile deviating from that of normal chromatin (Fig.1). When isolated nucleosomes from such a chromatin were tested,no

163

differences between the two strands were revealed. These data are compatible with an asymmetric interaction of the two DNA strands with the histone cores when the nucleosomes are organized in chromatin structures.

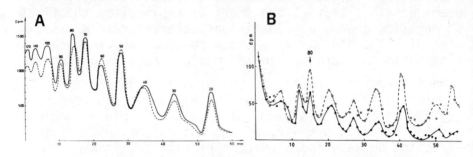

Fig.1
DNase I digestion pattern of normal chromatin (A) and of chromatin from cycloheximide-treated cells (B). ●——● - DNA strands labelled in vivo with 14C-TdR for 48h; o---o - DNA strands labelled in vitro with 3H-TdR for 90 min in the presence of cycloheximide(27).

The asymmetric interaction of DNA with the histones may be important for the segregation of different types of nucleosomes to the two daughter cells and also for the liberation of the coding DNA strand during transcription.

The sequential addition of histone complexes to replicating DNA and the late addition of H1 (15) suggest that the properties of replicating chromatin should differ from those of bulk chromatin. This difference was revealed only during the very early stages of replication,and is characterized by an increased sensitivity to nuclease digestion,altered lengths of the linkers and the presence of tight dimers close to the replication fork (cf.16,17, 21;28). On the other hand,the only electron microscopic pictures of replicating chromatin in Drosophila embryos (29) did not reveal any difference between the nucleosomal structure of replicating and of bulk chromatin.
The disagreement between the biochemical and the electron microscopic evidence led us to undertake an ultrastructural study on chromatin replication in early Droso-

phila embryos. Observations on 100 replication figures(30) showed that as a rule their structure differed from that of nonreplicating chromatin: a/In very small replication "eye-forms" the nucleosomal density was about half the normal value (Fig.2a); b/Histone cores were often found free,dissociated from the replicating DNA (Fig.2b); c/In small replicating eye-forms some of the linker DNA was sensitive to S1 nuclease (Fig.2c); d/In most cases the nucleosomes in the replication fork were irregularly arranged,revealing linkers with varying size and tight dimers (Fig.2b,d).

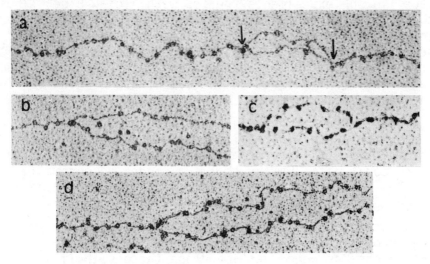

Fig.2
Electron micrographs of replication figures in chromatin of early Drosophila embryos.a - small eye-form with a strongly reduced nucleosome density; b - replication fork with free particles, presumably dissociated histone cores; c - small eye-form treated on the grid with S1 nuclease; d - Replication fork with irregularly arranged nucleosomes(30).

These ultrastructural features are in full agreement with the biochemical data.They are to be expected if new nucleosomes lack H1 (15) and DNA can be partially uncoiled,thus facilitating nucleosome sliding and dissociation. Another factor may be that in early embryos with a very fast rate of replication the unwinding of DNA may go ahead of DNA synthesis,as found in the sea urchin embryo (31). Thus,pictures like those in Fig.2a and 2c may well represent DNA unwinding. The possibility of single-stranded DNA associating with histone cores has been demonstrated (32).

The difference between our data and those previously published (29),may be explained by the possibility that the irregular spacing and loose binding of nuclesome cores in replicating chromatin become evident due to shearing forces and interaction of the chromatin with the grid surface (in our experiments treated with Alcian Blue). Thus, these differences may be revealed or not,depending on the conditions of chromatin preparation and spreading. It seems that under our experimental conditions the lability of the immature nucleosome structure of replicating chromatin is visualized due to the same factors which provide the biochemical evidence.

Higher order structures should also be strongly affected by the process of replication since they can not be formed before H1 is added. This is supported by electron microscopic data showing that the condensed chromatin undergoes an ordered cycle of localized disaggregation and reaggregation associated with DNA replication (33).

The behaviour of the third level of chromatin folding - the chromatin loops - is less clear. The existence of such loops has been questioned and the possibility was suggested that the internal nuclear matrix may be an artifactual aggregate of proteins induced by the high salt concentration (34). This aggregate could entangle DNA which then necessarily will have to loop out of it.There are data,however,which indicate that the loop organization of DNA is not an artifact. The size of the DNA domains determined by biochemical methods are of the same order as the size of the loops (cf.3). On the other hand electron microscopic observations show that interphase nuclei spread at low ionic strength also have their chromatin organized in loops attached to proteinous structures (4). Our unpublished experiments confirm this result for both interphase nuclei and mitotic chromosomes (Fig.3).

166

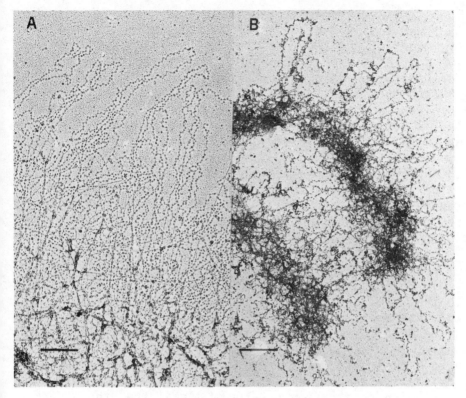

Fig.3
Electron micrographs of chromatin loops
attached to a proteinous skeleton in the
spread interphase nucleus of a Friend cell
/A/ and in spread mitotic chromosomes of
an early Drosophila embryo /B/.Bar is
0.34 μm in A and 0.60 μm in B.

It is interesting that we have found the same loop organization of DNA in the mature sperm of ram,trout and
mussel (35-37). The lack of RNP network in the nucleus of
the mature sperm permits one to visualize the attachment
sites of the DNA loops. In all three species they represented ringshaped granular bodies 30 to 70 nm in size,
resistant to high salt extraction and built of nonhistone
proteins mainly in the region between 60 and 80 kD.
The similarity of the structures organizing DNA in

167

loops in three evolutionary so distinct species indicates that the loop organization of DNA may be functionally very important and the loops may be inheritable DNA domains. The possibility that the loops are structures transmitted to the progeny is also suggested by data that the same DNA sequences (38) and tightly bound proteins (39) are involved in the attachment sites both in interphase nuclei and in metaphase chromosomes. On the other hand we have demonstrated in a variety of cellular types the existence of metabolically stable nonhistone proteins transmitted to the progeny during many cellular divisions (cf.21).

The attachment of the chromatin loops to nuclear structures is associated with their supertwisting. This imposes some torsional constraint on DNA and makes it similar to the circular DNA. There are indications that this supercoiling of DNA might be involved in the regulation of replication and is important for its proper initation (40). On the other hand a number of reports have indicated that replication of DNA is associated with its skeletal attachment sites (cf.41). If so,these sites should be different from the permanent attachment sites discussed above. In high salt treated nuclei replication figures have been located distal from the nuclear matrix (42). In low salt spread nuclei we also have observed chromatin loops with replication eye-forms distal from the attachment sites (Fig.4). Thus,either the association of replication with the nuclear matrix is an artifact of preparation,or these sites are weak and easily dissociated.

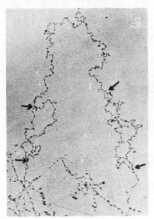

Fig.4
Electron micrograph of a chromatin loop of the nucleus from an early Drosophila embryo,exhibiting two symmetrical replication figures distal from its attachment sites (30).

The elucidation of the functional role of the chromatin loops,the possible existence of different types of attachment sites,the localization of genes with respect to the strong attachment sites,the transmittance of this pattern to the progeny - unchanged or altered during cell differentiation - are unsolved problems which might be important for understanding the organization and regulation of the eukaryotic genome.

REFERENCES

1.McGhee,J.D.& Felsenfeld,G.A.(1980)Annu.Rev.Biochem.49, 1115-1156.
2.Finch,J.T.& Klug,A.(1976)Proc.Natl.Acad.Sci.USA,73, 1897-1901.
3.Igo-Kamenes,S.,Hörz,W.& Zachau,H.G.(1982)Annu.Rev.Biochem.51,89-121.
4.Rattner,J.B.& Hamkalo,B.A.(1979)J.Cell Biol.81,453-457.
5.Adolph,K.W.,Cheng,S.M.,Paulson,J.R.& Laemmli,U.K.(1977) Proc.Natl.Acad.Sci.USA,74,4937-4941.
6.Hancock,R.(1969)J.Mol.Biol.40,457-466.
7.Russanova,V.,Venkov,C.& Tsanev,R.(1980)Cell Differ.9, 339-350.
8.Tsanev,R.& Russev,G.(1974)Eur.J.Biochem.43,257-263.
9.Russev,G.& Tsanev,R.(1979)Eur.J.Biochem.93,123-128.
10.Freedlander,E.F.,Taichman,L.& Smithies,O.(1977)Biochemistry,16,1802-1808.
11.Jackson,V.,Grainger,D.& Chalkley,R.(1976)Proc.Natl. Acad.Sci.USA,73,2266-2269.
12.Seale,R.L.(1976)Proc.Natl.Acad.Sci.USA,76,2270-2274.
13.Hancock,R.(1978)Proc.Natl.Acad.Sci.USA,75,2130-2134.
14.Crémisi,C.,Chestier,A.& Yaniv,M.(1978)Cold Spring Harbor Symp.Quant.Biol.42,409-416.
15.Worcel,A.,Han,S.& Wong,M.L.(1978)Cell,15,969-977.
16.Crémisi,C.(1979)Microbiol.Rev.43,297-319.
17.DePamphilis,M.L.& Wassarman,P.M.(1980)Annu.Rev.Biochem. 49,627-666.
18.Senshu,T.,Fukuda,M.& Ohashi,M.(1978)J.Biochem.84,985-988.
19.Seidman,M.M.,Levine,A,J.& Weintraub,H.(1979)Cell,18, 439-449.
20.Riley,D.& Weintraub,H.(1979)Proc.Natl.Acad.Sci.USA,76, 328-332.

21.Tsanev,R.(1982)Replication of chromatin.In:Progress in Mutation Research (Natarajan,A.T. et al.,eds.),vol.4, Elsevier/North Holland,Amsterdam,pp.131-145.
22.Pospelov,V.,Russev,G.,Vassilev,L.& Tsanev,R.(1982)J.Mol. Biol.156,79-91.
23.Russev,G.& Hancock,R.(1982)Proc.Natl.Acad.Sci.USA,79, 3143-3147.
24.Annunziato,A.T.& Seale,R.L.(1983)Molec.Cellul.Biochem. 55,99-112.
25.Leffak,I.M.,Grainger,R.& Weintraub,H.(1977)Cell,12, 837-845.
26.Richmond,T.J.,Finch,J.T.,Rushton,B.,Rhodes,D.& Klug,A. (1984)Nature,311,532-537.
27.Chipev,C.& Tsanev,R.,unpublished.
28.Levy,A.& Jacob,K.(1978)Cell,14,259-267.
29.McKnight,S.L.& Miller,O.L.(1977)Cell,12,795-804.
30.Tsanev,R.& Semenov,E. ,unpublished.
31.Baldari,C.T.,Amaldi,F.& Bonjiorno-Nardelli,M.(1978) Cell,15,1095-1107.
32.Palter,K.B.,Foe,V.E.& Alberts,B.M.(1979)Cell,18,451- 467.
33.Setterfield,G.,Sheinin,R.,Dardick,I.,Kiss,G.& Dubsky,M. (1978)J.Cell Biol.77,246-263.
34.Hadlaczky,G.,Sumner,A.T.& Ross,A.(1981)Chromosoma(Ber- lin)81,557-567.
35.Tsanev,R.& Avramova,Z.(1981)Eur.J.Cell Biol.24,139-145.
36.Tsanev,R.& Avramova,Z.(1983)Eur.J.Cell Biol.31,143-149.
37.Avramova,Z.,Zalensky,A.& Tsanev,R.(1984)Exp.Cell Res. 152,231-239.
38.Razin,S.V.,Mantieva,V.L.&Georgiev,G.P.(1979)Nucl.Acids Res.7,1713-1735.
39.Razin,S.V.Chernokhvostov,V.V.,Roodin,A.V.,Zbarsky,I.B. & Georgiev,G.P.(1981)Cell,27,65-73.
40.Mattern,M.R.& Painter,R.B.(1979)Biochim.Biophys.Acta, 563,293-305;306-312.
41.Berezney,R.(1979)Dynamic properties of the nuclear matrix.In:The cell nucleus (Busch,H.,ed.),vol.7,Acad. Press,New York,London,pp.413-456.
42.Hancock,R.& Hughes,M.(1982)Biol.Cell,44,201-212.

Symposium X

PROTEIN BIOSYNTHESIS

STRUCTURE AND FUNCTION OF BACTERIAL ELONGATION FACTOR EF-Tu

B.F.C. CLARK, T.F.M. LA COUR, K.M. NIELSEN, J. NYBORG &
S. THIRUP
Division of Biostructural Chemistry, Dept. of Chemistry,
Aarhus University, 8000 Aarhus C, Denmark

INTRODUCTION

The interactive recognition of nucleic acids by proteins
is a central process in the regulation of gene expression.
In order to explain such interactions, we require a knowledge of the appropriate three-dimensional structures and
biochemical functional information. One convenient object
for study is the strong and specific interaction between
aminoacyl-tRNA (aa-tRNA) and the bacterial elongation factor
EF-Tu, in a ternary complex which also contains GTP. The
ternary complex is a central feature in carrying aa-tRNA
to the ribosomal A-site for decoding the mRNA and thereby
placing the amino acid in the correct order during its
incorporation into a polypeptide chain [1]. A knowledge of
the recognitory interaction of aa-tRNA with EF-Tu should
help to explain other types of nucleic acid-protein interactions and may allow general principles to be postulated
concerning regulatory mechanisms for gene expression.

Clearly, the direct way of obtaining information about
the nucleic acid-protein recognition in a ternary complex
would be to solve the three-dimensional structure to high
resolution (about 25 nm), using X-ray crystallography. No
suitable crystals large enough for X-ray studies exist at
present, so we decided on an indirect approach to the
problem. Since the three-dimensional structure for yeast
tRNA^{Phe} is known and is thought to be a good general model
for tRNAs, and since there is good evidence that the structure of tRNA does not change significantly on aminoacylation to aa-tRNA, we have analysed the structure of EF-Tu
by X-ray crystallography and have studied the ternary
complex by biochemical and chemical methods as a prelude
to model-building studies for the ternary complex.

Here we wish to report current progress in these studies.
First we shall describe how a high-resolution electron

Proceedings of the 16th FEBS Congress
Part B, pp. 173–181
© 1985 VNU Science Press

density map (0.29 nm) of EF-Tu has enabled us to locate functionally important residues in the three-dimensional structure. Secondly, we shall describe how foot-printing studies of aa-tRNA in ternary complex have allowed us to propose a convenient model in terms of a 0.5 nm model tRNA^{Phe} for which parts of the tRNA are in contact with the protein.

THREE-DIMENSIONAL STRUCTURE OF EF-Tu

EF-Tu is the most abundant protein in *Escherichia coli*, constituting up to 6% of the total protein, depending on the growth conditions [2]. Interestingly, this relatively high concentration (~0.3 mM) in the bacterial cell is about the same as the aa-tRNA concentration. The role of EF-Tu may well be therefore to sequester the aa-tRNA during protein biosynthesis to prevent the easy chemical hydrolysis of the bond between the amino acid and the tRNA. This action would conserve energy in the form of ATP, the hydrolysis of which is needed to re-form aa-tRNA. When we decided to determine the three-dimensional structure of EF-Tu, no primary structure was known, so we completed the primary structure with the help of Dr. S. Magnusson's group [3]. We were rather fortunate in that it was possible to elucidate the structure of the protein isolated as a mixture of two gene products. It was known that the *tufA* gene was expressed about 3.5 times as much as the *tufB* gene [4], and only one ambiguity was observed in the peptides produced after the protein's degradation, in that the C-terminal Gly was found in three times the amount of C-terminal Ser. We proposed therefore that the Gly-containing product arose from the *tufA* gene and the Ser-containing product from the *tufB* gene. The determined DNA sequences of the *tufA* gene [5] and the *tufB* gene [6] confirmed this. Actually, the two genes contained 12 other base differences, which were not expressed as different amino acids. The problem of differential gene expression and its regulation has not been explained so far from knowledge of the gene sequences and their flanking regions.

EF-Tu has a molecular weight of about 43000 daltons from 393 amino acids. It starts with a blocked amino acid, acetyl Ser, and ends with either Gly or Ser, depending on which gene the product arises from, as described above. Interestingly, Lys 56 was methylated to about 60% to give monomethyl Lys, depending on the cellular growth conditions. Trp 184 is the only Trp in the protein, so it could be useful as a probe for physical chemical studies. There are three Cys residues: Cys 81 is thought to be concerned with aa-tRNA binding, Cys 137 with GDP/GTP binding, and Cys 255 is buried [7]. His 66 is also thought to be concerned with the aa-tRNA binding site [8]. Ala 375 is the residue which is replaced in a kirromycin resistant strain, for example by Thr [9, 10] or Val [11]. More details of the important residues have been described earlier [12].

During our EF-Tu crystallization studies, the protein becomes nicked at Arg 58 (also perhaps later at Arg 44) when good crystals are produced, giving evidence perhaps of a strained or exposed polypeptide stretch.

The binary complex EF-Tu:GDP, either intact or enzymically digested, crystallizes readily in a variety of different forms. So far, no useful crystals of EF-Tu:GTP have been obtained. In our laboratory, we have experienced that a spontaneously nicked form of EF-Tu:GDP gives the most useful crystals for data collection and heavy metal derivatization. The preliminary results of our studies with this orthorhombic crystal form describing data collection to 0.26 nm, a low-resolution model (0.5 nm) [13] and further refinement allowing an extended chain tracing in one domain [14] have already been published.

When we produced the first high-resolution electron density map, we were not able to correlate secondary structure with sequences, because only part of the primary structure was known. However, we were able to locate the bound GDP with respect to elements of secondary structure. Improvements in the method of analysis and the determination of the primary structure enabled us to locate about 70% of the structure in space. Because of lack of isomorphism of the heavy atom derivatives, the range of data was reduced to 0.29 nm in a determination of a revised map [14]. With the revised map, it was possible to describe the structure conveniently in terms of three domains I, II, and III, [15] respectively, based on the amount of secondary structure they each contain. A simplified drawing is shown in Fig. 1, which also places some highlighted residues in the spatial

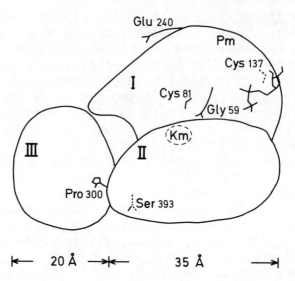

Fig. 1: *A simplified drawing of the overall shapes of the domains of EF-Tu:GDP.* The position of GDP is shown by the skeletal structure. Connecting amino acids and biochemically important positions are indicated. K_m = amino acid site 375 which is concerned with kirromycin effect; P_m = proposed puromycin binding site. The dotted surround indicates that the site is behind the surface shown. The domains I, II, and III are also referred to as the tight, the loose, and the floppy.

structure. An end-on view of this simplified spatial structure is shown in Fig. 2. Progress in amino acid assignments in the spatial structure has come from refinement of the structure and molecular model building in a molecular graphics system helped by a collaboration with the Molecular Structure Group at Uppsala University's Biomedical Center.

With our revised map, it has been possible to assign amino acids 60 to 240 to the tight domain I, which contains a high amount of secondary structure and contains the GDP binding site, shown by the skeletal structure in Figs 1 and 2. The correctness of the map assignment is supported by location of the heavy atoms Hg, Pt and Pb at the expected amino acid residues Cys, Met and acidic amino

176

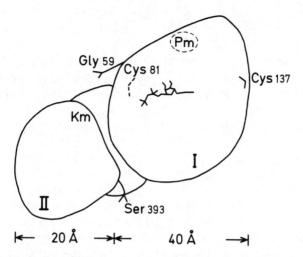

Fig. 2: *A drawing of the overall shapes of the domains I, II, and III of EF-Tu:GDP* viewed at 90° from the GDP binding end to the view shown in Fig. 1. Amino acids and GDP are indicated as in Fig. 1.

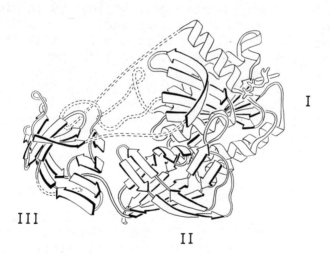

Fig. 3: *A cartoon illustrating the secondary structural elements describing the total structure of EF-Tu.* Flat arrows show β-strands, end flat helical bands show α-helices. The dotted lines show parts of the structure (about 30 amino acids) not yet delineated.

acids, respectively. The folding pattern of domain I [14] shows a 5-stranded parallel β-sheet, which is extended by a sixth anti-parallel strand. The β-strands are connected by 6 α-helices via loops that are short except in one case. The β-sheet forms a central hydrophobic core with a relatively large left-handed twist. Surrounding this core, the α-helices provide an efficient interface with the solvent in a compact arrangement. The positions of Cys 81 and Cys 137 associated with aa-tRNA cofactor binding are also shown in Figs 1 and 2. An almost complete chain tracing from a recent map interpretation is shown in Fig. 3. Domain II contains about 100 residues (approx. 300-393), which form a number of β-strands but no α-helices. This loose domain is in contact with helices I and II of the tight domain. The location of the C-terminal amino acid (in this case Ser 393) is shown in the cleft between domains I and II (Figs 1, 2 and 3). At present, the only covalent connection between domains I and II appears to be via the strand 44-58, which may be missing in the crystal, whereas the rest of the contacts are due to hydrophobic forces and salt bridges. Residue 59 in Figs 1 and 2 shows where the chain tracing ends in our model building. The electron density in domain III is still difficult to trace due to some less well defined electron density for residues 1-58 and 240-300 and the presence of only short stretches of β-strands. This floppy domain may be aptly named, because it may be flexible in the absence of aa-tRNA. The connection between domains II and III is presumably around residue 300 (see Fig. 1), and the chain tracing is again lost at Glu 240.

Biochemical properties related to the structure

There are indications that the interface between domains I and II is involved in allosteric changes, which are observed when EF-Tu exerts some of its functions. Some mutants of EF-Tu have been shown to be resistant towards the antibiotic kirromycin, which is an inhibitor of protein biosynthesis. Two of these mutants have been shown to contain Thr and Val, respectively, in position 375 instead of Ala 375 in the wild type [9-11]. In our interpretation of the electron density near the C-terminal end of the polypeptide chain, we have located residue 375 in the cleft formed between domains I and II and not far below the putative position of strand 44-58 [10] (see K_m site in Figs 1 and 2). Binding of the antibiotic causes a significant change of the affinities of the protein towards both GDP and GTP and alters the GDP binary complex to bind aa-tRNA. This allows us more confidently to use the structure of EF-Tu:GDP in our model building studies for the ternary complex. Although EF-Tu:GDP does not normally bind aa-tRNA, under the special conditions described above it can. Thus it seems likely that the disposition of the domains will change going from the GDP to the GTP form of EF-Tu, but structures within the domains will probably remain the same.

Work is continuing to improve the interpretability of our electron density map, especially to locate the atomic environment and bonding for the bound cofactor GTP. Clearly the conserved region around Cys 137 for GTP binding proteins [16] is concerned with the GDP site in some way. Cys 137 is not necessarily directly involved, because not all EF-Tu sequences contain a Cys in this position. Our present model building fails to show a hydrophobic pocket for binding the guanine base of GDP. So far it seems that Leu 175 is concerned with hydrophobic binding in the pocket and Ser 173 and Asn 135 is H-bonded to O_6 of the guanine. It appears the Asn 135 is crucially conserved in several GDP binding proteins. It is difficult to see how the sugar is bound, but the ring oxygen is closest to the protein with the 2'-, 3'-hydroxyl groups free and pointing into the solvent. Arg 230 and the loop 275-278 are probably involved in binding to the phosphate groups. Magnesium is also involved. The stereochemistry appears to be different from a normal nucleotide binding domain.

There are several lines of biochemical evidence that aa-tRNA binding to EF-Tu involves the N-terminal region of EF-Tu, at any rate around Cys 81 [7, 17] and His 66 [8]. However, Cys 81 must be involved as a structural determinant in an indirect way, because other species of EF-Tu, for example *Thermus thermophilus*, not containing an equivalent to Cys 81, still bind aa-tRNA [18].

179

The tight domain I has also been implicated in binding the 3'-end of aa-tRNA in preliminary experiments by J.R. Rubin in this laboratory. By treatment of EF-Tu:GDP crystals with the analogue puromycin (which resembles tyrosyl-adenosine), subsequent X-ray data collection and difference Fourier analysis, changes in the electron density above helix VI were observed. Assuming that puromycin binds at the correct aa-tRNA binding site, this locates the 3'-end of the tRNA on the top surface of domain I approx. above the guanine base of GDP as shown in Figs 1 and 2.

Further work is necessary to complete the EF-Tu three-dimensional structure. One approach is to soak oligonucleotides corresponding to short pieces of tRNA into EF-Tu crystals in an attempt to fix the flexible floppy domain.

The regions of tRNA which are in contact with EF-Tu:GTP have been reviewed earlier [12]. In addition to the aa-stem and T-stem, the extra loop region appears to be involved. Again more work is necessary to delineate atomic details of the interactions.

ACKNOWLEDGEMENTS

We gratefully acknowledge financial support from the Danish Natural Science Research Council (J.no. 11-3906). We wish to thank Dr. D.L. Miller for cooperation and advice and Orla Jensen, Arne Lindahl and Lisbeth Heilesen for help in the production of the manuscript.

REFERENCES

[1] Clark, B.F.C. (1980). Trends Biochem. Sci., 5, 207-210.
[2] Furano, A. (1975). Proc. Natl. Acad. Sci. USA, 72, 4780-4784.
[3] Jones, M.D., Petersen, T.E., Nielsen, K.M., Magnusson, S.M., Sottrup-Jensen, L., Gausing, K. & Clark, B.F.C. (1980). Eur. J. Biochem., 108, 507-526.
[4] Reeh, S. & Pedersen, S. (1978). In: Gene Expression, B.F.C. Clark, H. Klenow & J. Zeuthen (eds). Vol. 43 of FEBS Symp., Pergamon Press, pp. 89-98.
[5] Yokota, T., Sugisaki, H., Takanami, M. & Kaziro, Y. (1980). Gene, 12, 25-31.

[6] An, G. & Friesen, J.D. (1980). Gene, 12, 33-39.
[7] Laursen, R.A., Nagarkatti, S. & Miller, D.L. (1977). FEBS Letters, 80, 103-106.
[8] Johnson, A.E., Miller, D.L. & Cantor, C.R. (1978). Proc. Natl. Acad. Sci. USA, 75, 3075-3079.
[9] Duisterwinkel, F.J., De Graaf, J.M., Kraal, B. & Bosch, L. (1981). FEBS Letters, 131, 89-93.
[10] Duisterwinkel, F.J., Kraal, B., De Graaf,J.M.,Talens, A., Bosch, L., Swart, G.W.M., Parmeggianni, A., la Cour, T.F.M., Nyborg, J. & Clark, B.F.C. (1984). EMBO J., 3, 113-120.
[11] Swart, G.W.M., Kraal, B., Bosch, L. & Parmeggiani, A. (1982). FEBS Letters, 142, 101-106.
[12] Clark, B.F.C., la Cour, T.F.M., Nielsen,K.M.,Nyborg, J., Petersen, H.U., Siboska, G.E. & Wikman, F.P. (1984). In: Gene Expression, B.F.C. Clark & H.U. Petersen (eds). Alfred Benzon Symp. 19, Munksgaard, Copenhagen, pp. 127-148.
[13] Morikawa, K., la Cour, T.F.M., Nyborg, J., Rasmussen, K.M., Miller, D.L. & Clark, B.F.C. (1978). J. Mol. Biol., 125, 325-338.
[14] Rubin, J.R., Morikawa, K., Nyborg, J., la Cour, T.F.M., Clark, B.F.C. & Miller, D.L. (1981). FEBS Letters, 129, 177-179.
[15] Clark, B.F.C., la Cour, T.F.M., Fontecilla-Camps, J., Morikawa, K., Nielsen, K.M., Nyborg, J. & Rubin, J.R. (1982). In: Cell Function and Differentiation, Vol. 66 of FEBS Symp., Part C, Alan R. Liss Inc., New York, pp. 59-64.
[16] Leberman, R. & Egner, U. (1984). EMBO J., 3, 339-341.
[17] Jonák, J., Petersen, T.E., Clark, B.F.C. & Rychlík, I. (1982). FEBS Letters, 150, 485-488.
[18] Kaziro, Y. (1978). Biochem. Biophys. Acta, 505, 95-127.

STRUCTURE FUNCTION RELATIONSHIP IN THE tRNA^{Asp} ASPARTYL-tRNA SYNTHETASE SYSTEM FROM YEAST

J.P. EBEL, P. DUMAS, R. GIEGE, B. LORBER, D. MORAS, P. ROMBY, J.C. THIERRY and E. WESTHOF
Institut de Biologie Moléculaire et Cellulaire, 15, rue René Descartes 67084 STRASBOURG, FRANCE

I. INTRODUCTION

Transfer RNAs (tRNAs) participate in numerous biological processes. The function which has been the most extensively studied is their role in the mRNA mediated protein biosynthesis (for a review, see Schimmel et al., 1979). In that process their function is to carry amino acids to the ribosomes, to decode the messenger RNAs and to incorporate the correct amino acid into the protein sequence. These functions lead tRNAs to many interactions with different proteins and nucleic acids. With aminoacyl-tRNA synthetases, enzymes which attach the correct amino acid to the 3'-end of their cognate tRNAs, the molecular recognition must be highly specific. The same is true for the decoding of the genetic code at the messenger RNA level. However, with the elongation factor, which carries the aminoacylated tRNAs to the ribosome and also with the ribosomal components which are involved in peptide bond synthesis, the common partners imply common features. In this study, we will concentrate on two interactions which are examples of the first situations and which have been extensively studied in our laboratory : the highly specific interaction of tRNAs with aminoacyl-tRNA synthetases and with messenger RNA.

Proceedings of the 16th FEBS Congress
Part B, pp. 183–197
© 1985 VNU Science Press

II. STRUCTURE OF tRNA

The three-dimensional structures of two tRNAs, yeast tRNA(Phe) and tRNA(Asp), have been solved at high resolution. Both are elongator tRNAs with a short extra-loop. In this section, we will focus on the structure tRNA(Asp) with reference to that of tRNA(Phe).

1. Primary structure

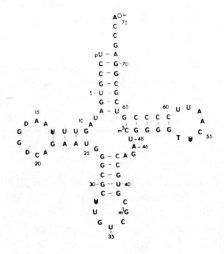

Figure 1 : The nucleotide sequence of yeast tRNA^{Asp}. For convenience the numbering system of the nucleotides is that of yeast tRNA(Phe) ; in the 75-nucleotide long tRNA(Asp), position 47 in the variable loop has been omitted. Non-classical Watson-Crick base pairs are indicated by broken lines.

The nucleotide sequence of yeast tRNA(Asp), shown on Figure 1, presents some characteristic features

184

(Gangloff et al., 1971). It contains a high number of G-C base pairs, except in the D-stem where two G-U base pairs are present. The variable loop is made of four nucleotides versus five in tRNA(Phe) (for convenience of comparisons we kept the same numbering, assuming a deletion at position 47). The D-loop has the same length as that of tRNA(Phe) but the two conserved Gs, which are crucial for D- and T-loops tertiary interactions, are at positions 17 and 18 instead of 18 and 19, thus making α and β regions of the D-loop quite symmetrical. Last but not least, the anticodon GUC presents the peculiarity to be self-complementary, with a slight mismatch at the uridine position. This feature was first noted by Grosjean et al. (1978) who showed the existence of a significant interaction in solution and suggested it to be a tempting model to study tRNA-mRNA recognition.

2. Crystal structure

For yeast tRNA(Asp) two structures have been solved from a multiple isomorphous replacement (MIR) X-ray analysis of two crystal forms (Moras et al., 1980). The transition between forms A and B is temperature dependent but it can also be induced around 20° by pH changes or the addition of some heavy atoms derivatives (Huong et al., 1984). The structure of one form, the lower temperature one, has been refined in reciprocal space using the restrained least-square method of Konnert and Hendrickson (1980) and in real space with the graphic modelling program FRODO (Jones, 1978). Both programs were adapted for nucleic acid handling.

Boomerang versus L-shape : A view of the tRNA^{Asp} molecule together with a similar view of tRNA(Phe) are shown on Figure 2. The topological organization of the cloverleaf sequence is similar with that first found for yeast tRNA(Phe). This gives the L-shaped structure formed by two units : vertically the anticodon and the

185

D-stems, horizontally the T- and the amino acid
accepting stems. However in the case of tRNA(Asp) the
two branches forming the L are more open (by more than
10°) than in tRNA(Phe) conferring to this tRNA a
boomerang-like shape. This results in a different
positioning of the anticodon and of the T-stems and
loops with respect to fixed acceptor and D-stems which
superpose well to the corresponding part of tRNA(Phe)
(Moras et al., 1980).

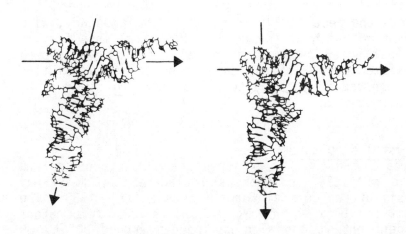

Figure 2 : Two views of the three-dimensional
structures of yeast tRNA(Asp) (left) and tRNA(Phe)
(right). The coordinates of tRNA(Asp) correspond to the
refined low temperature form ; the R-factor for these
data is presently 23.5% at 3Å resolution. The CCA-end
part however is not yet fully defined and was set in
the standard helical conformation. The coordinates of
yeast tRNA(Phe) are those of the orthorhombic crystal
form (Quigley et al., 1975)

Anticodon-anticodon interaction : In the orthorhombic
crystal lattice (space group $C222_1$) tRNA(Asp) molecules
are associated through a two-fold symmetry axis
parallel to the crystallographic **b** direction by
anticodon-anticodon interactions. Figure 3 represents

the local conformation (Westhof et al., 1983). The GUC anticodon triplets of symmetrically related molecules form complementary hydrogen bonded base pairs, arranged in a normal helical conformation. This small helix is stabilized by stacking of the modified base m^{1}G37 on both sides. This packing confers a great stability to the dimeric structure and explains the good quality of the electron density map in the anticodon region. A contact between the anticodon loops of two tRNAs also exists in the orthorhombic form of yeast tRNA(Phe). In that case, however, the G$_m$AA anticodons cannot be base paired and they are arranged in a stacked conformation.

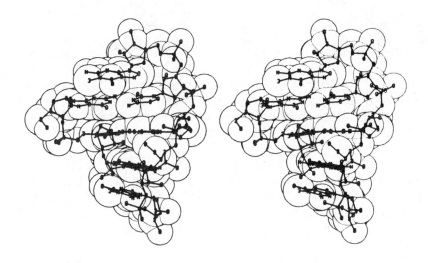

Figure 3 : Stereo views of the anticodon triplet (GUC) base pairing in yeast tRNA(Asp).

Dynamic aspects : Crystallographic refinement leads to the determination of the so-called Debye-Waller temperature factor. Although temperature factors contain various components, it has been shown (Frauenfelder et al., 1979 and Artymiuk et al., 1979) that their variation along a macromolecular backbone has some physical meaning. In Figure 4 are represented the temperature factors of each phosphate along the polynucleotide chain in tRNA(Asp) and in tRNA(Phe).

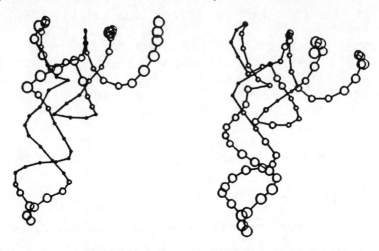

Figure 4 : Thermal vibration of the backbones. Two views of yeast tRNA(Asp) (left) and tRNA(Phe) (right) are shown. Each phosphate group is presented by a ball proportional to the value of the temperature factors.

For tRNA^{Asp}, it is apparent that the stems are more rigid than the loops, except for the end of the amino acid acceptor stem. This variation is not so apparent for tRNA(Phe), although the effect is present. Also, in tRNA(Asp), the T-loop presents higher temperature factors than the anticodon loop. This is in marked contrast to the situation in tRNA(Phe), where the anticodon loop presents the highest temperature factors and the T-loop the lowest ones. There is a similar but less pronounced reversal in the region of the P10-loop, where P10 is at a minimum in tRNA(Asp) and at a maximum in tRNA(Phe). The origins of these differences are difficult to pinpoint. We think that the different behaviour of the "flexibility" of the tRNA molecule in the two crystals arises from the different packing of the molecules in crystals of tRNA(Asp) and of tRNA(Phe), since there is anticodon-anticodon base-pairing in the former crystals and not in the latter ones.

To summarize we can say that the structure of tRNA(Asp) shows the conformational state of a tRNA on the ribosome. In the crystals one GUC triplet from one tRNA molecule mimicks a codon of mRNA interacting with the GUC anticodon of a second molecule. This interaction might act as a signal and trigger conformational changes elsewhere. The open structure of the tRNA might be a result of such a mechanism. Influence on the D and T-loop association is strongly suggested by thermal factors. The structure of tRNA(Phe) would be that of a free tRNA, with flexible anticodon stem and loop.

III. INTERACTION BETWEEN tRNA and AMINOACYL-tRNA SYNTHETASE

1. Crystallization of the tRNA^{Asp}-aspartyl tRNA synthetase complex

Both tRNA(Asp) and aspartyl-tRNA synthetase could be crystallized in various media including low salt conditions (Giegé et al, 1977; Dietrich et al, 1980). The best diffracting crystals, however, could only be grown in the presence of amonium sulfate at 62% saturation for tRNA(Asp) and at 54% for the synthetase. For the complex, crystallization was observed to occur only under high salt conditions, between 48 and 53% saturation of ammonium sulfate depending upon the concentration of macromolecular components and the temperature. The optimal crystallization conditions for the different components of the aspartic acid system are summarized in table I. A full account of the crystallization procedure was reported by Giegé et al (1980) and Lorber et al (1983).

Molecules	tRNA^{Asp}	AspRS	Complex
Molecular weight	24,160	125,000	175,000

Precipitant
  Nature
  Concentration
	62%	(NH4)2 SO4
		54%
			50%

Macromolecular
concentrations
  tRNA
  Enzyme
	3-5
	-
		mg.ml^{-1}
		
		-
		4
			1-5
			3-12

pH	6.8	6.7	7.0-8.0
Crystal form	Orthorhombic	Quadratic	Cubic
Space group	C222$_1$	P4 2$_1$2$_1$	P432

Table 1 : Crystallization conditions of tRNA^{Asp} aspartyl-tRNA synthetase and the complex formed between these two macromolecules.

For the complex one of the most important factors in crystal formation is the stoechiometry of the components. No crystals can be grown for a molecular ratio tRNA/enzyme inferior to 1.8 and the quality of the crystals degrades when that ratio increases to more than 2.2. These values only reflect the experimental uncertainty of the concentration measurements; the best crystals are obtained when the mother liquor contains two tRNA molecules for one dimeric enzyme.

The first problem to solve in the presence of putative complex crystals is to ascertain the coexistence, within the crystal, of both the nucleic acid and the protein. The presence of tRNA(Asp) and aspartyl-tRNA synthetase was tested by gel electrophoresis and by biochemical activity assays. All experiments were done with crystals carefully washed so that the possibility of contamination by non-crystallized material could be eliminated. The presence of aspartyl-tRNA synthetase was demonstrated by the aminoacylation of exogeneous tRNA added to the medium. For the tRNA two different experiments allowed to demonstrate its presence. With and without addition of exogeneous enzyme it was possible to recover equivalent amount of trichloroacetic acid precipitable radioactivity, clearly establishing the aspartylation of a significant amount of tRNA.

Crystals belong to the cubic system with a unit cell parameter of 354Å. The systematic absence of hkl for $h+k+l=2n+1$ leads to the space group I432, with 48 asymmetric units cell. Assuming one molecule of enzyme and two molecules of tRNA per asymmetric unit the value of Vm (crystal volume per unit of macromolecular weight) is 5.3Å /dalton, outside the standard range for proteins (1.68 to 3.53). For a partial specific volume of 0.7 $cm^3.g^{-1}$ the solvent content of the crystal would then be 78%, a large value consistent with the particular softness of the crystals. For the best crystals, diffracted intensities extend up to 7.5Å resolution but routinely the limit of resolution is 8.5Å.

2. Solution studies

One way to determine the part of two macromolecules interacting with each other is to compare the accessibility of these molecules to a chemical probe in the free and complexed states. This can easily be done on tRNA, a molecule for which many specific chemical

191

reagents are available which can attack functional groups on the individual nucleotides. The regions interacting with the probe in the free tRNA but not in the complexed molecule can be considered in close contact with the interacting macromolecule, an aminoacyl-tRNA synthetase for example, and thus protected by it.

Here we present results obtained with ethylnitrosourea, an alkylating reagent which essentially ethylates the phosphate residues of nucleic acids (Kusmierek and Singer, 1976 ; Vlassov et al., 1981). The principle of the method derives from the chemical sequencing methodologies of nucleic acids and relies on statistical and low yield modification at each phosphate, in such a way that each tRNA undergoes less than one modification. The tRNA molecules labelled at their 3'- or 5'-end with radioactive ATP are then specifically split at the modified position and the resulting end-labelled oligonucleotides are analyzed by high voltage electrophoresis on sequencing gels followed by autoradiography. Assignment of bands is done by comparing their migrations to ladders obtained after limited T1 RNase digestion or alkaline hydrolysis. In such a way it is possible to probe the entire tRNA molecule in one experiment. In the presence of aminoacyl-tRNA synthetases, experimental conditions must allow both chemical reactivity and good complex formation. Therefore samples are incubated for 3h at pH 8.0 and at 20°C in the presence of magnesium at a rather low ionic strength and with concentrations of tRNA (1.5 µM) and enzyme (5 µM) in the range where the complex formation is guaranteed. Detailed experimental procedures were published for experiments with tRNA(Asp) and tRNA(Phe) (Vlassov et al., 1983).

A typical alkylation experiment of 5'-labelled tRNA(Asp) is shown on figure 5. This experiment allows to probe the phosphate groups located between positions 6 to 55. Similar assays with 3'-labelled tRNA probing the phosphates from the 3'- to the 5'-side of the molecule were also carried on. In the presence of aspartyl-tRNA synthetase the splitting at some phosphate positions is nearly suppressed or is strongly reduced (for instance P27 to P33), suggesting that these groups are protected from alkylation by the enzyme and thus most likely are in close contact with the protein. The results are summarized on figure 5 in which the protected phosphate groups are indicated by arrows on the cloverleaf structure of yeast tRNA(Asp). Among the parts of the molecule not tested it is clear that the CCA-end or at least the terminal adenosine is also in contact with the enzyme for catalytic necessity.

If one compares the protected phosphates in tRNA[Asp] with results obtained by the same approach in the phenylalanine and valine systems (Vlassov et al., 1983) the striking feature which emerges is the large difference between contact areas. In the three systems, the only common contact areas, beside the terminal adenosine, are the variable loop and the neighbourhood of P9. Not surprinsingly these regions are very close in space. Biochemical experiments have also emphasized the involvement of U8 in a contact interaction of tRNAs with their cognate synthetase (Starzik et al., 1982).

For tRNA(Asp) one side of the L-shaped molecule is clearly involved in protein-nucleic acid association. This face includes the variable loop, the 5'-end of the anticodon stem and part of the 3'-end of the aminoacid arm. The surface involved is quite important and this observation is consistent with neutron diffraction results which lead to the existence of large contact areas between the protein and the nucleic acid (Moras et al., 1983). This interaction differs significantly from the one proposed for tRNA(Phe) derived from cross-linking experiments (Rich and Schimmel, 1977). If one assumes a similar folding for tRNA(Asp), another type of interaction between the enzyme and the tRNA must be postulated.

These observations underline the differences which are

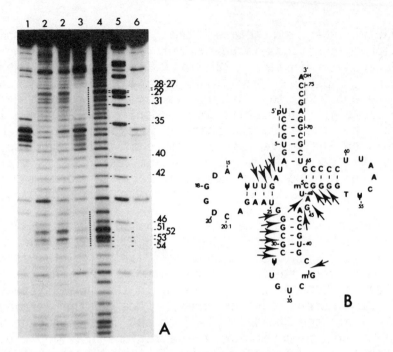

Figure 5 : A. Autoradiogram of 15% acrylamide gel of a phosphate alkylation experiment with ENU of 3'-end labelled tRNA(Asp) from yeast in the presence of yeast aspartyl-tRNA synthetase. Lanes 1,6 : control incubations in the absence of reagent (lane 6) and in the presence of enzyme (lane 1) ; lanes 2,4 : alkylation at 20°C (lane 2) and 80°C (lane 4) in the absence of enzyme ; lane 3 : alkylation at 20°C in the presence of aspartyl-tRNA synthetase ; lane 5 : partial ribonuclease T1 digest. The phosphates protected against alkylation in the tRNA complexed with its synthetase (lane 4) are indicated by diamonds. B. Cloverleaf structure of yeast tRNA(Asp) (Gangloff et al., 1971) with positions of the phosphates strongly protected by yeast aspartyl-tRNA synthetase against ENU. Full arrows show the phosphates protected by the aspartyl-tRNA synthetase, regions not tested for technical reasons (Vlassov et al., 1983) are indicated by dashed lines.

likely to exist in the recognition between tRNAs and their cognate synthetases. It is worthwhile noticing that the oligomeric structure of the aminoacyl-tRNA synthetases in the aspartic acid, phenylalanine and valine systems are quite different : aspartyl-tRNA synthetase is a dimer (α_2) of MW$\approx$ 125,000 daltons which can bind two tRNA molecules, whereas phenylalanyl-tRNA synthetase is an $\alpha_2\beta_2$ tetramer (MW$\approx$ 270,000) which also binds two tRNA(Phe) molecules and valyl-tRNA synthetase is a large monomer (MW $\approx$ 130,000) which binds one tRNA(Val) molecule.

IV. CONCLUSION

The best understood biological role of transfer RNAs is their participation in ribosome-mediated protein synthesis. This function leads tRNAs to many interactions with different proteins and nucleic acids. With aminoacyl-tRNA synthetases, the molecular recognition must be highly specific. The same is true for the decoding of the genetic code at the messenger RNA level. In this report using both biochemical and crystallographic approaches, we have presented experimental results on yeast tRNA(Asp) which illustrate these two types of specific interactions.

REFERENCES

ARTYMIUK, P.J., BLAKE, C.C.F., GRACE, D.E.P., OATLEY, S.I., PHILLIPS, D.C. and STERNBERG, N.J.E., (1979). Crystallographic studies of the dynamic properties of lysozyme. Nature **280**, 563-566.
DIETRICH, A., GIEGE, R., COMARMOND, M.B., THIERRY, J.C. and MORAS, D., (1980). Crystallographic studies on the aspartyl-tRNA synthetase-tRNA(Asp) system from

yeast. J. Mol. Biol. **138**, 129-135.

FRAUENFELDER, H. PETSKO, G.A. and TSERNOGLOU, D., (1979). Temperature-dependent X-ray diffraction as a probe of protein structural dynamics. Nature **280**, 558-560.

GANGLOFF, J., KEITH, G., EBEL, J.P. and DIRHEIMER, G., (1971). Structure of aspartate-tRNA from brewer's yeast. Nature New Biol. **230**, 125-127.

GIEGE, R., MORAS, D. and THIERRY, J.C., (1977). Yeast transfer RNA(Asp) : a new high resolution X-ray diffracting crystal form of a transfer RNA. J. Mol. Biol. **115**, 91-96.

GIEGE, R., LORBER, B., EBEL, J.P., THIERRY, J.C. and MORAS, D., (1980). Cristallisation du complexe formé entre l'aspartate de levure et son aminoacyl-tRNA synthétase. C.R. Séances Acad. Sci. (Paris) Série D **291**, 393-396.

GROSJEAN, H., DE HENAU, S. and CROTHERS, D.M., (1978). On the physical basis in the genetic coding interactions. Proc. Natl. Acad. Sci. USA **75**, 610-614.

HUONG, P.V., AUDRY, E., GIEGE, R., MORAS, D., THIERRY, J.C. and COMARMOND, M.B., (1984). Conformational changes in tRNA(Asp) : laser Raman and X-ray crystallographic studies. Biopolymers **23**, 71-81.

JONES, T.A., (1978). A graphics model building and refinement system. J. Appl. Cryst., **11**, 268-272.

KONNERT, J.H. and HENDRICKSON, (1980). A restrained-parameter thermal factor refinement procedure. Acta Cryst. **A36**, 344-350.

KUSMIEREK, J.T. and SINGER, B., (1976). Sites of alkylation of poly(U) by agents of varying carcinogenicity and stability of products. Biochim. Biophys. Acta **142**, 536-538.

LORBER, B, GIEGE, R., EBEL, J.P., BERTHET, C., THIERRY, J.C. and MORAS, D., (1983). Crystallization of a tRNA-aminoacyl-tRNA synthetase complex. J. Biol. Chem. **258**, 8429-8435.

MORAS, D., COMARMOND, M.B., FISCHER, J., WEISS, R., THIERRY, J.C., EBEL, J.P. and GIEGE, R., (1980).

Crystal structure of yeast tRNA(Asp). Nature **286**, 669-674.

MORAS, D., LORBER, B., ROMBY, P., EBEL, J.P., GIEGE, R., LEWITT-BENTLEY, A. and ROTH, M., (1983). Yeast tRNA(Asp) aspartyl-tRNA synthetase : the crystalline complex. J. Biomol. Str. Dyn. **1**, 209-223.

QUIGLEY, G.J., SEEMAN, N.C., WANG, A.H.T., SUDDATH, F.L. and RICH, A., (1975). Yeast phenylalanyl transfer RNA : atomic coordinates and torsion angles. Nucl. Acids. Res. **2**, 2329-2339.

RICH, A. and SCHIMMEL, P.R., (1977). Structural organization of complexes of tranfer RNAs with aminoacyl-tRNA synthetases. Nucleic Acids Res. **4**, 1649-1665.

SCHIMMEL, P.R., SOLL, D. and ABELSON, J.N. Eds, (1979), Transfer RNA Structure, Properties and Recognition, Cold Spring Harbor Lab.

STARZYK, R., KOONTZ, S. and SCHIMMEL, P., (1982). A covalent adduct between the uracil ring and the active site of an aminoacyl-tRNA synthetase. Nature **298**, 136-140.

VLASSOV, V.V., GIEGE, R. and EBEL, J.P., (1981). Tertiary structure of tRNAs in solution monitored by phosphodiester modification with ethylnitro-sourea. Eur. J. Biochem. **119**, 51-59.

VLASSOV, V.V., KERN, D., ROMBY, P., GIEGE, R. and EBEL, J.P., (1983). Interaction of tRNA(Phe) and tRNA(Val) with aminoacyl-tRNA synthetases : a chemical modification study. Eur. J. Biochem. **132**, 537-544.

WESTHOF, E., DUMAS, P. and MORAS, D., (1983). Loop stereochemistry and dynamics in transfer RNA. J. Biomol. Str. Dyn. **1**, 337-355.

AMINO ACID ANALOGS AS A TOOL IN ELUCIDATION OF PROOF-READING MECHANISMS OF AMINOACYL-tRNA SYNTHETASES

Sabine Englisch, Friedrich von der Haar*, Friedrich Cramer

Max-Planck-Institut f. experimentelle Medizin, Abt. Chemie
Hermann-Rein-Str. 3, 3400 Göttingen, Fed.Rep.Germany
*Present Address: B. Braun Melsungen AG, Postfach 110,120,
3508 Melsungen, Fed.Rep.Germany

To maintain life, several key reactions have to be performed with extraordinary precision. Activation of amino
acids as building blocks for enzymes is such a reaction.
The aminoacyl-tRNA synthetases (E.C.6.1.1.-) link specific
amino acids with their corresponding tRNA. The overall
error rate of this reactions is less than one in about
10^4-10^5. In view of the structural similarity of the
amino acids, this accuracy has attracted the interests
of biochemists for a long time.

One example studied particularly well is isoleucyl-tRNA
synthetase. This enzyme activates isoleucine, but also
valine. The preference for isoleucine in this reaction
is twohundred-fold greater. The binding forces of the
additional methylene group in isoleucine, as compared to

Proceedings of the 16th FEBS Congress
Part B, pp. 199–204

valine, should be large enough to account for a twenty-fold selectivity. In view of this, it was logical to conclude that the lack of presision in binding had to be corrected by a second so-called proofreading reaction on the level of activation and transfer to tRNA. Our mechanistic understanding was greatly improved when we learned that a tRNA^{Ile} lacking the 3'terminal OH accepted the misactivated valine without proofreading, Val-tRNA^{Ile}-C-C-3'dA being produced.

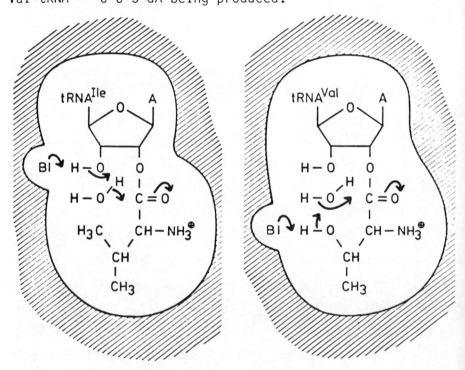

Figure 1: Schematic display of the mechanism of chemical proofreading: Val-tRNA^{Ile} proofread by isoleucyl-tRNA synthetase (left) and Thr-tRNA^{Val} proofread by valyl-tRNA synthetase (right).

In combination with other results we proposed the proofreading mechanism shown in figure 1. Misactivated valine is transfered transiently to tRNA^{Ile}. The space of the methyl group of isoleucine, which is missing in valine, is occupied by a water molecule in case of mis-activation of valine. This water molecule is activated by an enzymatic group.

A similar mechanism is able to explain how threonine which is activated by valyl-tRNA synthetase and tran-siently transfered to tRNA^{Val} is finally hydrolysed from the tRNA^{Val} (figure 1).

This mechanistic explanation which we have termed **"chemical proofreading"** deserved further experimental support. To evaluate meaningfull experiments, the follo-wing hypothesis was worked out.

HYPOTHESIS

Stereochemically isoleucine in a first approximation is very similar to -hydroxyvaline. In γ-hydroxyvaline a water molecule is linked to valine. If the proposed mecha-nism, shown in figure 1, is correct, isoleucyl-tRNA synthetase should catalyse tansformation of γ-hydroxy-valine into the corresponding lactone consuming stoichio-metric amounts of ATP. These amino acids with branched side chains containing OH groups, might yield meaningfull mechanistic information. Consequently such amino acids were synthesised and tested.

RESULTS

The four diastereomeres of the analogue γ-hydroxyvaline were synthesized, L allo-; L-iso-; D-allo-; and D-iso-γ-hydroxyvaline. Much to our surprise none of them was substrate for isoleucyl-tRNA synthetase in any step of the the enzyme. This was true for the enzyme from Escherichia coli as well as from yeast. γ-hydroxyvaline was chosen as an analogue because it resembles isoleucine. Inspection of space-models gave a hint that the hydroxy group might be fixed via a hydrogen bridge to the carboxy group. In such a model γ-hydroxyvaline looks much more like valine than like isoleucine. Valyl-tRNA synthetase seems to share this opinion, L-iso- γ-hydroxyvaline as well as L-allo-γ-hydroxyvaline are substrates in all partial reactions for valyl-tRNA synthetase from yeast as well as from E.coli. The Michaelis-Menten-constant is about 10-fold that of valine for both substrates in the ATP/PP$_i$ exchange reaction, and 40-fold in AMP-forming assay. The presence of tRNA is absolutley necessary indicating a transfer to tRNA^{Val} prior to proofreading.

In the AMP-forming assay γ-hydroxyvaline is transformed into the corresponding lactone. This is the strongest indication that the mechanism described in figure. 1 is basically correct.

γ-hydroxyvaline is partially escaping the proofreading and stable γ-hydroxyvalyl-tRNA^{Val} is released from the enzyme. This tRNA can be subjected to AMP/PP$_i$ independent hydrolysis. In this reaction the amino acid is transformed into the lactone.

The events described above can all be seen from the back titration: γ-hydroxyvaline is transferred to tRNA^{Val} and partially escaping the proofreading reaction. As a consequence, the free tRNA^{Val} accessible for aminoacylation with radioactively labelled valine decreases. With time the continuous AMP consumption due to proofreading exhausts the ATP pool. AMP/PP$_i$ independent hydrolysis starts and mischarged tRNA is diminishing, which results in increasing amounts of free tRNA^{Val} for backtitration.

Homocysteine and γ-hydroxyisoleucine behave similarly to valyl-tRNA synthetase from yeast and E.coli as does γ-hydroxyvaline. γ-hydroxyisoleucine behaves different as indicated by AMP formation and back-titration reaction. Proofreading with this analogue is about a factor of 10 less efficient, if AMP formation is taken as a criterium.

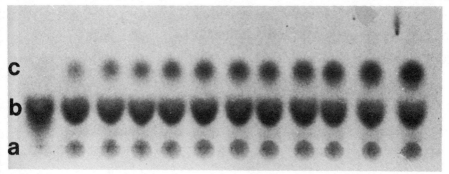

Figure 2: Thinlayer chromatogram (silica-gel) of an aminoacylation assay with valyl-tRNA synthetase of E.coli, γ-hydroxyvaline and tRNA^{Val}. (a) start, (b) γ-hydroxyvaline, and (c) lactone of γ-hydroxyvaline.

As a consequence, mischarging of tRNA^{Val} with the enzyme leads to a relative stable product as can be seen by back titration.

The procedure allows to differeniate between different types of mechanisms: The iso-forms of γ-hydroxyisoleucine are activated by isoleucyl-tRNA synthetase from E.coli as well as from yeast. Whereas we were not able to detect any transfer of the misactivated amino acid to tRNA^{Ile}, a large amount of AMP according to could be detected in absence as well as in presence of tRNA. These results are typical for a **pretransfer proofreading** situation.

-hydroxyleucine is misactivated by leucyl-tRNA synthetase from E.coli as well as from yeast. With the yeast enzyme, AMP formation occured in absence of tRNA. In contrast, AMP formation with the E.coli enzyme took place only in presence of tRNA suggesting a **post-transfer-proofreading** mechanism.

δ-hydroxyisoleucine as well as δ -hydroxyleucine incubated with leucyl-tRNA synthetase from yeast show a third pathway. We could neither observe AMP-formation nor transfer to tRNA in any experimentel situation created. As far as we imagine, this result can only be explained by assuming that no stable aminoacyl-AMP intermediate is formed. Consequently we conclude, that for these analogues a kinetic type of proofreading may be applicable.

(Experimentel details, graphic displays, and citations please find in S.Englisch, Diplomarbeit and Ph.D.thesis.)

EXPRESSION OF TRANSLATIONAL INITIATION FACTOR
GENES IN ESCHERICHIA COLI

MARIANNE GRUNBERG-MANAGO, JACQUELINE A. PLUMBRIDGE,
CHRISTINE SACERDOT, MATHIAS SPRINGER, JOHN W.B. HERSHEY[+],
GUY FAYAT*, JEAN-FRANCOIS MAYAUX*, AND SYLVAIN BLANQUET*
Institut de Biologie Physico-chimique, 13 rue Pierre et
Marie Curie, 75005 Paris, France; [+]Department of
Biological Chemistry, School of Medicine, University of
California, Davis, California 95616, USA; *Laboratoire de
Biochimie, Ecole Polytechnique, 91128 Palaiseau, France

The initiation of protein synthesis in bacteria requires
the cooperative interaction of three initiation factors
IF1, IF2, and IF3. IF3 and IF1 shift the equilibrium from
70S ribosomes towards dissociation into 30S and 50S subunits while IF2 directs fMet-tRNA binding to the 30S subunit. IF3 also stimulates the interaction of mRNA with
the 30S ribosome.

The expression of the genes for initiation factors is
subject to different types of control: their synthesis is
coordinated with that of ribosomes, is proportional to
growth rate (so-called "metabolic control"), and at least
one is inhibited in vitro by ppGpp (stringent control)
[1]. In addition, the expression of translational components is subject to specific individual control mechanisms
which regulate their respective concentrations.

Our aim is to analyze the structure and expression of
these genes in order to provide information on specific
mechanisms of gene control and on how global coordination
of their expression with all of the protein biosynthetic
apparatus is achieved.

ORGANIZATION AND EXPRESSION OF THE IF3 GENE CLUSTER

Transcriptional Units

The isolation of a λ transducing phage (λp2) permitted the
localization of infC, the gene for IF3, at 38 min on the
E. coli chromosome. This phage also carries four other

Proceedings of the 16th FEBS Congress
Part B, pp. 205–212
© 1985 VNU Science Press

genes in the following order: thrS infC rplT pheS pheT
which correspond respectively to the genes for threonyl
tRNA synthetase (an α2 type dimeric enzyme), initiation
factor IF3, ribosomal protein L20, and the small and large
subunits of phenylalanyl tRNA synthetase (tetrameric enzyme α2β2) (Fig. 1). A 10.5 kb E. coli DNA fragment of

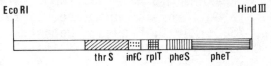

Fig. 1: Gene organization around intiation factor IF3

λp2 was cloned in pBR322 giving a plasmid pB1 which ex-
presses these 5 genes. All these genes are transcribed in
the same direction, anticlockwise from thrS to pheT [2,3]
    In order to characterize the transcriptional units pre-
sent in this region, several different techniques have
been used: i) cloning of selected restriction fragments
into different bacteriophages and plasmid vectors under
conditions which reveal promoter activities; ii) DNA
sequencing of most of the E. coli DNA insert of pB1 and
identification of putative promoter and termination
sequences; iii) S1 nuclease mapping of the in vitro transcription products and sequencing the 5' ends of mRNA.
The results of these experiments form a coherent picture
of transcription [3,4].
    Five promoters have been identified (Fig. 2). One,
situated upstream of thrS but not yet precisely localized,
is responsible for thrS expression. The thrS and infC
genes are contiguous, separated by only three nucleotides
and thus any transcripts for thrS must continue into infC.
Most noteworthy is the unusual initiation codon for IF3:
AUU. The strong Shine/Dalgarno sequence GGAGG upstream
from AUU is localized in the thrS structural gene. A promoter P₀ situated in the middle of thrS is active in vitro, synthesizing transcripts which enter the infC gene.
It seems likely that infC can be expressed either from a
polycistronic messenger for thrS and infC or from an independent transcript initiating within the thrS structural
gene.

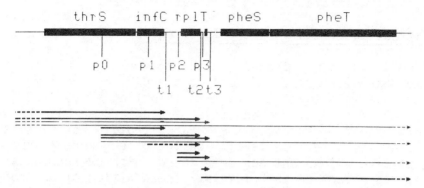

Fig. 2: Transcriptional units in IF3 cluster. Transcripts indicated by horizontal arrows, with thickness
roughly proportional to their relative synthesis.

An in vitro transcript starting 15 nucleotides from the
initiation codon AUG of rplT (P_2 promoter) covers rplT.
In addition, a promoter P_1 situated within the infC gene
also directs in vitro transcription towards the rplT
region. A promoter, P_3 is located 368 nucleotides in
front of pheS. This promoter is active in vivo and in
vitro. No promoter has been found between pheS and pheT;
thus pheS and pheT constitute an operon.
Three rho independent terminators have been identified.
t1 and t2 are situated downstream of infC and rplT respectively while the third terminator t3 is part of an attenuator located between the pheS,T promoter P_3, and the
pheS,T structural genes. The t1 and t2 terminators are
not very efficient: 80% of the in vitro transcripts originating at the P_1 site read through t1 and extend into
the rplT structural gene. This raises the possibility
that rplT can be expressed not only from its own promoter
but also from the thrS or infC promoters. The structural
part of rplT ends in the region composing the terminator
t2 (8 nucleotides before the G + C rich region of the dyad
symmetry). In vitro and in vivo data indicate that about
70% of the transcripts from P_2 continue past t2. It thus
seems that initiation and termination signals are arranged
to yield a set of overlapping transcripts and that differ-

ential regulation of the genes may occur at the level of transcription through the utilization of multiple transcription initiation and termination sites.

Expression of the thrS and infC region

In order to study the expression of thrS and infC in vivo, thermosensitive mutants were obtained by P_1-localized mutagenesis. Quantitative immunoblotting shows that a subset of thrS thermosensitive strains and an auxotrophic thrS mutant overproduce the mutated protein but synthesize IF3 at the wild type level. On the other hand, a thermosensitive IF3 mutant has been found which overproduces IF3 with no effect on thrS levels. The addition of one copy of infC from a wild type strain inhibits the overproduction of IF3 in accordance with the idea that wild type IF3 inhibits its own synthesis.

In order to further elucidate the expression of thrS and infC, we constructed recombinant phages where the lacZ gene was fused to various points of the thrS-infC operon. Autoregulation of thrS at the level of translation was indicated with a thrS-lacZ protein fusion (but not an operon fusion) in which the β-galactosidase translational initiation site is replaced by the thrS initiation site and promoter; the synthesis of β-galactosidase was derepressed in a mutant thrS background. A possible autoregulation of infC at the level of transcription was suggested by the observation that in strains carrying a mutated infC, β-galactosidase was derepressed with an operon fusion in which the thrS and infC promoters were fused to the complete lacZ gene with its initiation sequences. Thus it is possible to differentially regulate these two adjacent genes. S_1 mapping of mRNA in vivo and quantitation of mRNA by hybridization with specific probes are still in progress but indicate that the infC region is transcribed more frequently than thrS. This reinforces the view that infC has its own promoter.

ORGANIZATION AND EXPRESSION OF THE IF2 GENE CLUSTER

The gene for initiation factor IF2 (infB) was identified

in a cosmid library of E. coli DNA because the presence of
the infB gene on a multicopy cosmid increased the cellular
concentration of IF2 [5]. IF2 is present in two forms in
the cell: IF2α(100,000) and IF2β(80,000). Both forms are
coded by infB and are overproduced in cells carrying
multicopies of the gene. The gene maps at 69 min and is
quite close to the argG, nusA, rpsO and pnp genes coding
respectively for arginino-succinate synthetase, pNusA
involved in transcription termination, ribosomal protein
S15 and polynucleotide phosphorylase (Fig. 3). In addition to these genes, the work of Kurihara and Nakamura

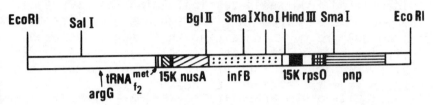

Fig. 3: Gene organization around initation factor IF2

[6] and Ishii et al. [7] indicate that at least three
other genes are contained in this cluster: metY coding
for a minor form of the initiator tRNA, a gene coding for
a protein (P15a) of 15 kDa and a gene coding for another
protein (P15b), also of 15 kDa. The order of these genes
is: argG metY P15a nusA infB P15b rpsO pnp. The genes
metY to pnp are transcribed in the same direction anticlockwise on the E. coli map.
   The expression of the genes from the IF2 cluster appear
to be subject to complex regulation. The major promoter
for nusA has been located before metY [7]. After metY are
two rho independent transcription termination signals, at
which 90% of the transcripts are terminated in vitro.
Expression of nusA and infB is the result of readthrough
at these terminators. The work of Nakamura's group (personal communication) and the sequence determination and S_1
mapping by our group indicate that P15a, NusA, IF2 and
P15b may be in the same operon. On the other hand, the
genes rpsO and pnp do not appear to be expressed from the
metY promoter. In addition, possible minor promoters for
nusA and infB have been detected. This operon is remark-

209

able because both tRNA and protein genes are found in a single transcriptional unit. Furthermore, the fMet-tRNA is a substrate of IF2 during the initiation of protein biosynthesis. Whether an interaction between IF2 and the tRNA in the transcript plays a role in the regulation of the expression of metY and infB is presently under investigation.

The two forms of IF2 appear to be synthesized from the same mRNA. The initiator codon for IF2α is AUG, whereas the IF2β initiator codon is GUG and is found 471 base pairs downstream in the same reading frame. These sites were identified from the N-terminal amino acid sequences of the proteins and from in vitro synthesis of dipeptides. A 9.41 kb DNA fragment containing these genes has been entirely sequenced: (metY 15Ka nusA) [8]; infB 15Kb S15 pnp [9, P. Regnier, C. Portier and J. Sands, unpublished]. Downstream from the coding sequence of IF2 is a sequence which resembles a transcription terminator; the efficiency of this terminator remains to be investigated. There is an AUG 15 bp after the terminator which is the beginning of the P15b.

From the point of view of protein structure, IF2 shows some remarkable features. In the N-terminal region, IF2α shows a clearly defined periodicity which may confer a regular helical conformation. The structure is likely flexible in the absence of long-range interactions, but could assume a fixed conformation as a result of interaction with ribosomes or tRNA. An association of this region with RNA is strongly suggested by the presence of electrostatic dipoles which could interact with nucleic acid phosphates. The middle part of IF2 shows striking homologies with the N-terminal region of elongation factor EFTu and lesser homologies with EFG. A second region of homology between IF2 and EFTu is situated in the region of the GTP binding site, and putative secondary structures are similar. The homology between the EFTu and IF2 genes is likely highly significant from an evolutionary point of view. The common functions of tRNA recognition and ribosome-dependent GTPase activity appear to have been conserved during the evolution of these genes.

CONCLUSION

Whereas the three initiation factor genes are coordinately expressed, their loci are separated on the E. coli genome. Both the infB and infC genes have been cloned, sequenced and characterized. Each is surrounded by other genes coding for components involved in gene expression, such as those for aminoacyl-tRNA synthetases, ribosomal proteins, transcriptional factors and tRNA. The striking feature of the organization and expression of the gene clusters is their complexity. Both initiation factor genes are expressed at least in part as polycistronic mRNAs, and yet each appears to have its own promoter as well. The occurance of multiple promoters and variable read-through of terminators generates many possibilities for the control of these genes. Detailed studies continue on the transcription of the gene clusters in vitro and in vivo. We also seek to determine whether autoregulation is a major mechanism for controlling infB and infC expression. What remains unclear at the moment is how the initiation factor operons are coordinated with those for ribosomal components. Nomura and coworkers [10] suggest that non-translating ribosomes prevent further expression of rRNA and tRNA operons by directly recognizing some rRNA or tRNA-like structure. It is, therefore, noteworthy that the infB operon begins with a tRNA gene; furthermore thrS translation is inhibited by ThrRS, suggesting that a tRNA-like structure may exist in the transcript. It is therefore reasonable to speculate that rRNA or tRNA-like structures are also involved in coupling the synthesis of initiation factors and aminoacyl tRNA synthesis to that of ribosomes.

REFERENCES

1. Howe, J.G., and Hershey, J.W.B. (1983). Initiation factor and ribosome levels are coordinately controlled in E. coli growing at different rates. J. Biol. Chem. 258, 1954-1959.
2. Plumbridge, J.A., Springer, M., Graffe, M., Goursot, H., and Grunberg-Manago, M. (1980). Physical

localization and cloning of the structural gene for E. coli initiation factor IF3 from a group of genes concerned with translation. Gene 11, 33-42.

3. Fayat, G., Mayaux, J-F., Sacerdot, C., Fromant, M., Springer, M., Grunberg-Manago, M., and Blanquet, S. (1983). Escherichia coli phenylalanyl-tRNA synthetase operon region. Evidence for an attenuation mechanism. Identification of the gene for the ribosomal protein L20.

4. Mayaux, J-F., Fayat, G., Fromant, M., Springer, M., Grunberg-Manago, M. and Blanquet, S. (1983). Structural and transcriptional evidence for related thrS and infC expression. Proc. Natl. Acad. Sci. USA 80, 6152-6156.

5. Plumbridge, J.A., Howe, J.G., Springer, M., Touati-Schwartz, D., Hershey, J.W.B., and Grunberg-Manago, M. (1982). Cloning and mapping of a gene for translational initiation factor IF2 in E. coli. Proc. Natl. Acad. Sci. USA 79, 5033-5037.

6. Kurihara, T., and Nakamura, Y. (1983). Cloning of the nusA gene of E. coli. Mol. Gen. Genet. 190, 189-195.

7. Ishii, S., Kuroki, K., and Imamoto, M. (1984). tRNA metf2 gene in the leader region of the nusA operon in E. coli. Proc. Natl. Acad. Sci. USA 81, 409-413.

8. Ishii, S., Ihara, M., Maekawa, T., Nakamura, Y., Uchida, H. and Imamoto, F. (1984). The nucleotide sequence of the cloned nusA gene and its flanking region of E. coli. Nucleic Acid Research 12, 3333-3342.

9. Sacerdot, C., Dessen, P., Plumbridge, J.A., Hershey, J.W.B., and Grunberg-Manago, M. (in press). Initiation factor IF2: Unusual protein features and homologies with elongation factors. Proc. Natl. Acad. Sci. USA.

10. Nomura, M., Gourse R., and Baughman, G. (1984). Regulation of the synthesis of ribosomes and ribosomal components. Ann. Rev. Biochem. 53, 75-117.

INVESTIGATION OF THE INTERACTION OF tRNA AND mRNA WITH RIBOSOMES BY AFFINITY LABELLING

DMITRY G. KNORRE
Institute of Bioorganic Chemistry, Siberian
Division of the Academy of Sciences of USSR
630090 Novosibirsk, prospekt Lavrent'eva 8

INTRODUCTION

Ribosomes consist of a great variety of proteins and several ribonucleic acids and elucidation of the functional role of each protein
and each domain of rRNA molecules is essential
for understanding of the translation mechanism.
Ribosomes interact specifically with mRNA at
least with two and maybe with three molecules
of tRNA, with a number of translation factors,
with a set of antibiotics. Therefore a lot of
functionally significant sites are located at
the ribosome surface. One of the most informative approaches to localization of these sites
is affinity labelling. Using the reactive derivatives of specific ligands one may bind them
covalently to respective areas and thus localize proteins and rRNA domains forming these
areas.
The present paper deals with the results which
were obtained in the last few years in the institute headed by the author by d-r G. Karpova
and coworkers using reactive derivatives of
oligoribonucleotides and tRNA derivatives with
reactive group attached to its internal part.

AFFINITY LABELLING OF THE mRNA BINDING AREA

The most part of these investigations was performed using oligouridilate derivatives bearing
reactive p-N-2-chloroethyl-N-methylaminophenyl
group attached either to 3'- or to 5'-terminal

Proceedings of the 16th FEBS Congress
Part B, pp. 213–218
© 1985 VNU Science Press

nucleotide residue.This group is able to alky-
late nucleophilic centers of proteins and nucleic acids and is further referred as RCl resi-
due.The former of the above mentioned derivatives containes RCl moiety attached via acetal
bond to 2',3'-cis-diol group and is easily produced by treatment of oligo(U) with aldehyde
HCORCl in dimethylformamide in the presence of
trifluoroacetic acid and 2,2-dimethoxypropane
(1)

$$(pU)_n + HCORCl = (pU)_n CHRCl \quad (I-n)$$

The latter may be obtained by condensation of
oligouridilate with respective amine

$$(pU)_n + ClRCH_2NH_2 = ClRCH_2NH(pU)_n \quad (II-n)$$

and contains the reactive ClR moiety attached
via phosphamide bond (2).
Using I-5 ÷ I-8 and II-4 ÷ II-7 with ^{14}C label
it was found that all the reagents form ternary
complexes with 70S ribosomes and phenylalanine
specific tRNA.Incubation of the complexes resulted in covalent attachment of the label to
ribosomes.Distribution of the label between
subunits and within subunits between rRNA and
total protein was determined.Labelled proteins
were identified by 2D-electrophoresis.Details
of the experiments may be found in (2,3).The
extent of alkylation varied within 0.1-0.4 mol
of covalently bound reagent per mol ribosomes.
Only 30S subunits were modified with the most
short reagents I-5 and II-4 as well as with I-7
whereas all other reagents alkylated both 30S
and 50S subunits at similar extent.This means
that although mRNA binding area is located at
30S subunit it is not far from the region of
intersubunit contact.Alkylation of 16S rRNA
strogly predominated over that of 30S proteins
in most cases.In 50S subunits reversed ratio
was observed.Significant level of alkylation
of30S proteins was found for I-7 (30%),II-4
(30%),II-6 (40%) and II-8 (90% of the total

214

label incorporated in the subunit).The most
significantly modified proteins were found to
be S9,S18 with I-7,S3,S4 with II-4,S3,S9,S11,
S13 with II-6 and S5,S11,S13 with II-7.
16S E.coli rRNA modified within ternary complex
with I-7 was subjected to detailed investiga-
tion.It was shown that the label was removed
at pH 4 (70% for 60 min at 40°).At pH 9 (20min
20°) 16S rRNA isolated from alkylated ribosomes was partially splitted in two definite re-
gions.Using gel-electrophoresis of treated 16S
rRNA with attached radioactive pCp at 3'-end
it was demonstrated that the regions of splitting were located at 480 and 110 nucleotides
from 3'-end.The results suggest that respective internucleotide phosphates were specifically alkylated in the ternary complex (4).
It is seen that in the case of E.coli ribosomes modification points are rather ambiguous.
One of the reasons of such an ambiguity is the
dimensions and the mobility of spacer group
separating oligonucleotide from reactive center.
The other one is the absence of Phe-tRNA in the
A site in the course of affinity labelling.To
eliminate the first reason we tried to attach
oligonucleotide directly to ribosome using the
treatment of ternary complex with N-cyclohexyl-
N'-2-(N-methylmorpholinium)ethylcarbodiimide.
Experiments performed by d-r O.Gimautdinova
in conditions of saturation of P site with
specific tRNA with vacant A site have demonstrated that in this case heptauridilate bearing
5'-phosphate binds in some measurable extent
to proteins of both subunits S7,S8,L23 and L25
being preferentially modified.However when additionally A site was saturated with Phe-tRNA
in the presence of EF-Tu and GTP only 30S subunit was phosphorylated and modification of S3
protein strongly predominated.This result clearly demonstrates the significance of overall
state of the complex for appropriate location

of mRNA fragment.

AFFINITY LABELLING OF THE tRNA BINDING REGIONS

Reactive moieties may be easily bound to 3'-end
of tRNA either via aldehyde groups formed by
periodate oxydation of 3'-terminal cis-diol or
via aminoacyl residue.Some minor bases may be
used as photoreactive moieties or as the points
of attachment of reactive groups.However to get
sufficient information concerning contact area
of ribosomes with tRNA it seemed necessary to
elaborate some method which supplied various
tRNA regions with reactive groups.In (5) it was
proposed to use tRNA derivatives with photoreactive groups scattered statistically over numerous guanine residues.This may be realized
by treatment of tRNA with restricted amount of
p-N-2-chloroethyl-N-methylaminobenzylamine with
subsequent arylation of the introduced strongly
basic amino groups with 2,4-dinitro-5-azidoflu-
orobenzene.Derivatives with no more than 2-3
reactive residue per tRNA chain remain active
in enzymatic aminoacylation as well as in the
EF-Tu dependent binding to programmed ribosomes
When phenylalanine specific E.coli tRNA is alkylated in the absence of Mg ions the reactive
groups are scattered over 15 residues.In the
presence of Mg ions residues G-15,G-53,G-57,G-
63 and G-65 remain unmodified.The derivatives
prepared in these two conditions will be further referred as azido-tRNA-I and azido-tRNA-II.
An attempt was done to restrict the number of
alkylation points in tRNA by reversible attachment of alkylating amine via phosphamide bond
to 5'-phosphate of deoxyribooligonucleotide
d(pApApCpCpA).It was demonstrated by d-r D.Grai-
fer that in this case only G-24 is alkylated to
significant extent.Oligonucleotide moiety may
be removed in mild acid conditions and arylazi-
dogroup may be then introduced in this part of

tRNA molecule.

Derivatives are photoreactive at wave-length exceeding 300nm not damaging proteins and RNA. Azido-tRNA in the complex with ribosomes and poly(U) binds covalently to ribosomes under irradiation.Both subunits are labelled.There is no labelling of rRNA.Modified proteins may be identified by 2D-electrophoresis after nuclease treatment to remove tRNA moieties.The details of experiment are given in (6).Below are given the results obtained with the following azido-tRNA states:1)Azido-tRNA-I at P site,A site is vacant; 2)The same with azido-tRNA-II; 3)At A site oligo(Phe)-tRNA,at P site azido-tRNA; 4)At A site AcPhePhe-azido-tRNA,at P site tRNA (two pretranslocational states with reactive derivative at either P or A site).Proteins labelled in definite state are marked by "+".

State number	S2	S5	S7	S9	S11	S12	S13	S14	S19	S20	S21
1)		+		+	+	+	+		+	+	+
2)				+	+	+	+				+
3)		+	+	+	+	+	+	+			
4)	+	+	+								+

proteins of 50S subunit

State	L2	L11	L13	L14	L23	L24	L27	L31	L32	L33
1)				+		+	+	+		+
2)				+			+	+		
3)	+		+			+	+	+	+	
4)		+			+					

It is seen that azido-tRNA-II with restricted set of reactive groups modifies smaller number of proteins than azido-tRNA-I.In similar state tRNA with single reactive group at G-24 doesn't react at all.Comparison of the states 1 and 3 demonstrates that the presence of AcPhePhe-tRNA at A site changes significantly the contact area between ribosome and azido-tRNA at P site. However there are eight common proteins in the set of modified proteins in these states.Only

two common proteins are labelled with azido-
tRNA in either P or A site when similar states
3 and 4 are compared. Thus the approach seems
to be highly informative when used to follow
the dynamic behaviour of tRNA on ribosomes.

REFERENCES

1. Ryte,V.K.,Karpova,G.G.,Grineva,N.I.(1977).
Conformation of 2',3'-O-(4-(N-2-chloroethyl-
-N-methylamino)benzylidene)oligocytidilates
and properties of their complexes with poly-
inosinic acid. Bioorg.Khym.,3,31-38.
2. Gimautdinova,O.I.,Karpova,G.G. and Kozyre-
va,N.A.(1982). Affinity labelling of ribosomes from Escherichia coli with 4-(N-2-chloro-
ethyl-N-methylamino)benzyl-5'-phosphamides of
oligouridilates of different length. Moleku-
lyarn.biol. 16, 752-762.
3. Gimautdinova,O.I.,Karpova,G.G.,Knorre,D.G.
and Kobets,N.D. (1981). The proteins of the
messenger RNA binding site of Escherichia
coli ribosomes. Nucl.Acids Res. 9,3465-3481.
4. Karpova,G.G.,Kobets,N.D.,Silina,S.A. and
Godovicov,A.A. (1981). Affinity labelling of
16S rRNA in E.coli ribosomes by heptauridy-
late analogue bearing a chemically reactive
group at 3'-end. Bioorg.Khym. 7, 1503-1511.
5. Vlassov,V.V.,Lavrik,O.I.,Khodyreva,S.N.,
Chiszikov,V.E.,Shvalie,A.F. and Mamaev,S.V.
(1980). Chemical modification of the phenylalanyl-tRNA synthetase and ribosomes of Escherichia coli with derivatives of tRNA^{phe} carrying photoreactive group on guanine residues.
Molekulyarn.Biol. 14, 531-538.
6. Babkina,G.T.,Bausk,E.V.,Graifer,D.M.,Karpo-
va,G.G. and Matasova,N.V. (1984). The effect
of aminoacyl- or peptidyl-tRNA at the A site
on the arrangement of deacylated tRNA at the
ribosomal P site. FEBS Letters 170, 290-294.

RIBOSOMAL COLLAPSE TRIGGERED BY A DNA OLIGONUCLEOTIDE

ERIC HENDERSON and JAMES A. LAKE

Molecular Biology Institute and Department of Biology
University of California, Los Angeles
California 90024

INTRODUCTION

Recent descriptions of enzymatic activities innate to
specific RNA species (1,2) suggest that ribosomal RNA
(rRNA) may have a more central role in protein synthesis
than previously thought. In general, one finds a strong
correlation between functionally important regions of
rRNA from highly divergent species (see eg. 3). One
highly conserved sequence in 23S (bacterial) and 28S
(eucaryotic) rRNA which may participate in protein
synthesis is the region including nucleotides 2654-2667
in E. coli. Ribosomes are inactivated when this sequence
is specifically cleaved by the cytotoxin alpha-sarcin
(4). This strongly conserved sequence displays approximately 90% homology between E. coli, chloroplast and
eukaryotes (including yeast, rat, frog and rabbit) (5).
Cleavage of a single phosphodiester bond in this sequence
in rat 28S rRNA (between nucleotides 4325 and 4326) inactivates 60S ribosomal subunits and precipitates an
event that can be described as "ribosomal collapse" and
involves the dislocation of 5.8S rRNA from the ribosome
(6).

    In the course of surveying probes that could be useful
for mapping specific rRNA sequences by DNA hybridization
microscopy (7) we observed an unexpected effect. A
large shift in large ribosomal subunit conformation can
be produced by the binding of a synthetic DNA fragment
complementary to the alpha-sarcin sensitive sequence.

Proceedings of the 16th FEBS Congress
Part B, pp. 219–228
© 1985 VNU Science Press

Upon binding of this DNA fragment the sedimentation coefficient is reduced from 50S to about 43S, a specific
set of ribosomal proteins and 5S rRNA are lost from the
altered ribosomal particle (referred to as the alpha-
sarcin particle). In addition, 23S rRNA is cleaved at
several sites generating at least three 3' 23S rRNA end
fragments. One of these fragments (about 350 nucleotides
long) hybridizes to the alpha-sarcin site specific DNA
probe. A second fragment does not hybridize to the
alpha-sarcin site specific probe and is of the appropriate size (about 250 nucleotides) to place the cleavage
site at or near the alpha-sarcin sensitive sequence in
23S rRNA.

RESULTS

Large ribosomal subunits were incubated with synthetic DNA
probes that were complementary to the alpha-sarcin sensitive sequence (nucleotides 2654-2667 in E. coli).

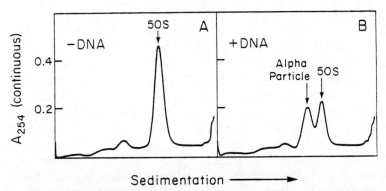

Figure 1. Production of alpha-sarcin particles by the
15-alpha DNA probe. 45 pmole of 50S subunits were incubated with 350 pmole 15-alpha DNA in a buffer containing 20mM Tris-HCl (pH. 7.5 at room temperature), 1mM
$MgCl_2$, 600mM NH_4Cl, 1mM DTT and 0.1mM EDTA in a total reaction volume of 10 μl. Reaction mixtures were incubated
for 30 minutes at 51° C and analyzed by centrifugation
through a 15% to 30% (w/v) sucrose gradient, containing

the reaction buffer, for 30 minutes at 3° C and 50,000
RPM in a Beckman VTi 65 rotor. Panel A shows the gradient profile of mock treated 50S subunits (no DNA added).
The gradient profile in Panel B shows the production of a
subribosomal particle, the alpha-sarcin particle, upon
incubation of 50S subunits with 15-alpha DNA. Gradients
were fractionated on an Isco fractionator. The top of
the gradient is at the left of each panel.

This probe will be referred to as the 15-alpha probe. A
dramatic consequence of incubation of 50S ribosomal subunits with either of the probes is the production of a
sub-ribosomal particle, the "alpha-sarcin particle", with
a sedimentation coefficient less than that of 50S ribosomal subunits (about 43S). As shown in figure 1, a
molar excess of 15-alpha DNA efficiently converts 50S
subunits to a slower sedimenting species, alpha-sarcin
particles (see figure legend for incubation conditions).

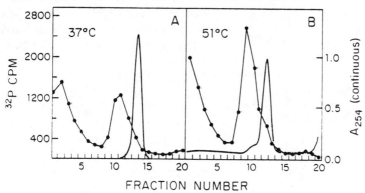

Figure 2. Binding of ^{32}P labeled 15-alpha DNA to 50S
subunits (alpha-sarcin particles) analyzed by sucrose
gradient centrifugation. Approximately 30 ng of ^{32}P 3'
end labeled 15-alpha DNA were incubated with 45 pmole of
50S subunits, at either 37° or 51° C (panels A and B respectively), and analyzed by sucrose gradient centrifugation as described in the legend to figure 1. Reaction
mixtures were as described in figure 1. Radioactive
content of gradient fractions was determined by scintillation counting.

221

The DNA probe does not sediment with the 50S peak in a sucrose gradient, but sediments with the alpha-sarcin particle (figure 2). In addition, the binding of the 15-alpha probe to the alpha-sarcin particle, as well as the production of the particle are increased at elevated incubation temperatures (51° C vs 37° C) (figure 2). In control experiments, 50S subunits incubated under identical conditions in the absence of the 15-alpha probe (figure 1, panel A), with a non-complementary probe, or with a probe complementary to another 23S rRNA sequence (nucleotides 1087-1103, data not shown) no alpha-sarcin particle production was observed.

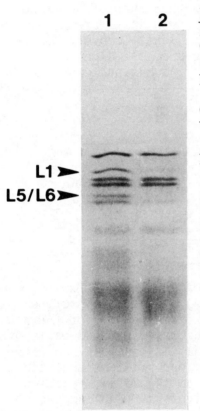

Figure 3. SDS polyacrylamide gel electrophoretic analysis of protein content of alpha-sarcin particles (lane 2) compared to control 50S subunits (lane 1). Alpha-sarcin particles and control 50S subunits were prepared as described in the legend to figure 1 and pelleted for 16 hours in a SW 50.1 rotor at 35,000 RPM and 3° C. The pellets were resuspended in loading buffer and electrophoresed through a 12.5% polyacrylamide gel as described (9). Ribosomal proteins missing from the alpha-sarcin particles are indicated.

The purified alpha-sarcin particle lacks a specific set of ribosomal proteins, and 5S rRNA, and contains 23S rRNA that is degraded in a characteristic fashion.

Figure 3 shows the protein composition of control 50S subunits and of alpha-sarcin particles analyzed by SDS polyacrylamide gel electrophoresis. The alpha-sarcin particles have lost a specific set of ribosomal proteins. These include: L1, L5/L6 and several smaller proteins, possibly including L7/L12.

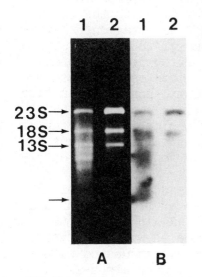

1 2 1 2

23S→
18S→
13S→

→

A   B

Figure 4. Agarose gel electrophoretic analysis of rRNA species associated with alpha-sarcin particles and control 50S subunits (panel A). Samples were prepared as described in the legends for figures 1 and 3, and suspended in gel loading solution containing 40% (w/v) sucrose and 0.5% (w/v) SDS and loaded onto a 1.5% agarose gel containing 89mM Tris, 89mM Borrate and 1mM EDTA. The samples were electrophoresed for 2 hours at 7° C and 6.5 volts/cm in TBE plus 1 ug/ml ethidium bromide and visualized by UV illumination. Lane 1 contains alpha-sarcin particle rRNA and lane 2 contains control 50S subunit rRNA. The RNA from the gel was transferred to a nitrocellulose filter (panel B) in 20X SSC (1X SSC is 150mM NaCl, 15mM Na Citrate, pH 7.5) and probed with 3' end labeled 15-alpha DNA for 20 hours at 37° C in 6X NET (1X NET is 150mM NaCl, 15mM Tris-HCl (pH 7.5) and 1mM EDTA), 0.5% SDS and 5X Denhardt's solution (10). The filter was washed as described in 6X SSC (11) except at 170° C, dried and placed against x-ray film. The rRNA fragment present only in the alpha-sarcin particles which hybridized to the 15-alpha DNA probe is indicated by an arrow.

Figure 4 shows an electrophoretic analysis of rRNA prepared from alpha-sarcin particles and mock treated 50S subunits. The rRNA from the alpha-sarcin particles is extensively cleaved whereas, in contrast, control 50S subunits contain only amounts of smaller rRNA fragments that are normally found in ribosome preparations (figure 4A). The rRNA digestion occurring in the alpha-sarcin particles results in the formation of specific bands in the gel as well as some less specific background fragments. When rRNA subfragments from the alpha-sarcin particle are transferred from an agarose gel to nitrocellulose and hybridized with radiolabeled 15-alpha DNA, as shown in figure 4B, the probe hybridizes to the intact rRNA (also to 18S rRNA, a 23S rRNA sub-fragment that is normally found in E. coli ribosomes), to a background of many smaller fragments, and most extensively to one small fragment. This rRNA subfragment migrates to a position in a non-denaturing agarose gel corresponding to a size greater than 5S rRNA (130 nucleotides) and less than the 13S rRNA subfragment (about 1100 nucleotides) giving it an approximate size of 350 nucleotides. This fragment must contain the alpha-sarcin sensitive sequence. To deter-

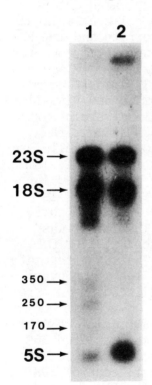

Figure 5. 3' end fragments of 23S rRNA generated by treatment of 50S subunits with 15-alpha DNA. 50S subunits were labeled with ^{32}P cytidine bis-phosphate and incubated with 15-alpha DNA to produce alpha-sarcin particles. The rRNA from these (lane 1) and control 50S subunits (lane 2) was electrophoresed as in figure 4. The gel was dried and placed against x-ray film. Three 3' end fragments are found in the alpha-sarcin particles with lengths of roughly 350, 250 and 170 nucleotides. The loss of 5S rRNA from the DNA treated 50S subunits mentioned in the text is evident.

mine is this fragment was generated by a single excision
event, the 3' end of 23S rRNA was radiolabeled in 50S ribosomal subunits using T4 RNA ligase and ^{32}P-cytidine bis-
phosphate. The 3' end-labeled 50S subunits were then incubated with the 15-alpha probe. Ribosomal RNA was prepared from these subunits and from mock treated radiolabeled subunits and these were analyzed by gel electrophoresis. Figure 5 shows that the fragment containing
the alpha-sarcin sensitive sequence which is produced
upon incubation of 50S subunits with the 15-alpha probe
includes the native 3' end of 23S rRNA. Two smaller fragments are also generated which contain the native 23S rRNA
3' end but do not contain the complete alpha-sarcin sensitive sequence. Assuming that the electrophoretic migration characteristics under non-denaturing conditions
are indicative of the length of the fragment, we estimate that the point of excision is approximately 100 nucleotides upstream from the alpha-sarcin sensitive sequence. Figure 5 also illustrates that 5S rRNA, also 3'
labeled, is removed from the DNA treated 50S subunits.

The 15-alpha probe is unable to cause the cleavage of
naked 23S rRNA under the conditions in which 50S subunits
are converted to alpha-sarcin particles. When the 15-
alpha probe was incubated with naked rRNA in low magnesium
concentration (1mM) no obvious differences were observed
between the +DNA and -DNA experiments (data not shown).
Since these conditions are identical to those which produce alpha-sarcin particles we conclude that the RNA scission is not produced by a contaminating enzymatic activity present in the synthetic DNA.

DISCUSSION

It is remarkable that a DNA fragment only 15 nucleotides
long could alter so extensively a complex macromolecule
nearly 320 times larger. These effects are illustrated
in Figure 6. Alpha DNA binds to a site located on the
large ribosomal subunit. The three dimensional location
of this site is unknown but it is schematically shown at
the center of the subunit. Binding releases a set of

225

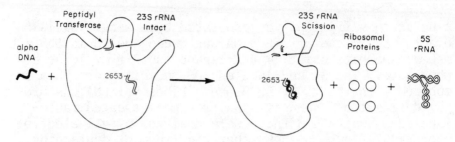

Figure 6. A diagramatic representation of the events
that are triggered by binding of the alpha-sarcin DNA
probe to the large ribosomal subunit. These include
changes in ribosomal conformation, scission of 23S rRNA,
loss of r-protein and loss of 5S rRNA.

ribosomal proteins and 5S rRNA, and rRNA is cleaved at a
number of sites, but preferentially at a site located
near the peptidyl transferase. In addition, electron
micrographs of the alpha sarcin particle indicate a disrupted ribosome structure (data not shown).

In some ways the 15-alpha DNA fragment mimics the
effects of alpha-sarcin upon large ribosomal subunits.
The rRNA structure is severely perturbed upon interacting
with the 15-alpha probe in a fashion similar to that
elicited by alpha-sarcin treatment (5). Unlike alpha-
sarcin treatment, DNA treatment produces a background of
rRNA fragments in addition to specific bands. Also in
contrast to alpha-sarcin treatment, DNA treatment releases 5S rRNA. Of the three specific DNA induced rRNA
bands containing the native 3' end of 23S rRNA, only one
hybridizes to the 15-alpha probe. The position of this
cleavage is about 100 nucleotides 3' distal to the alpha-
sarcin sensitive site in 23S rRNA. The other two 3' end
fragments are of roughly the appropriate size to result
from cleavage of 23S rRNA at or near the alpha-sarcin
sensitive sequence. If one of these two cleavages were
within the alpha-sarcin sensitive sequence, under the
conditions of stringency used the rRNA fragment produced would not be expected to hybridize to the DNA probe.
Hence one of these two fragments, although not hybridiz-
ing with the 15-alpha probe, could still correspond to
alpha-sarcin fragment of eukaryotic ribosomes.

As shown by Northern hybridization of the 15-alpha probe to rRNA subfragments, the rRNA cleavage observed in our experiments is moderately specific. This could be consistent with either exogenous or endogenous RNase activity being the cause of the rRNA scissions. We do not think that the RNase activity is a contaminant of the DNA since extensive care was taken to remove possible RNase contaminants from the DNA probes. In addition, the alpha-sarcin DNA did not degrade naked 23S rRNA under conditions identical to those which produce the alpha-sarcin particle from 50S subunits. The effects of the alpha-sarcin probe upon 50S subunits have not been observed with a synthetic DNA probe prepared the same way as the 15-alpha probe but complementary to nucleotides 1087-1103 of the large ribosomal subunit rRNA. Our experiments with naked 23S rRNA do not rule out the possibility that the effect could be an auto-catalytic property of the 23S rRNA (1,2) since our experiments on naked rRNA were performed at 1 mM $MgCl_2$ and in the absence of guanine ribonucleotide phosphates. In comparison, the experiments of Krugev et al. (1)and Guerrier-Takada et al. were performed at higher magnesium, 5mM and 60mM respectively, and Cech and coworkers had found that guanine ribonucleotides were critical for the autocatalysis of Tetrahymena rRNA. Alternatively they do not rule out the possibility that the cleavage is a property of ribosomal proteins or ribosomal associated proteins.

The observation that a synthetic oligonucleotide probe complementary to a particular 23S rRNA sequence can cause such drastic alterations in ribosome subunit structure was unexpected. This suggests that probes to this and other rRNA sequences may prove useful in understanding some of the functional roles of rRNA in protein synthesis. Since these probes can be designed so precisely, such experiments may provide details at the resolution of individual nucleotides.

ACKNOWLEDGEMENTS

We are grateful to Michael W. Clark, Melanie Oakes and Andrew Scheinman for helpful discussion and criticsm. This work was supported by grants to J.A.L. from the National Science Foundation (PCM 76-14710) and the National Institute of General Medical Science (GM-240341). E. H. was supported by a NIH Cell and Molecular Biology training grant.

LITERATURE CITED

1 Kruger,K., Grabowski,P.J., Zaug,A.J., Sands,J., Gottschling, D.T. and Cech, T.R. (1982) Cell 31, 147-157.
2 Guerrier-Takada,C., Gardiner,K., Marsh,T., Pace,N. and Altman,S. (1983) Cell 35, 849-857.
3 Noller,H. (1984) Annual Review of Biochemistry, (Richardson,C., Boyer,P. and Meister,A., eds.), in press.
4 Endo,Y., Huber,P.W. and Wool,I.G. (1983) J. Biol. Chem. 258(4), 2662-2667.
5 Chan,Y-L., Endo,Y. and Wool,I.G. (1983) J. Biol. Chem. (258(21), 12768-12770.
6 Walker,T.A., Endo,Y., Wheat,W.H., Wool,I.G. and Pace,N.R. (1983)J. Biol. Chem. 258, 333-338.
7 Oakes,M., Clark,M., Henderson,E. and Lake,J.A. (1984) J. Cell Biol. (Abstr.).
8 Miyoshi,K.I., Miyake,T., Hozumi,T. and Itakura,K. (1980) Nuc. Acids Res. 9(22), 5473-5489.
9 Laemmli,U. (1970) Nature 227, 680.
10 Denhardt,D.T. (1966) Biochem. Biophys. Res. Comm. 23(5), 641-646.
11 Itakura,K., Miyake,T., Kawashima,E.H., Ike, Y., Ito,H., Morin,C., Reyes,A.A., Johnson,M.J., Schold,M. and Wallace,R.B. (1981). In: Recombinant DNA, Proceedings of the Third Cleveland Symposium of Macromolecules, A.G. Walton (ed), Elsevier Scientific Publishing Company, Amsterdam.

OPTIMAL ACCURACY, MAXIMAL GROWTH

C.G. KURLAND, M. EHRENBERG, T. RUUSALA, D. ANDERSSON, K. BOHMAN, P. JELENC.

Molecular Biology Institute, BMC, Box 590, S-751 24 Uppsala, Sweden.

Introduction

We have discovered an unexpected relationship between the accuracy of gene expression and the growth rates of bacteria. Thus, it would surprise noone to discover that high error rates in the biosynthesis of proteins lower the efficiency of a biological system. However, what has been quite unforseen is our finding that extreme accuracy of translation has precisely such an inhibitory effect. This finding has led us to formulate an hypothesis that relates the accuracy of gene expression to growth rates in terms of a trade-off between the negative consequences of errors on the one hand and the costs of accuracy in protein biosynthesis on the other. Briefly, we suggest that the error rates are set at a level that maximizes the growth rate of bacteria. This optimum is reached at an error rate for which further increase of the accuracy would improve the kinetic efficiency of the proteins to an extent that is insufficient to compensate for the increased kinetic cost to the biosynthetic pathways.

Evidence to support the notion of an optimum rather than a maximum accuracy for the translation apparatus has been available for quite some time but not appreciated in this way until very recently. Thus, there are easily obtained ribosome mutants that are resistant to antibiotics such as streptomycin (Sm), which greatly raise the translational error rate. It has been well established that at least a subset of these mutants restrict translation errors even in the absence of antibiotics (1). Since most of the evidence for hyperaccurate Smresistant (SmR) mutants was obtained by the analysis of nonsense suppression frequencies, we felt obliged to see if the same restriction pattern could be observed for missense substitutions. Hence we measured missense frequencies at

Proceedings of the 16th FEBS Congress
Part B, pp. 229–238
© 1985 VNU Science Press

defined positions in two proteins in the absence of Sm. Our data confirmed the existence of missense restriction by mutant ribosomes of the smR phenotype and it also indicated that in the wild-type ribosomes could normally be viewed as the major source of errors in gene expression (2).

Thus, the missense errors at two different codon positions are between three and seven-fold higher in wild-type compared to these of an SmR mutant with an alteration in ribosomal protein S12. If these observations are representative, they suggest that at least three fourths of the missense substitutions in proteins produced by wild-type bacteria occur at the ribosome. In other words, these data would suggest that the errors of RNA polymerase and amino acyl-tRNA synthetases may be negligible compared to those of ribosome function. We make use of this conclusion below, and we initiate the present argument with a simple question: Why haven't wild-type ribosomes evolved so that they are at least as accurate as some SmR variants?

Growth rates and Accuracy
We take as our starting point the assumption that the wild-type form of E. coli that has been maintained in laboratories for decades is an organism that has been selected for its ability to grow at a maximum rate in artificial culture media. If this is so, we might guess that the reason that wild-type bacteria are less accurate protein synthesisers than SmR mutants is that the latter grow less rapidly than do wild-type bacteria. Indeed, direct comparisons by competition in unlimited batch culture shows that this guess is correct (Andersson and Kurland, unpublished data). Indeed, it is possible to order according to their growth rates a variety of SmR mutants with varying degrees of enhanced accuracy of translation in vivo or in vitro. This rank order of growth rates is the same as that which is obtained by ranking the bacteria according to their error rates. In other words, error-restrictive mutants tend to grow slower than the wild type.

At this point it is important to stress that the correlation between error rate and growth rate does not extend into mutants that are less accurate than wild type. Thus, a variety of Ram mutants that result from alterations expressed in ribosomal protein S4, are significantly less accurate than wild type, but these mutants also grow slower than do wild-type bacteria (3). On the surface it would seem that the rates of growth are maximized at an optimal accurcy which is close to that of the wild type.

Now, the S4 alterations that are responsible for the Ram phenotype are highly pleiotropic. One relevant effect of S4 alteration is that expressed in the lowered affinity of the mutant protein for its 16S RNA binding site (4), which will account for the 30S ribosomal assembly defect that S4 mutants of the Ram phenotype display (5, 6). Since the assessment of the impact of the Ram phenotype of the S4 mutations on the growth rate is complicated by that of the correlated ribosome assembly defect, we are obliged to focus our attention only on the restrictive mutants.

There are at least three well defined types of restrictive mutants that we have studied, all are due to alterations in the protein S12 (7, 8, 9). One group are SmR mutants that are indifferent to the presence or absence of Sm; another are the SmP mutants that grow in the absence of antibiotic, but are significantly stimulated by it; and, finally there are the SmD mutants that have an absolute requirement for Sm or a comparable agent in order to grow. When the ribosomes from this collection of mutants are analyzed in vitro it is observed that they can be ordered according to their accuracy of translation as wild type $\ll$ SmD $<$ SmP $<$ SmR (10). Why should dependence on an error-inducing antibiotic for growth be correlated with an increased accuracy of function of ribosomes in the absence of antibiotic? If we assume for the movement that, as will be substantiated below, this correlation is not entirely fortuitous, it would seem that there is something associated with extreme accuracy of ribosome function that is inhibitory for growth. In order to see what that might be, we will look next at the mechanism of aminoacyl-tRNA selection on ribosomes.

The proofreading costs

The key to our hypothesis is that the precision of translation is obtained at a metabolic cost that increases to
growth inhibitory levels in hyperaccurate mutants. Such
an expandable metabolic cost is implicit in the ideas of
Hopfield (11) and Ninio (12). They have suggested that
aminoacyl-tRNA's are matched with their cognate codon-
programmed ribosomes in a multi-step editing process that
is called proofreading. The relevant characteristic of
proofreading mechanisms is that they provide a way in
which the accuracy of the substrate selection can be
amplified at the cost of an excess dissipative loss. It
is this excess dissipative loss that we identfy with a
metabolic cost.

A proofreading mechanism for aminoacyl-tRNA selection
would involve an initial selection step in which a limited accuracy in matching the ternary complex with the
codon at the ribosomal A-site would be obtained by a
fully reversible binding interaction: The premise of Hopfield (11) and Ninio (12) is that this initial selectivity is inadequate and that one or more subsequent
steps are required to amplify the accuracy. The latter
are envisioned as irreversible steps which follow the
hydrolysis of the GTP introduced by the ternary complex.
In these irreversible editing steps there is a preferential discard of the noncognate aminoacyl-tRNA's and a
preferential forwarding of the cognate species towards
peptide bond formation: Since the preferential discard of
noncognate species occurs at the expense of prior GTP
hydrolysis, the accuracy enhancement is associated with
an excess dissipation of ternary complexes.

Soon after the appearence of this hypothetical mechanism experiments were described by Thompson and Stone (13)
who claimed to to have identified the putative proofreading step for aminoacyl-tRNA in single cycle experiments with ternary complexes and mRNA programmed ribosomes in vitro. Since alternative explanations of their
results with single cycle experiments were and still are
possible (14), we developed a steady state in vitro system that synthesises polypeptides at rates and accuracies
not very different from those observed in vivo in order

to study this problem. We have used this system to study the kinetics of the EF-Tu cycle during polypeptide bond synthesis (17). On the basis of such data we could develop two specific assays to determine whether or not during polypeptide synthesis there is an excess dissipation of ternary complexes which is preferential for noncognate aminoacyl-tRNA species (18, 19, 20).

The data obtained in the high performance, steady state system are persuasive: There is a requirement in a poly(U)-programmed reaction for 50-150 EF-Tu ternary complex cycles in order to insert a single leucine into a peptide chain compared to a little more than one cycle to insert a phenylalanine; the average number of ternary complex cycles depends on which Leu-tRNA isoacceptor species is competing with the cognate Phe-tRNA (18). Antibiotics such as kanamycin and streptomycin that stimulate the error rate also suppress the proofreading flows (21, 22). Ribosomes with the Ram phenotype are defective proofreaders, which accounts for their higher error rates (23). In contrast, ribosomes from restrictive mutants with the SmR, SmP and SmD phenotypes all have proofreading activities that are more vigorous than wild type, and this will account for their greater accuracies of function both in vivo as well as in vitro (10, 19).

We will consider these mutant phenotypes again below, but for the moment we present their altered kinetic characteristics as evidence for the existence of a ribosome-mediated proofreading function: What is important here is the conclusion that the efficiency of translation can vary accordingly to the vigor of the proofreading flows. In particular ribosomes that are more accurate due to enhanced proofreading are less efficient in terms of ternary complex consumption. Indeed, the proofreading flows are so disturbed in the extreme case of SmD mutants that it takes more than two ternary complex cycles on average to insert a cognate amino acid into a polypeptide chain (10). With this observation we are now in a position to close our argument relating translational accuracy and growth rate by considering the impact on the cell of changes in the efficiency of ternary complex usage.

The growth optimum

There are two conclusions that we now wish to relate to each other. The first is the inference that there is something growth inhibitory associated with extreme translational accuracy. The second is the demonstrable decrease in the efficiency of ternary complex usage by hyperaccurate mutant ribosomes. In order to show that the latter can explain the former we must set the flows for protein biosynthesis within the context of the metabolic constraints on bacterial growth.

The necessarily brief description to be presented here is a synopsis of a more complete discussion of growth constraints found in our previous studies (24, 25). There we identify the primary limitation on the growth rate with the limited speed with which substrates in the media can be mobilized and converted into more bacteria. Thus, the substrate flows into the bacteria should tend to be maximized, and these maxima will determine the maximum growth rate in a medium of given composition. Furthermore, each particular substrate flow will be partitioned between different biosynthetic pathways: For example, ATP can be used to synthesize RNA or protein. According, these two major pathways will be "competing" for the ATP.

Such competitive partitioning of limited substrate flows will require optimal allocations of the different substrate flows to different metabolic compartments. In this context a significant change in the efficiency of ternary complex consumption could have a rather pronounced inhibitory effect on the substrate flows into other metabolic pathways, which would tend to decrease the growth rate. For example, the increased consumption of GTP associated with polypeptide formation by ribosomes that are abnormally vigorous proofreaders might be sufficient to suppress the rate of other GTP requiring processes such as nucleic acid synthesis. Hence, excessive GTP consumption by the ribosome could inhibit growth to the extent that this consumption exceeds the maximum rate of GTP production by the bacteria.

This is not the only conceivable inhibitory effect of the enhanced proofreading flows. Thus, in order to an optimal partitioned substrate flow pattern, the macromolecular components of the system must also be accumulated in optimal amounts. In other words, there are optimal amounts of ribosomes, EF-Tu and EF-Ts for maximum growth on a given medium. Accordingly, a preciptious increase of the proofreading flows would require a greater number of ternary complex cycles per peptide bond, and if the amounts of EF-Tu or EF-Ts present are not sufficient to meet this requirement, protein synthesis will be retarded. Likewise, the increased discard of aminoacyl-tRNA's at the proofreading steps on the ribosome can lead in the extreme to a kinetic situation in which the rate of ribosome function is significantly decreased. Here, the effective saturation level of the ribosomes could be decreased by excessive proofreading of the amonoacyl-tRNA species (10).

In summary, there are at least three kinetic consequences of excessive proofreading that could lead to depressed growth rates: one is by limitation of GTP production, another is limitation by the cycle time of the EF-Tu-EF-Ts compartment; and finally, there is the limitation of protein synthesis by lower saturation levels of ribosomes. Opposed to these kinetic effects that would tend to lower the efficiency of the system is the increased efficiency of all of the proteins in the system that results from the concomittant higher accuracy of ribosome function. Acordingly we suggest that the optimum accuracy is simply that at which these kinetic tendencies are just balanced against each other.

One test of this hypothesis is provided by the SmP and SmD mutants. These mutants produce ribosomes that according to our interpretation are excessive proofreaders. According these mutants should be made to grow faster if their translational accuracy is lowered by agents that reduce their proofreading flows. This expectation has been demonstrated both with antibiotics and suppressor mutations. Hence, the SmP and SmD bacteria are much more accurate than wild type and their maximum growth rates are supported by concentrations of Sm that raise their translational error frequencies to levels equal to or greater than wild type in the absence of antibiotic (10). Similarly, double mutants containing SmD alleles of S12

235

and Ram alleles of S4 have translational acuracies as well as growth rates similar to those of wild type (Andersson and Kurland, unpublished data). The growth stimulatory effects of both Sm and the Ram allele on the SmP or SmD mutant ribosomes can be shown by in vitro experiments to be associated with a suppression of the excessive proofreading flows (10, Andersson and Kurland, unpublished data).

In other words, we have demonstrated that there is not a monotonic relationship between growth rate and translational accuracy. It now remains for us to demonstrate in vivo that there is not a monotonic relationship between growth rate and proofreading. We are nevertheless confident that our ideas concerning the optimization of the growth inhibitory and growth-stimulatory tendencies of ribosomal proofreading will account in large measure for the interactions of the classical S4 and S12 mutant alleles. And, we close this discussion with a curious observation: although our recent data correlate excessive accuracy of translation with growth inhibition, there is to our knowledge no unambiguous demonstration of the analogoues effect of generally decreased accuracy of translation.

1) Gorini, L. (1974) Streptomycin and misreading of the genetic code. In "Ribosome". M.Nomura, A. Tissieres, and P. Lengy, editors. pp. 791-804.

2) Bouadloun, R., Donner, D., and Kurland, C.G. (1983) Codon-specific missense errors in vivo. The EMBO Journal 2 No.8, 1351-1356 (1983).

3. Andersson, D.I., Bohman, K., Isaksson, L.A., and Kurland, C.G. (1982). Translation Rates and Misreading Characteristics of rpsD Mutants in Escherichia coli. Mol. Gen. Genet. 187, 467-472 (1982).

4. Green, M., Kurland, C.G. (1971). Mutant ribosomal protein with defective RNA binding site. Nature New Biology 234, 273-275.

5. Olsson, M., Isaksson, L.A., Kurland, C.G. (1974). Pleiotropic Effects of ribosomal protein S4 studied in E. coli mutants. Mol. Gen. Genet. 135, 191-202.

6. Olsson. M., Isaksson, L.A. (1979). Analysis of rpsD Mutations in Escherichia coli I: Comparison of Mutants with Various Alterations in Ribosomal Protein S4. Molec. Gen. Genet. 169, 251-257.

7. Birge, A.E., Kurland, C.G. (1969). Altered protein in streptomycin dependent E. coli. Science 166, 1282-1284.

8. Ozaki, M., Mizushima, S., Nomura, M. (1969). Identification and functional characterization of the protein controlled by the streptomycin resistant locus in E. coli Nature 222, 338-339.

9. Zengel, J. M., Young, R., Dennis, P.P., Nomura, M. (1977).Role of ribosomal protein S12 in peptide chain elongation J. Bact. 129, 1326-1329.

10. Ruusala, T., Andersson. D., M. Ehrenberg., and Kurland, C.G. (1984) Hyper-Accurate Ribosomes Inhibit Growth. EMBO J.

11. Hopfield, J.J. (1974). Kinetic Proofreading. Proc. Natl. Acad. Sci. USA 71, 4135-4141.

12. Ninio, J. (1975). Kinetic amplification of enzyme discrimination. Biochimie 57, 487-595.

13. Thompson, R.C., and Stone, P.J. (1977). Proofreading of the codon-anticodon interaction on ribosomes. Proc. Natl. Acad. Sci. 74, 198-202.

14. Kurland, C.G. (1978). The role of Guanine Nucleotide in Protein Biosynthesis. Biophys. J., 22, 373-392.

15. Jelenc. P.C., and Kurland, C.G. (1979). "Nucleoside Triphosphate regeneration decreases the frequency of translation Errors". Proc. Nat. Acad. Sci USA, 76, 3174-3178.

16. Wagner, E.G.H., Ehrenberg, M., and Kurland, C.G. (1982). Suppression of Translational Errors by (p)ppGpp. Mol. Gen. Genet. 185, 269-274.

17. Ruusala, T., Ehrenberg, M., and Kurland, C.G. (1982). Catalytic effects of elongation factor Ts on polypeptide synthesis. The EMBO Journal 75-78.

18. Ruusala, T., Ehrenberg, M., and Kurland, C.G. (1982) Is there proofreading during polypeptide synthesis? The EMBO Journal 741-745.

19. Bohman, K., Ruusala, T., Jelenc, P.C., and Kurland, C.G. (1984). Kinetic Impairment of Restrictive Streptomycin Resistant Ribosomes. Mol. Gen. Genet. in press.

20. Ehrenberg, M., Kurland, C.G., and Ruusala, T. (1985). Biochemie submitted.

21. Jelenc, P.C., and Kurland, C.G. (1984). Multiple Effects of Kanamycin on Translational Accuracy. Mol. Gen. Genet. in press.

22. Ruusala, T., and Kurland, C.G. (1984). Streptomycin Peturbs Preferentially Ribosomal Proofreading. Mol. Gen. Genet., in press.

23. Andersson, D.I., and Kurland, C.G. (1983). Ram Ribosomes are Defective Proofreaders. Mol. Gen. Genet. 191, 378-381.

24. Ehrenberg, M., and Kurland, C.G. (1984). Costs of accuracy determined by a maximal growth rate constraint. Quart. Rev. Biophys., in press.

25. Kurland, C.G., and Ehrenberg, M. (1984). Optimization of Translational Accuracy. Progress in Molecular Biology and Nucleic Acid research.

REGULATION OF RIBOSOME BIOSYNTHESIS IN ESCHERICHIA COLI

MASAYASU NOMURA
Institute for Enzyme Research and Departments of
Genetics and Biochemistry, University of Wisconsin,
Madison, Wisconsin 53706

INTRODUCTION

The synthesis of ribosomes in E. coli is regulated so
that the cellular concentration of ribosomes is
roughly proportional to the growth rate. In addition,
the synthesis rates of all the ribosomal components
are balanced and, like the synthesis of ribosomes,
respond coordinately to changes in environmental
conditions. This second aspect of the regulation can
now be explained by the translational feedback
regulation of ribosomal protein (r-protein) synthesis.
When r-protein synthesis rates exceed those needed for
ribosome assembly, certain "free" ribosomal proteins
act as translational repressors on their respective
mRNAs to inhibit further translation. In order to
explain the first aspect of the regulation, the growth
rate dependent regulation of ribosome biosynthesis, we
have previously proposed that products of rRNA
operons, presumably non-translating ribosomes,
feedback inhibit rRNA (and tRNA) synthesis. We call
this model "ribosome feedback regulation model."

In this article, I shall first summarize some
essential features of translational regulation of
r-protein synthesis, and then briefly discuss some new
experimental results related to the mechanisms
involved in this regulation. Finally, I shall discuss
the ribosome feedback regulation model, and explain a
probable mechanism that is responsible for determining
the total amount of ribosomes in response to
environmental growth conditions.

Proceedings of the 16th FEBS Congress
Part B, pp. 239–248
© 1985 VNU Science Press

TRANSLATIONAL FEEDBACK REGULATION OF r-PROTEIN SYNTHESIS.

The translational feedback regulation model of r-protein synthesis was originally proposed based on experiments which analyzed the effect of gene dosage on the synthesis rate of r-protein mRNA and the synthesis rates of r-proteins (1). We found that the rate of r-protein mRNA synthesis increases in proportion to the increase in gene dosage, yet the rates of synthesis of corresponding r-proteins do not increase in proportion to gene copy. To explain these results, we suggested that r-protein synthesis and ribosome assembly is coupled so that when the r-protein synthesis rates exceed those needed for ribosome assembly, "free" r-proteins not incorporated into ribosomes inhibit their own synthesis.

Subsequent experiments using both in vitro and in vivo approaches identified several specific r-proteins as translational repressors and demonstrated that the proposed translational feedback regulation is essentially correct (for reviews, see 2, 3). In addition, these studies have revealed some interesting details of this regulatory system. I will summarize here what we now know to be the essential features of the translational regulation of r-protein synthesis: (1) only certain r-proteins (e.g., S4, S7, S8, L1, L4 and L10), but not all r-proteins, are translational repressors; (2) there are units of translational regulation and each unit contains the gene for its own unique translational repressor. There may be one or more regulatory units within each transcription unit, but these regulatory units do not overlap; (3) a translational repressor r-protein acts at a single target site on the polycistronic mRNA to affect the translation of all the proteins encoded within the regulatory unit. The target site is at or near the translation initiation site for the first protein in the regulatory unit; (4) interaction of the repressor with the target site directly blocks translation of the first cistron encoded in the regulatory unit. The translation of downstream cistrons is coupled with and dependent on that of the first cistron in the unit (called "translational coupling" or "sequential translation"), and this is the basis of the regulation of multicistronic units by a single translational repressor; (5) the mechanism of translational repression involves competition between structurally similar regions of rRNA and mRNA for the binding of r-proteins. Repressor r-proteins bind preferentially to rRNA and interact with the mRNA target site only when synthesized in excess of the amount needed for ribosome assembly. In fact, significant structural homology has been found in some cases between repressor target sites on mRNA and corresponding r-protein binding sites on rRNA; and (6) repressor r-proteins act in trans as well as in cis at least in the case of S4 and probably in all cases. The experimental evidence that supports these conclusions has been extensively discussed in several reviews as well as original papers (for references to the original papers, see reviews by 2, 3). I shall just mention some recent progress made on this subject using the L11-L1 operon system (4, 5).

The L11 ribosomal protein operon in Escherichia coli consists of the genes for proteins L11 and L1, and is feedback regulated by the translational repressor L1. Our earlier studies showed that the mRNA target site for this repression is located close to the translation initiation site of the first L11 cistron. We have recently constructed hybrid deletion plasmids carrying these two genes with decreasing amounts of the leader mRNA under lac transcriptional control. We measured mRNA and protein synthesis directed by these plasmids in vitro and in vivo and demonstrated that the regulation of this operon is indeed post-transcriptional. For example, induction of transcription with a lac operon inducer, isopropyl-thiogalactoside (IPTG), increased the mRNA synthesis rate about 10-fold without any significant increase in the synthesis rate of L11 or L1. A deletion or a

single base alteration in the r-protein repressor-
target site on the mRNA abolished this regulation and
led to a large overproduction (up to 10-fold) of these
r-proteins, corresponding to the mRNA overproduction.
These experiments convincingly demonstrate that E.
coli cells are able to balance the synthesis rate of
at least some and probably most or all r-proteins
without regulating the synthesis rates of their mRNA.
Thus, regulation at the level of translation is very
effective and able to prevent overproduction (or
underproduction) over a wide range of transcriptional
activities of r-protein genes. In addition, through
the deletion analysis (4) and site directed
mutagenesis studies using synthetic oligonucleotides
(5), we identified a region of the mRNA, preceding the
proximal L11 gene, important for successful feedback
inhibition of L11 and L1 synthesis by L1. In the
mutagenesis experiments, we specifically examined the
importance of a presumptive double-stranded stem
structure which is common among L1 binding sites on
rRNA from a variety of organisms and in the L11 mRNA.
Mutational alterations that disrupt the stem structure
were found to abolish translational regulation as
analyzed both in vitro and in vivo. Two of the
mutations were combined so that the stem structure is
restored but with a different primary nucleotide
sequence. This double mutant was shown to restore the
original phenotype, the ability to be translationally
regulated by L1. These experiments demonstrate the
importance of the stem structure, but not its primary
sequence, for the interaction of L1 with the mRNA, and
support the concept that mRNA target sites share some
structural features with the corresponding r-protein
binding sites of rRNA.
  From the various experimental results, it is now
clear that the final synthesis rates of r-proteins are
determined not by transcriptional mechanisms, but by
the translational feedback mechanism and are balanced
with the synthesis rate of ribosomes. It thus follows
that the synthesis rates of r-proteins are ultimately

determined by the synthesis rate of a single component that is rate-limiting. We believe that this rate-limiting component is rRNA under normal growth conditions (except under slow growth conditions).

THE RIBOSOME FEEDBACK REGULATION MODEL OF rRNA SYNTHESIS.

As mentioned above, the regulation of the synthesis of rRNA is probably the most important factor in determining the synthesis rate of ribosomes under normal growth conditions (except slow growth conditions, see below). How is the synthesis of rRNA (and hence ribosomes) regulated in response to growth conditions so that the amount of ribosomes synthesized is appropriate for the growth rate achieved in a given growth condition? In order to explain the growth-rate-dependent regulation of ribosome synthesis we have recently proposed a simple feedback model called "the ribosome feedback regulation model" and carried out a series of experiments to test the model (6). We suggest that bacterial cells regulate the ribosome synthesis rate (that is, the rRNA synthesis rate that is rate-limiting) as a result of a feedback mechanism that involves excess, non-translating "free" ribosomes, rather than as a direct response to environmental conditions. We imagine that cells are inherently prone to make excess ribosomes relative to other gene products which provide substrates and energy for macromolecular synthesis; overproduced non-translating ribosomes monitor the outcome of ribosome biosynthesis and prevent further unnecessary synthesis of ribosomes by inhibiting rRNA synthesis (and/or the synthesis of some other rate-limiting ribosome component). In this way, cells are able to adjust the amount of ribosomes so that the protein-synthetic capacity is just sufficient to maintain the growth rate while the free non-translating ribosome concentration is kept small.

A prediction of the ribosome feedback regulation model described above is that cells with an increased number of rRNA operons will not increase rRNA synthesis in proportion to the increase in gene copy numbers; rather, cells will maintain approximately the same (actually slightly higher) total rRNA synthesis rate by reducing rRNA synthesis from individual rRNA operons. These predictions were essentially confirmed. In strains carrying extra rRNA operons on multicopy plasmids, the rate of total rRNA synthesis was about the same or only slightly higher compared to the control strains, and the reduction of transcription of individual rRNA operons was confirmed by monitoring the synthesis of tRNA encoded by chromosomal rRNA operons.

We also carried out control experiments using strains carrying extra rRNA operons which have large deletions within the rRNA coding region. In this case, we found that the intact chromosomal rRNA genes were regulated normally to produce enough rRNA for the normal complement of ribosomes. In addition, the defective rRNA genes on the plasmids produced extra (non-functional) rRNA at a rate that simply reflected gene dosage, as predicted from the ribosome feedback regulation model.

In the course of these gene dosage experiments, we discovered that, in strains carrying extra rRNA operons on multicopy plasmids, the synthesis of tRNAs which are not encoded in rRNA operons was inhibited as well as the synthesis of tRNAs encoded by chromosomal rRNA operons. When the plasmid-encoded rRNA operons contained deletions within the rRNA coding region, no such inhibition was observed. Thus, the synthesis of most, if not all, tRNAs is subject to the same regulation by products of rRNA operons as are the rRNA operons themselves. Apparently, cells do not have regulatory systems that monitor production of tRNAs directly and regulate it to maintain the "normal" synthesis rate appropriate for given growth conditions. In agreement with this conclusion, the regulation of the synthesis of tRNAs that are not encoded in rRNA operons is similar to that of rRNA, e.g., with respect to growth-rate-dependent control, but, in contrast to the rRNA operons, the synthesis rate of any of these tRNAs individually is gene-dosage-dependent; that is, there is no feedback regulation by overproduced tRNAs.

In the above gene dosage experiments, decreases in the efficiency of individual rRNA promoters observed in cells carrying extra intact rRNA operons take place, according to the ribosome feedback regulation model, as a result of an increased level of free non-translating ribosomes in the cellular pool. By using double isotope labeling techniques, we have, in fact, found that the amounts of polysomes and "70S ribosomes", which constitute the majority of the ribosomes in cell extracts, were approximately the same in extracts from cells with or without extra rRNA operons, while the amount of both 30S and 50S ribosomal subunits in the extract from cells with extra rRNA operons was almost 2-fold higher than that in the extract from control cells. The amount of RNA in the tRNA fraction of the extract from the plasmid carrying strain was about half of that found for the control cells as expected (Y. Takebe and M. Nomura, unpublished experiments). These results are consistent with those expected from the ribosome feedback regulation model, and give additional support to the validity of this model.

Further experimental support of the model was also recently obtained in our laboratory. The tandem rRNA promoters were removed from the rrnB operon on a plasmid and replaced by the lambda P_L promoter. This hybrid operon contains intact coding and adjacent regions required for rRNA processing and is heat inducible in strains carrying temperature sensitive lambda cI repressor genes. A control plasmid was also prepared which is identical to this hybrid plasmid but a large part of the rRNA coding region is deleted. In preliminary experiments, the strains carrying these

245

plasmids were grown at 30°C, and then shifted to 42°C. Induction of the synthesis of extra rRNA and ribosomes was successfully achieved in this way, and the expected strong inhibition of the transcription of chromosomal rRNA operons (measured by follownig the synthesis of tRNAs encoded by these operons) and tRNA operons was demonstrated in experimental, relative to control strains (R. L. Gourse, Y. Takebe, R. Sharrock and M. Nomura, unpublished experiments). We expect that the new experimental system will be very useful in analyzing intermediate steps between the induction (initiation of the excess transcription of rRNA) and the final regulatory events (increased inhibition of transcription of chromosomal rRNA and tRNA operons).

Finally, I would like to mention that there are several other observations made in vivo which support indirectly the postulated feedback regulation model (for further discussion and references, see Nomura et al., 1984). As already discussed, the model predicts that the conditions which lead to a decrease in free non-translating ribosomes in the cellular pool would cause preferential stimulation of rRNA (and tRNA) synthesis, and alternatively, that conditions which lead to an increase in free ribosomes in the cellular pool would cause preferential inhibition of the synthesis of rRNA (and tRNA). First, we as well as other earlier workers observed that cold-sensitive, ribosome assembly defective mutants overproduce rRNA and tRNA at low temperatures. Similarly, we used conditions where ribosome assembly was inhibited by overproduction of repressor r-proteins from an inducible promoter, presumably because of unbalanced r-protein synthesis. Under these conditions, cells continued linear growth and a significant stimulation of rRNA (and tRNA) synthesis rate was in fact observed. Second, earlier work showed that stimulation of rRNA synthesis takes place in cells treated with inhibitors of protein chain elongation such as fusidic acid and chloramphenicol. We interpret that this stimulation is caused by a decrease in the amount of free ribosomes in the pool under the conditions where the protein chain elongation is reduced without reducing the rate of chain inititaion. Third, Mg^{++} starvation causes degradation of cellular ribosomes. It is known that preferential stimulation of rRNA and r-proteins takes place during the recovery period from such ribosome-deficient conditions. Finally, preferential and immediate stimulation of rRNA (and r-protein) synthesis upon nutritional shift-up can be explained by the present model. We suggest that a stimulation of protein synthesis upon nutritional shift-up mobilizes the small amount of non-translating ribosomes in the pool, thereby causing a burst of derepressed synthesis of rRNA and hence ribosomes.

The ribosome feedback regulation model discussed here has now a considerable amount of experimental support. In addition, as mentioned above, it can explain various known observations in the regulation of ribosome biosynthesis. However, it is not known whether free non-translating ribosomes inhibit transcription of rRNA (and tRNA) genes directly or indirectly through other effectors. Identification of the real repressor participating in this important regulation must await future studies.

ACKNOWLEDGEMENT
I thank my present, as well as my previous, coworkers, who participated in the work described in this article. The work in this laboratory was supported by grants from the National Institutes of Health (GM-20427) and from the National Science Foundation (PCM 79-10616), and by the College of Agriculture and Life Sciences, University of Wisconsin-Madison.

REFERENCES

1. Fallon, A. M., C. S. Jinks, G. D. Strycharz and M. Nomura. (1979). Regulation of ribosomal protein synthesis by selective mRNA inactivation in Escherichia coli. Proc. Natl. Acad. Sci USA 76, 3411-3415.

2. Nomura, M., S. Jinks-Robertson and A. Miura. (1982). Regulation of ribosome biosynthesis in Escherichia coli. In: Interaction of Translational and Transcriptional Controls in the Regulation of Gene Expression, J. Grunberg-Manago and B. Safer (eds). Elsevier Science Publishing, New York, pp. 91-104.

3. Nomura, M., R. Gourse and G. Baughman. (1984). Regulation of the synthesis of ribosomes and ribosomal components. Ann. Rev. Biochem. 53, 75-117.

4. Baughman, G. and M. Nomura. (1983). Localization of the target site for translational regulation of the L11 operon and direct evidence for translational coupling in Escherichia coli. Cell 34, 979-988.

5. Baughman, G. and M. Nomura. (1984). Translational regulation of the L11 ribosomal protein operon of Escherichia coli: Analysis of the mRNA target site using oligonucleotide-directed mutagenesis. Proc. Natl. Acad. Sci. USA, in press.

6. Jinks-Robertson, S., R. L. Gourse and M. Nomura. (1983). Expression of rRNA and tRNA Genes in Escherichia coli: Evidence for feedback regulation by products of rRNA operons. Cell 33, 865-876.

STRUCTURAL DYNAMICS OF THE RIBOSOME

A. S. SPIRIN, V. D. VASILIEV and I. N. SERDYUK
Institute of Protein Research, Academy of Sciences
of the USSR, Pushchino, Moscow Region, USSR

INTRODUCTION

The process of translation (elongation) on the ribosome
is composed of the repeating cycles, each consisting of
three successive steps: aminoacyl-tRNA binding, transpeptidation and translocation [1,2]. The translocation
step includes significant intraribosomal displacements of
a template and the products of the transpeptidation reaction: the release of deacylated tRNA, the transport of
peptidyl-tRNA from one site to the other and the shift of
the template polynucleotide by one codon.
    The question arises: is any step of the elongation
cycle, and particularly the translocation step, accompanied by mechanical alteration of the ribosomal particle?
The experimental answer to this question was found to be
not simple. First of all, physical measurements of functioning ribosomes require *all* the particles of the sample
under study to be active in elongation and present in the
same functional state. This is not the case for routine
ribosomal preparations where the particle population is
heterogeneous and only a fraction of it manifests full
activity.

PREPARATION OF ACTIVE ONE-FUNCTIONAL-STATE RIBOSOMES

To solve this problem, a special technique was deviced
for the isolation of translationally active ribosomes by
using columns with poly(U) coupled to Sepharose through
splittable disulfide bridges [3,4]. This technique allows
to obtain translating ribosomes stopped either in the
pre-translocation or in the post-translocation stage of
the elongation cycle and capable of continuing the cycle
and elongation at any moment when substrates and proper
temperature are provided.

Proceedings of the 16th FEBS Congress
Part B, pp. 249–255
© 1985 VNU Science Press

The content of translationally active particles in the ribosome samples prepared in such a way was not less than 95% [5]. The fraction of the particles in a given functional state (either post-translocation, i.e. puro-mycin-competent, or pre-translocation, i.e. puromycin-incompetent ones) was not less than 75-80%.

ELECTRON MICROSCOPY

A gallery of electron micrographs of the translating 70S ribosomes in the pre-translocation (a) and post-trans-location (b) states, as well as of the non-translating 30S·50S couples for comparison (c), is presented in Fig.1.

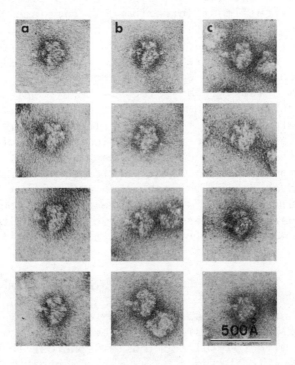

Fig. 1. A gallery of electron microscopy images of the pre-translocation state ribosomes (a), post-translocation state ribosomes (b), and non-translating 30S·50S couples (c) in the overlap projection.

Analysis of the images of about 1000 particles in each case has shown that the translating 70S ribosomes in the two functional states do not differ from the non-translating particles and from each other in respect to the mutual subunit orientation and the L7/L12 stalk position within the resolution limits of about 20 Å [6].

SEDIMENTATION

Fig. 2, with the sedimentation runs at different rates, shows that the pre-translocation state ribosomes sedimented somewhat faster than the post-translocation state particles. The difference of sedimentation coefficients of about 1S was observed at all three speeds used. Post-translocation state ribosomes look slightly less compact than ribosomes of the preceding (pre-translocation) stage. The difference seems to be small, however, it is not surprising that it could not be revealed by electron micro-

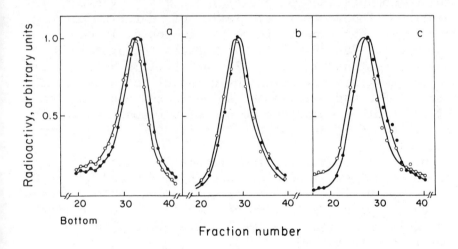

Fig. 2. Co-sedimentation of [^{14}C]pre-translocation (-o-) and [^{3}H]post-translocation (-●-) state ribosomes in sucrose gradient containing 20 mM tris·HCl, pH 7.5, 20 mM MgCl$_2$, 100 mM NH$_4$Cl, 4°C. (a): 20,000 r.p.m., (b): 30,000 r.p.m., (c): 40,000 r.p.m.

scopy. At the same time, another interpretation of the sedimentation experiments cannot be ruled out: pre-translocation state ribosomes sediment somewhat faster because of the presence of two tRNA residues per particle, instead of one tRNA residue in the post-translocation ribosome.

NEUTRON SCATTERING

Thus, the next problem in physical studies of functioning ribosomes arises. Indeed, the functional states (e.g. pre-translocation and post-translocation ones) are characterized by *different numbers* (e.g. two or one tRNA, respectively) and *different positions* of the RNA ligands on the ribosome.

For solution of this problem, the method of contrast variations in neutron scattering [7-10] was applied. Contrast-matched conditions can be achieved by placing the ribosome in various $H_2O/^2H_2O$ mixtures when one of the components (RNA or protein) becomes "invisible" for neutrons. Theoretical calculation of deuterium exchange and experiment show that the RNA component is contrast-matched in $\approx 70\%$ ^2H_2O [11,12], whereas the protein is contrast-matched in 40 to 42% ^2H_2O [8,12]. Hence, basing on the contrast variations by using different proportions of H_2O and ^2H_2O in the solvent, the contribution of the protein component change of a ribonucleoprotein particle can be estimated, *independently of RNA component changes*.

The Guinier plots for the translating ribosomes at different contrasts (H_2O, 16% ^2H_2O, 83% ^2H_2O and 97% ^2H_2O) are straight lines within the scattering vector range of 0.006 $Å^{-1}$ to 0.027 $Å^{-1}$. No noticeable rise of scattering intensities at the very small angles used ($\mu \sim 0.007$ $Å$) was observed both in H_2O and ^2H_2O.

The results of calculations of the neutron radii of gyration from Guinier plots are summarized in the Table. The values of the normalized intensity $I(0)_{normal}$ obtained by extrapolation of the Guinier plots to the zero scattering angle and divided by concentration of the ribosomal particles (reduced intensity) are also presented here.

TABLE
Radii of gyration of the ribosomes in pre-translocation and post-translocation states as measured by neutron scattering

Fraction of ^2H_2O in the $^1H_2O/^2H_2O$ mixture, vol.%	Radius of gyration, Å	
	Pre-translocation	Post-translocation
16	86.8 ± 0.4	87.3 ± 0.4
0	87.9 ± 0.8	88.3 ± 0.7
97	95.1 ± 0.3	96.4 ± 0.3
83	98.4 ± 0.8	101.0 ± 0.9

(Increase of protein contribution)

As seen from the Table, the neutron radii of gyration of the ribosomal particles in the post-translocation state are systematically greater than those of the pre-translocation state particles at all the contrasts used. At the same time, the value of the reduced normalized intensity of the neutron scattering (at zero scattering angle), which is proportional to a molecular mass, is found to be almost the same for the ribosomes in the two functional states (see Table). Hence, the small difference in R_g observed is not due to a contribution of an additional protein or RNA in one of the states. This observation leads to the conclusion that the difference in compactness of the ribosomes in the two functional states is a result of translocation.

Fig. 3 demonstrates the dependence of the radii of gyration of the particles on the contrasts, in coordinates R_g^2 versus $1/\Delta\rho$, for the preparations of the pre-translocation and post-translocation state ribosomes. It is seen that the difference in compactness increases as the scattering contribution of the protein component becomes greater, attaining the maximum ΔR_g value of about 3 to 5 Å at the contrast where the contribution of the RNA component is negligible.

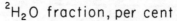

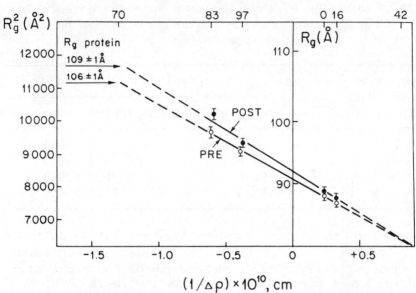

Fig. 3. Dependence of radius of gyration of pre-translocation (-o-) and post-translocation (-●-) state ribosomes on the contrast in Stuhrmann coordinates [R_g^2 vs $1/(\overline{\Delta\rho})$] (see [8]). Vertical segments indicate error values ($\pm 1.5\sigma$).

These experimental results are the first to demonstrate that translocation is accompanied by a relative spatial displacement of some parts of the ribosome with an amplitude of several angstroms. The question as to which parts are involved in the movements, and whether a shift of one ribosomal subunit relative to the other is responsible for the difference in the compactness of the ribosomes of two functional states is still open.

These studies were done with the participation of V.Baranov (preparation of translating ribosomes, functional analyses and sedimentation experiments) and O.Selivanova (electron microscopy), Institute of Protein Research. Neutron scattering experiments were conducted in collaboration with Dr. Roland May, Institut Laue-Langevin, Grenoble.

REFERENCES
1. Watson, J.D. (1964). The synthesis of proteins upon ribosomes. Bull. Soc. Chim. Biol. 46, 1399-1425.
2. Lipmann, F. (1969). Polypeptide chain elongation in protein biosynthesis. Science, 164, 1024-1031.
3. Belitsina, N.V., Elizarov, S.M., Glukhova, M.A., Spirin, A.S., Butorin, A.S. and Vasilenko, S.K. (1975). Isolation of translating ribosomes with a resin-bound poly-U column. FEBS Lett. 57, 262-266.
4. Baranov, V.I., Belitsina, N.V. and Spirin, A.S. (1979). The use of columns with matrix-bound polyuridylic acid for isolation of translating ribosomes. In: Methods in Enzymology, K.Moldave and L.Grossmann (eds.). Academic Press, New York, San Francisco, London, v.59, pp.382-398
5. Baranov, V.I. (1983). Preparation of translating ribosomes using columns with immobilized polyuridylic acid. Bioorgan. Khim. 9, 1650-1657.
6. Vasiliev, V.D., Selivanova, O.M., Baranov, V.I. and Spirin, A.S. (1983). Structural study of translating 70S ribosomes from Escherichia coli. FEBS Lett. 155, 167-172.
7. Engelman, D.M. and Moore, P.B. (1975). Determination of quaternary structure by small-angle neutron scattering. Ann. Rev. Biophys. Bioeng. 4, 219-241.
8. Ibel, K. and Stuhrmann, H.B. (1975). Comparison of neutron and X-ray scattering of dilute myoglobin solutions. J. Mol. Biol. 93, 255-265.
9. Jacrot, B. (1976). Study of biological structures by neutron-scattering from solution. Rep. Prog. Phys. 39, 911-953.
10. Ostanevich, Y.M. and Serdyuk, I.N. (1982). Neutronographic studies of biological macromolecule structures. Uspekhi Fiz. Nauk, 137, 85-116.
11. Serdyuk, I.N., Schpungin, J.L. and Zaccai, G. (1980). Neutron scattering study of the 13S fragment of 16S RNA and its complex with ribosomal protein L4. J. Mol. Biol. 137, 109-121.
12. Serdyuk, I.N. (1979). A method of joint use of electromagentic and neutron scattering: a study of internal ribosomal structure. In: Methods in Enzymology, K.Moldave and L.Grossman (eds.). Academic Press, New York, San Francisco, London, v.59, pp.750-775.

255

BIOENERGETICS

MECHANISM OF ATP SYNTHASE(FoF$_1$) STUDIED BY RECONSTITUTION

YASUO KAGAWA, NOBUHITO SONE AND MASASUKE YOSHIDA

Department of Biochemistry, Jichi Medical Shool,
Minamikawachi, Tochigi-ken, Japan 329-04

INTRODUCTION

The chemiosmotic hypothesis for proton motive ATP synthesis by ATP synthase (FoF$_1$) has received experimental support at the physiological level using reconstituted FoF$_1$-liposomes (1). FoF$_1$ is composed of a catalytic portion, F$_1$, and a proton channel portion, Fo. However, the mechamism of this process at the molecular level using reconstituted systems has yet to be described.

Complete reconstitution of F$_1$'s from mitochondria (MF$_1$) or chloroplasts (CF$_1$) from their five subunits ($\alpha,\beta,\gamma,\delta$ and ε) has not yet been achieved except for F$_1$'s obtained from thermophilic bacterium PS3 (TF$_1$) and Escherichia coli from their subunits after these had been isolated. The stability of TF$_1$ in denaturating agents is useful in the reconstitution study. The subunits of TF$_1$ were renatured from their primary structure when these agents were properly removed, and subunits α and β were both shown to bind AT(D)P after the renaturation. The properties of mesophilic F$_1$'s (CF$_1$, MF$_1$ and EF$_1$) are compared with those of TF$_1$ (Table I). The advantage of using TF$_1$ is not only its high reconstitutability, but also its simple interactions with ligands such as AT(D)P, divalent ions and inhibitors. Thus, the true substrate for TF$_1$ was shown to be the Δ,β,γ-bidentate ATP-Mg, and the 1:1:1 ADP-Mg-TF$_1$ complex was isolated. The details of recent studies have been reviewed in the light of genetic analysis and physicochemical properties of F$_1$(2).

Proceedings of the 16th FEBS Congress
Part B, pp. 259–264
© 1985 VNU Science Press

Table I. Properties of mesophilic and thermophilic F_1's.

Analytical Methods and Results	Mesophilic F_1	TF_1
Reconstitution of oligomers		
renaturation of subunits	impossible	possible
reassembly of minimum ATPase	$\alpha_3\beta_3\gamma$ (EF_1)	$\alpha_3\beta_3\gamma, \alpha_3\beta_3\delta$
Stereochemistry of reaction		
true substrate of F_1	? (no Cd)	Δ, β, γ-ATPMg
product, $[^{16}O, ^{17}O, ^{18}O]$-thioPi	inverted	inverted
Ligand binding		
endogenous F_1-bound AT(D)P	2-3, tight	none
1:1:1 ADP-Mg-F_1 complex	not clear	stable
total number of AT(D)P/F_1	6(3AMPPNP)	6($3\alpha, 3\beta$)
endogenous F_1-bound Mg	unremovable	none
aurovertin, quercetin etc.	inhibited	no effect
Conformation analysis		
^{1}H-^{2}H-exchange by Fourier IR	difficult	easy
α-helix and β-sheet estimation	calculation	by CD
^{31}P-NMR of F_1-nucleotide	not clear	clear, 50℃
crystallography dimension	3D (MF_1)	2D
Chemical modification		
8-azido ATP in Rossmann fold	yes in β	β and α
3'arylazido-8-azido ATP	α-β link	α-β link
DCCD binding site in the β (*)	GE*RTREGN	GNDXYHE*M
nonspecific agents	denatured	resistant
F_1-ATP synthesis from F_1-ADP-Pi		
without proton gradient	yes (CF_1, MF_1)	yes
Energization of FoF_1-liposomes		
ΔpH by acid-base transition	narrow ΔpH	wide ΔpH
$\Delta\Psi$ by high salt gradient	inactive	effective
$\Delta\Psi$ by external electric pulses	possible	possible
Genetic analysis		
nonspecific ts-mutation	inactivated	resistant
DNA sequencing of FoF_1 gene	EF_1, CF_1	in progress

For details, refer to (2). Subunit organization (3, 4), nucleotide-binding and metal-binding (6) and stereochemistry (8) of TF_1 are described previously.

THE MINIMUM ACTIVE COMPLEXES: $\alpha_3\beta_3\gamma$ AND $\alpha_3\beta_3\delta$

A solution of TF_1 (0.1 mg/1% trifluoroacetic acid) was chromatographed on a BioRad HiPore(C4) column with a Waters model 204 high performance liquid chromatography by eluting with solvents containing 0.1 % trifluoroacetic acid and 0 - 95 % acetonitrile at the flow rate of 1 ml/min. Proteins were monitored by the UV absorbance and the fractions were dried under the reduced pressure. The purity of each protein fraction was confirmed by polyacrilamide gel electrophoresis (PAGE) in the presence and absence of sodium dodecylsulfate (SDS). The dried pure subunits were dissolved in a solution containing 50 mM Tris-Cl (pH 7.3), 8 M urea and 2 mM $MgSO_4$, and dialyzed overnight against above buffer without urea at 40° C. ATPase activity was restored in the mixtures of $\alpha+\beta$ $+\gamma$ and $\alpha+\beta$ $+\delta$. Although weak interaction between α and β was confirmed, no ATPase activity was detected in the mixture lacking γ or δ. In order to exclude the possibility that ATPase activity of $\alpha+\beta+\delta$ was due to contaminations by the γ subunit, PAGE in the absence (Fig. 1) and presence (Fig. 2) of SDS were performed. In contrast to the $\alpha\beta\gamma$ complex, the $\alpha\beta\delta$ complex was heat labile, more active in alkali, and resistant to NaN_3. The staining intensities of each subunit after the SDS-PAGE, and UV absorption of each subunit during the liquid chromatography of isolated $\alpha+\beta+\gamma$ and $\alpha+\beta+\delta$ complexes suggested that the subunit stoichiometries were $\alpha_3\beta_3\gamma$ and $\alpha_3\beta_3\delta$, respectively. This is consistent with the subunit stoichiometry of TF_1 confirmed by ultracenrifugation (3), neutron scattering and small angle X-ray scattering (4). DNA sequencing of EF_1 already revealed that there is no repeating structure both in the γ and δ subunits (5), and thus these small subunits are connected to only one or two major subunits at one binding domain. The minor subunit must induce an asymmetric structure in the complex. It is interesting that the 1:1:1 TF_1-ADP-Mg complex which is also assymetric, was easily isolated (6). The strong negative cooperativity in nucleotide binding to TF_1 may be caused by the association of the γ or δ.

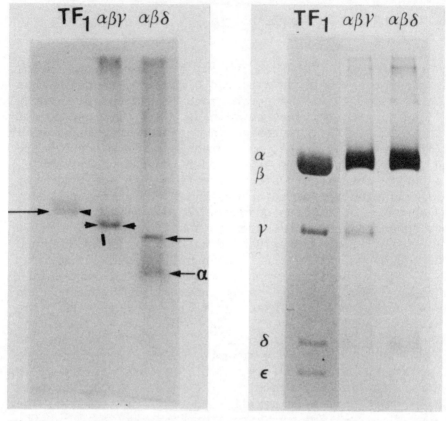

Fig. 1. PAGE of oligomers.   Fig. 2. SDS PAGE of subunit.

ACID-BASE CLUSTER HYPOTHESIS OF PROTON MOTIVE ATP-RELEASE

The formation of enzyme-bound ATP from ADP-Mg-Pi-TF$_1$,
without proton gradient suggested that the real energy
requiring step of ATP synthesis is the release of ATP-Mg
from F$_1$ (reviewed in ref. 2). There must be some device
in FoF which receives protons and changes the conformation of Rossmann fold at the interface of the α-β subunits (α-β cross-linking with 3'-arylazido-8-azido-ATP).
The acid-base cluster hypothesis was proposed (7), on
the basis of 3H$^+$/ATP stoichiometry, and the fact that

protons are transmitted through acid-base residues in a narrow area of FoF$_1$ junction, where potential gradient across the membrane is intensified. The conformation of acid-base cluster may respond to the proton flux, because CD spectra of a mixture of poly-Glu and poly-Lys were changed by pH shift in neutral range. The acid-base cluster selectively allows the passage of protons.

For the stereochemical analyses of F$_1$ reaction, TFoF$_1$ is suitable, because it does not contain tightly bound Mg^{2+} and nucleotides, and is active in Cd. The true substrate of F$_1$ was shown to be Δ,β,γ, bidentate ATP-Mg using Cd^{2+}- and Mg^{2+}- dependent diastereoisomer preference of TF$_1$(8). This result excluded the possibility of release of ATP-Mg (negatively charged) from F$_1$ by direct action of $\Delta\Psi$. Although ATPγS has been used to analyze the stereochemical course of ATPase reactions, it does not induce contraction of actomyosin. However ATPγS is a good substrate for TFoF$_1$ -liposome to translocate protons. The product of isotopically labeled (Rp) ATPγS was inverted [^{16}O, ^{17}O,^{18}O] thiophosphate (8). This result confirmed that ATP synthesis proceeds via in-line nucleo-philic displacement (SN2) and denied that the protons act directly on Pi to form metaphosphate (racemization, SN1).

The chemical modifications of one of the acid and base residues (Glu, Arg or Tyr) in the c subunit of TFo, abolished H$^+$ -translocating activity (2). Moreover, on specific removal of acid-base clusters in the b subunit, ATP-driven H$^+$-translocation was lost without impairment of passive H$^+$ -translocation or the F$_1$ binding capacity. Many of mutants defective in the acid-base clusters of FoF$_1$ were found to have lost H$^+$-translocation.

The FoF$_1$-liposomes were locally energized by imposing the external electric field (2). As shown by Witt, adenine nucleotides were released from F$_1$ by the electric pulses. In order to test the release of protons directly from TF$_1$, ion sensitive field effect transistors coated with organosilicate was improved. A novel, stable FoF$_1$ genetically modified for this purpose may be useful. DNA of thermophiles was found to be extremely rich in G+C, especially in the third position of the codon (9). The DNA of thermophilic FoF is now being sequenced with M13.

REFERENCES

1. Kagawa, Y. (1972). Reconstitution of oxidative phosphorylation. Biochim. Biophys. Acta 265, 297-338.
2. Kagawa, Y. (1984). Proton motive ATP synthesis. In: New Comprehensive Biochemistry, Bioenergetics, Ernster, L. (ed.). Elsevier Science Publishers, B.V., Amsterdam, pp. 149-186.
3. Yoshida, M., Sone, N., Hirata, H., Kagawa, Y. and Ui, N. (1979). Subunit structure of adenosine triphosphatase: comparison of the structure in thermophilic bacterium PS3 with those in mitochondria, chloroplasts and Escherichia coli. J. Biol. Chem. 254, 9525-9533.
4. Furuno, T., Ikegami, A., Kihara, H., Yoshida, M. and Kagawa, Y. (1983). Small-angle X-ray scattering study of adenosine triphosphatase from thermophilic bacterium PS3. J. Mol. Biol. 170, 137-153.
5. Kanazawa, H. and Futai, M. (1982). Structure and function of H^+-ATPase: what we have learned from Escherichia coli H^+-ATPase. Ann. N.Y. Acad Sci. 402, 45-64.
6. Yoshida, M. and Allison, W. S. (1983). Modulation by ADP and Mg of the inactivation of the F -ATPase from thermophilic bacterium PS3 with dicyclohexyl-carbodiimide. J. Biol. Chem. 258, 14407-14412.
7. Kagawa, Y. (1984). A new model of proton motive ATP synthesis: Acid-base cluster hypothesis. J. Biochem. 95, 295-298.
8. Senter, P., Eckstein, F. and Kagawa, Y. (1983). Substrate metal-adenosine 5'-triphosphate chelate structure and stereochemical course of reaction catalyzed by the adenosinetriphosphatase from the thermophilic bacterium PS3. Biochemistry 22, 5514-5518.
9. Kagawa, Y., Nojima, H., Nukiwa, N., Ishizuka, M., Nakajima, T., Yasuhara, T., Tanaka, T. and Oshima, T. (1984). High Guanine plus Cytosine content in the third letter of codons of an extreme thermophile. J. Biol. Chem. 259, 2956-2960.

MEMBRANE PROTEINS AS LIGHT ENERGY TRANSDUCERS

YURI A.OVCHINNIKOV

Shemyakin Institute of Bioorganic Chemistry, USSR Academy
of Sciences, ul. Vavilova 32, 117988 Moscow V-334, USSR

INTRODUCTION

Knowledge of the molecular mechanism of photoreception is
a key problem in the study of the visual process as a
whole. Rhodopsin, a basic protein component of disk membranes from outer segments of rods from the vertebrate
retina, plays a substantial role in photoreception initiating the visual perception. Therefore structure-functional investigations of rhodopsin are essential for
understanding physicochemical processes of vision.
Of much significance is the mechanism of light energy
transformation from the rhodopsin molecule which absorbed
light quanta to a cytoplasmic membrane and further to the
synaptic ending of the cell, viz. mechanism of photoreception.
Nowadays two possible mechanisms of the process are discussed, each suggests a mediator that regulates the
degree of polarization of the plasmic membrane. According
to the first the rhodopsin molecule participates in the
regulation of enzymic complex, controlling the amount of
cyclic nucleotide (c GMP) in cytoplasm. The second provides release of Ca^{2+} ions from the intradisk space (1).
Despite their ambiguity both the mechanisms propose considerable photoinduced conformational rearrangements in
the protein molecule. Obviously, molecular organization
of rhodopsin in the membrane might shed light on the interaction with the enzymic complex as well as the formation of transmembrane ion channel. That explains a keen
interest in deciphering of the rhodopsin primary structure and elucidation of peculiarities of its polypeptide
chain arrangement in the membrane.
Until recently rhodopsin was the only known light-trans-
ducing protein using retinal as a chromophore. The un-

Proceedings of the 16th FEBS Congress
Part B, pp. 265–278
© 1985 VNU Science Press

expected discovery, seemingly bearing no direct relation to visual excitation, gave a new impetus to these investigations (2).

Halophilic microorganisms of the *Halobacterium* family utilize the solar radiation energy due to the presence of bacteriorhodopsin, a light-driven primary proton translocase. Bacteriorhodopsin is a relatively small protein (about 250 amino acid residues) containing protonated aldimine of the retinal as a prosthetic group. In the cell membrane bacteriorhodopsin is concentrated in patches of *ca.* 0.5 μ, called purple membranes. Purple membranes are two-dimensional quasicrystals formed by hexagonally packed protein trimers, the space between them being filled with lipid molecules. Each working cycle of bacteriorhodopsin induced by the light quantum absorption is accompanied with transfer of at least one proton across the membrane, the retinal aldimine is reversibly deprotonated in the course of this cycle, as judged from spectral data. Bacteriorhodopsin makes up 75% of the total weight of the purple membrane, the remainder being a special set of phospholipids. By electron microscopic and diffraction methods Henderson and Unwin determined the three-dimensional structure of bacteriorhodopsin to a resolution of 7 Å within the membrane plane and about 14 Å perpendicular to the plane (3). According to these data the bacteriorhodopsin molecule consists of seven roughly parallel segments each spanning the membrane. Unwin and Henderson's three-dimensional model of bacteriorhodopsin left unresolved the question of the actual build up of its active site and arrangement of functional groups in the molecule.

RESULTS AND DISCUSSION

Our interest was focused on chemical and biochemical aspects of this unique membrane protein. No, doubt, such studies are necessary not only for elucidation of the mechanism of proton translocation by bacteriorhodopsin but also for understanding the dynamics of functioning of even more complex light energy transducing membrane proteins - visual pigments, halorhodopsin, etc.

A recent review from this laboratory (4) presents data concerning the structural basis for bacteriorhodopsin and rhodopsin function. A model which correlates the bacteriorhodopsin amino acid sequence and three-dimensional structure was elaborated. α-Helical rods appeared to have their hydrophobic sites facing the nonpolar lipid moiety, whereas more hydrophilic portions are in the molecule interior.

Comparison of the properties of native bacteriorhodopsin and bacteriorhodopsin with modified dimethylated lysine residues proves that retinal does not change its attachment site (Lys-216) during the photocycle, proton translocation and light-dark adaptation. Furthermore, ε-amino groups of the lysine residue do not play a key role in the coordinated pathway of proton translocation (5).

As judged from fluorescence, UV and CD data the chromophore is located 9 Å from the membrane surface. That was documented by retinal fluorescence quenching by lanthanide and Co^{++} ions as well as by the analysis of energy transfer between the retinyl of retinyliden moieties and 4-sulfophenylazo group at modified Tyr-64 or Tyr (NH_2)-64 side chain, respectively.

This paper summarizes recent advances in bacteriorhodopsin and rhodopsin studies.

The three dimensional picture of bacteriorhodopsin at atomic resolution will hopefully emerge from X-ray cristallography data. Leaving this for cristallographers we started a detailed immunological investigation of bacteriorhodopsin which proved to be useful in studying orientation and surface topology of the protein. Khorana et al. used this approach to identify distinct antibody binding sites on the cytoplasmic surface of bacteriorhodopsin (6) that allowed identification of a peptide loop between α-helical segments 3 and 4 and confirmation of the cytoplasmic location of the exposed C-terminal tail. In the course of immunological studies we obtained five hybridomas producing monoclonal antibodies to different membrane exposed parts of the polypeptide chain. Specificity of these antibodies was established using modified derivatives of bacteriorhodopsin and a number of overlapping peptides, derived from enzymatic or chemical cleavages of the protein.

The antigenic determinants are situated on the following exposed parts of bacteriorhodopsin Glu^1-Glu^9 with three N-terminal amino acids; Gly^{35}-Met^{56}, including Asp^{36} and/or Asp^{38} and Phe^{42}; Phe^{156}-Met^{163}, with Phe^{156}; Glu^{194}-Leu^{207}, including residue Glu^{194}; Pro^{200}-Leu^{207}. Thus bacteriorhodopsin fragments 4-65 and 156-231 have membrane exposed peptide regions. All the data, experimentally obtained and earlier available, concerning the membrane location of fragments 66-72 and 231-248, evidence that each of the sequence 4-65 and 156-231 traverses the membrane at least two times (Fig. 1).

Of even more importance is accessibility of Glu 194 to a monoclonal antibody. Upon the study of the chromophore orientation in bacteriorhodopsin by cross-linking using the photosensitive n-diaziridinophenyl analogue of reti-

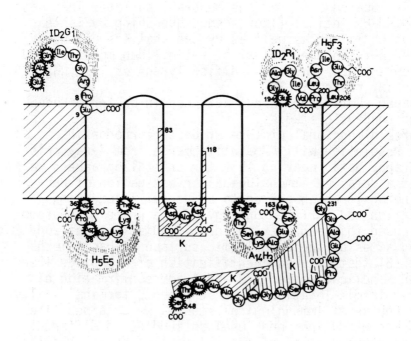

Fig. 1. Antigenic determinants of bacteriorhodopsin.

nal Ser[193] and Glu[194] were shown to be the sites of cross-linking with the diaziridine group located at the phenyl ring (7). Based on this finding a structural model with Glu[194] well in the membrane was put forward. Our result, on the contrary, proves that this residue, being a part of an antigenic determinant, should be located on the membrane surface. Obviously, only further studies will establish the real topography of bacteriorhodopsin and its chromophore in the membrane.

A charge movement and proton translocation across the purple membrane were investigated by various techniques. Upon comparing the kinetics of spectral, electrical and pH responses of bacteriorhodopsin induced by a 3 nanosecond laser flash the correlation was found between formation of the M 412 intermediate as well as proton extrusion and the microsecond stage of electrical potential generation. As to the M 412 decay and proton uptake, they correlate with the millisecond stage of the potential generation. The ratio of micro- and millisecond stages suggests that the outward proton conducting path is about four times shorther than the inward one.

Chemical enzymatic modification of the bacteriorhodopsin protein moiety can give important structure-functional information. As found removal of the C-terminal 17 amino acid residues did not affect efficiency of the proton transport in bacteriorhodopsin (8). However, according to the latest results the light induced proton release decreases by 50-70% in such preparations without affecting a photocycle. The data now available confirm our finding that removal of the C-terminal tail influences neither the rate nor the efficiency of the proton transport. An apparent decrease in the efficiency is due to aggregation of the protease treated membrane sheets, the effect being completely prevented by a detergent (9).

Bacteriorhodopsin reconstituted into artifical lipids is a useful model to study many chemical and biochemical aspects of proton translocation in membrane systems, to understand the principles of their denaturation and renaturation. The complete delipidation and reconstitution of the proton pumping activity were achieved in a pioneering work of Khorana (10-11). The completely delipidated bac-

teriorhodopsin was obtained by chromatography of a protein
sample solubilized in Triton X 100 on Biogel. The delipidated protein retained its spectral integrity. The vesicles
obtained from this preparation by adding different lipids
manifested the proton pumping activity. Rather important
were the experiments which demonstrated reconstitution of
the proton pumping activity from two separate and completely denaturated chymotryptic fragments of bacteriorhodopsin (12). These studies opened the way for purposeful
experiments which shed light on the structure functional
relashionships in bacteriorhodopsin. To clarify a possible role of each bacteriorhodopsin fragment the attemps
are made to obtain a hybrid system by exchanging the
fragments of bacteriorhodopsin and rhodopsin in reconstitution experiments.
Along with these studies we started an investigation into
the genetics of halobacteria searching for new ways to
approach the mechanism of the proton translocation.
Bacterioopsin genes were cloned in E. coli using pBr 322
as a vector plasmid. It made possible:
1) investigation of the gene structure and the nature of
gene-inactivating mutations;
2) creation of a basis for producing mutant bacteriorhodopsin by site-directed mutagenesis of the cloned gene;
3) investigation of a possibility for replication and
expression of H. halobium genetic material in E. coli
connected with fundamental problems of genetic engineering, as halobacterial DNA is far more alien to E. coli
enzymatic machinery than, say, human DNA;
4) investigation of prospects for production of such a
hydrophobic and unusual membrane protein as bacterioopsin
by E. coli cells.
Data on the primary structure of the wild type bacterioopsin gene obtained in our laboratory are consistent with
those published earlier by the Khorana group.
We found out that genes isolated bacterioopsin-deficient
strains contain inserts within its coding sequences. In
the case of H. halobium strain R1mR the bacterioopsin
gene contains an insert of 500 base pairs long. An insert
in the S1 strain is about 1700 base pairs long. The inserts are called ISH2 and ISH S1.
Primary structures of inserts ISH S1 and ISH2 were deter-

mined together with structures of surrounding opsin gene regions. In both cases there is a duplication of short stretches of opsin gene DNA at the element insertion site. These regions are represented only once in the wild type gene. Moreover, there are inverted nucleotide repeats at the ISH2 and ISH S1 termini. Both mentioned features are characteristic of a majority of known transposable elements in both prokariotes and eukaryotes.

The similar studies were simultaneously carried out by G.H.Khorana et al. Two insetion elements from bacterioopsin-deficient mutants were also found. The element from the R1mR strain is identical to the ISH2 element discovered by Khorana. We call our element ISH2. To avoid misunderstanding it should be noted that ISH S1 is another transposable element in halobacteria. The data accumulated clearly show that high frequency mutations in halobacteria are mediated in general by such transposable elements. Several recombinant plasmids were constructed to achieve the expression of bacterioopsin in E. coli.

To detect the level of expression we decided to exploit the well known fact that β-galactosidase of E. coli forms enzymatically functional hybrids if its several N-terminal amino acids are exchanged for some other polypeptide. It is easy to test expression of any forgeign protein in E. coli if its C-terminal part is fused to the gene coding β-galactosidase with a several N-terminal codons cut off. Such a hybrid gene placed under promoter control programs a synthesis of the hybrid protein possessing galactosidase activity and containing the polypeptide chain of the foreign protein of interest.

So, we fused the bacterioopsin gene to the lac Z gene (gene of β-galactosidase) and placed this hybrid gene downstream of the E. coli tryptophan promoter containing also the ribosome-binding site. This plasmid POG contains the full bacterioopsin gene. It means that this gene encodes an opsin precursor which is 13 amino acids longer than the mature opsin. Judging by β-galactosidase activity the level of expression was rather low.

So, we removed the signal peptide and changed the system of expression regulation. The POG 1 plasmid was reconstructed in a following way. The precursor region of opsin gene was removed and a strong promoter of phage λ 179 containing its own ribosome-binding site and initiating ATG-codon was placed upstream of the gene. High galactosidase activity implies a high level of hybrid protein expression (up to 1% to total cellular protein). The investigation into site-directed mutagenesis of bacterioopsin gene aiming at the production of mutated bacterioopsin and their functional investigations was started.

The nearer we are to understanding of the mechanism of bacteriorhodopsin functioning, the more surprising questions are posed whose solution requires new efforts and novel approaches.

Now let us see how can new ideas and experimental methods, created in the rapidly developing studies of bacteriorhodopsin, be applied to its analogue visual pigment-rhodopsin.

We determined the complete amino acid sequence of rhodopsin and showed that the polypeptide chain of the protein consists of 348 amino acid residues (4). Related results were obtained recently in the USA (13) by sequencing a structural gene of bovine rhodopsin. Nucleotide sequence analysis of the cloned DNA provided an intron-exon map of the gene. The mRNA homologous sequences in the 6.4 Kilobase gene is composed of the 96 base pairs, 5 untranslated regions, 1044 base pair coding region, and surprisingly long ~1400 base pair 3' untranslated region; they are divided into five exons by four introns that interrupt the coding region.

According to our data the characteristic feature of the amino acid sequence of the rhodopsin is the presence of extended regions of the polypeptide chain made up of nonpolar amino acid residues interrupted with comparatively small sites of polar residues. These hydrophobic extended regions compose the membrane part of the protein molecule.

The primary structure of rhodopsin was a basis for elucidation of the arrangement of the polypeptide chain in the membrane. The model building demands the combination of two approaches: a) analysis of the regions of the protein polypeptide chain located in the aqueous phase and accessible to the action of proteolytic enzymes;
b) localization of the protein molecule regions containing the least number of polar amino acid residues and

capable of spanning the lipid bilayer. Besides, two considerations are taken into account. First, membrane regions of the molecule have α-helical conformation and are situated perpendiculary to the membrane plane; secondly, the N- and C-terminal regions of rhodopsin are located on opposite sides of the membrane and, consequently, the polypeptide chain of the protein molecule should traverse the membrane uneven number of times. Now let us follow the path of the polypeptide chain in the membrane. Thirty amino acid residues in the N-terminal region of the protein molecule are accessible to the action of various proteolytic enzymes upon the treatment of inside-out photoreceptor disks. Consequently, the N-terminal region of 30 amino acid residues is localized in the intradisk space. The region accessible to the chymotrypsin action was identified on the outer surface of photoreceptor disks (residues Phe 146 - Arg 147). The region of 27 amino acid residues of the polypeptide chain in the α-helical conformation can traverse the lipid bilayer of the membrane (to span the entire membrane width 26-30 residues are necessary). Taking this finding into account in the analysis of distribution of polar and nonpolar residues of the polypeptide chain between two regions of proteinolysis (Tyr 30 - Phe 146), we identified three membrane segments separated with two small clusters of hydrophilic residues (regions 62-73 and 92-101). Consequently, regions Tyr 30 - Phe 146 of the polypeptide chain traverses the photoreceptor membrane three times. The region accessible to the papain action (Ser 186 - Cys 187) is located on the intradisk membrane surface. Apparently, the region of 40 amino acid residues can span the membrane only once; it contains membrane segment Ile 154 - Ser 176.

On the outer surface of photoreceptor disks there is rather extended region Gln 236 - Lys 245 accessible to the action of different enzymes. Since this region and the papain accessible one are on different membrane surfaces the polypeptide chain site between them (55 amino acid residues) spans the membrane uneven number of times. This region appeared to contain the only membrane segment (Phe 203 - Phe 228).

The C-terminal region of rhodopsin, is situated on the

outer disk surface, as is region Gln 236 - Lys 245. Consequently, the polypeptide chain part connecting these two regions traverses the membrane even number of times. At the study of distribution of polar and nonpolar amino acid residues of this part of the protein molecule (75 residues) two membrane segments (Met 253 - Phe 276 and Phe 283 - Met 309) were identified.

Thus seven segments of the polypeptide chain in the α-helical conformation, spanning the photoreceptor membrane width, compose the membrane moiety of the rhodopsin molecule. The N- and C-terminal regions are the largest sites exposed into the water phase.

There are three functionally important domains in the rhodopsin molecule: retinal-binding site, C-terminal region and polypeptide region connecting the V and VI membrane segments.

As retinal has the absorption maximum at about 380 nm, and rhodopsin - 498 nm, for such considerable bathochromic shift (120 nm) the charged groups should be incorporated into the retinal binding site. Besides, spectral investigations show that the Trp residue should be located in the active site of retinal. Lys 296, responsible for the retinal binding, is located in the VII segment in the middle of the lipid bilayer in accord with data obtained at the study of the energy transfer between the chromophore and terbium ions. Noteworthy Ala precedes the retinal binding Lys residue, in all the studied retinal binding proteins. The absence of the three dimensional model of the rhodopsin arrangement precludes localization of other amino acid residues in the active site of the protein. As known retinal is located at the 16-23⁰ angle to the membrane plane, i.e. almost parallelly to its surface. Upon studying various chromophore analogs the length of the retinal binding region was established to be 10.1-10.9 Å. The β-ionone ring of retinal, or at least its two methyl groups, are extremely important for the prosthetic group binding.

The study of the model compounds shows that bathochromic shift (120 nm) is possible if a carboxyl group of aspartic of glutamic acids is at the distance of 3 Å from the protonated Schiff base. The second negative charge should be localized within the region of double bond $C(II)-C(12)$

in the chromophore polyene chain. According to the propose model three negatively charged amino acid residues
Asp 83, Glu 113, Gln 122 are in the lipid matrix of the
photoreceptor membrane, one or two of them can regulate
the bathochromic shift of the visual pigment at the interaction with its chromophore. In addition, negatively
charged amino acid residues, such as Glu 134 or Glu 150,
located in the vicinity of the membrane surface, can be
included in the retinal binding site.
According to the model of the rhodopsin polypeptide chain
arrangement, four of five Trp residues (positions 126,
161, 175 and 265) are in the lipid matrix of the photoreceptor membrane.
Each of them can be involved in the active site of the
protein, however, Trp 265 located in the VI segment in
the vicinity of the aldimine bond seems to be the most
probable.
The active site of the protein includes the His residue,
its imidazole ring can be involved in the proton transfer
upon the rhodopsin functioning. In the lipid matrix of
the membrane the only residue, His 211, is situated. The
data on the tertiary rhodopsin structure, chemical modification of the protein, application of the photoaffinity
retinal analog provide detailed information on the retinal binding region of the visual pigment.
The second functionally important rhodopsin domain is the
C-terminal protein region exposed into the water phase.
This region of the polypeptide chain is phosphorylated
that results in inhibition of the action of the photolysed molecule of the visual pigment (see below). Determination of the primary structure of the C-terminal region
revealed seven possible sites of kinase action.
There exist data on participation of the C-terminal domain in formation of its complex with GTPase; except for
the finding that cleavage of the 12 membered peptide at
the short time thermolysine action (region Val 337 -
Ala 348) does not change the pigment-enzyme binding.
The C-terminal region of rhodopsin contains three of ten
Cys residues (positions 316, 322, and 323). Cys 316 is
accessible to the action of SH-blocking reagents upon the
treatment of the native protein in the photoreceptor membrane, whereas residues Cys 322 and Cys 323 are not modi-

fied even after the pigment bleaching. The study of the chemistry of rhodopsin sulfhydryl groups by covalent chromatography on the basis of thiol-disulfide exchange shows that after immobilization of the protein with reduced disulfide bonds and cyanogen bromide cleavage C-terminal fragment (containing residues Cys 322 and Cys 325) is covalently bound to the carrier. If disulfide bonds are not reduced, cyanogen bromide fragment forms no covalent bond with the carrier. Being isolated and incubated with dithiotreitol this peptide is capable of immobilization. The data obtained indicate the presence of the disulfide bond between residues Cys 322 and Cys 323 in the T-terminal region of the rhodopsin molecule. The study of the fragment by the resonance Raman spectroscopy in the region of the S - S valence vibrations supports this. That is the first case of discovering the disulfide bond between the adjucent Cys residues in the naturally occurring sample, since such a bond was found only in synthetic peptides.

Though the disulfide bond does not change upon the rhodopsin bleaching, its participation in the thiol-disulfide exchange when forming the pigment-GTPase complex is possible, as, for example, the receptor-insulin complex. Modification of GTPase with SH-blocking reagents precludes formation of the photolysed pigment - enzyme complex (the α-subunit of GTPase is modified).

The third functionally important domain is the polypeptide chain region connecting the V and VI membrane segments. Apparently, it participates in complex formation with GTPase, since at the thermolysin cleavage of this region into two membrane-bound fragments the photoreceptor disks considerably decrease its ability to the enzyme binding.

As mentioned above the C-terminal region of rhodopsin contains seven potential sites for the kinase action. However, 9 moles of Pi can be included into I mole of the protein upon its bleaching. One more region site of the kinase action is probably located on the polypeptide chain between the V and VI membrane segment containing three possible sites of the enzyme action, Ser 240, Thr 242, and Thr 243. If so, incorporation of two phos-

phate groups in this region after the pigment illumination may regulates the complex formation of photolysed
rhodopsin with GTPase.
Data available suggest that these peptide fragments provide interaction of photoexcited rhodopsin with the amplifier protein, GTPase (14). New structural information allowed us to start a detailed investigation of both rhodopsin and the protein components of a signal transducing
system. Our experiments were primarily aimed at the probing of the functional group located at the cytoplasmic
surface of rhodopsin and most probably involved in binding of the protein. Simultaneously we undertook the
study of the primary structure of GTPase subunits.
As the first step we determined the amino acid sequence
of the γ-subunit of GTPase. It consists of 69 amino acid
residues. Noteworthy there are two cystein residues in
positions 35 and 36.
The presence of a disulfide bridge in the C-terminal rhodopsin fragment and two adjacent Cys residues in the γ-
subunit of GTPase gives an idea that these groups provide
GTPase the activation via the thioldisulfide exchange
reaction.
There are still many questions to be answered and we hope
that a comparative study of bacteriorhodopsin and rhodopsin will stimulate further research of these and other
photosensitive proteins, and may help elucidate mechanisms
of light transduction.

REFERENCES

Uhe, R., Abrahamson, E.W. (1981) Chem. Rev. 81, 291-312.

Oesterhelt, D., Stoeckenius, W. (1971). Nature (New Biol.)
   233, 149-556.

Henderson, R., Unwin, P.N.T. (1975). Nature, 257, 28-32.

Ovchinnikov, Yu.A. (1980). FEBS Lett. 148, 179-191.

Abdulaev, N.G., Dencher, N.A., Dergachev, A.E., Fahr, A., Kiselev, A.V. (1984). Biophys. Struct. Mech. 10, 211-227.

Kimura, R., Mason, T.L., Khorana, H.G. (1982). J. Biol. Chem. 257, 2859-2867.

Huang, K.S., Radhakrishnam, R., Bayley, H., Khorana, H.G. (1982). J. Biol. Chem. 257, 13616-13623.

Abdulaev, N.G., Feigina, M.Yu., Kiselev, A.V., Ovchinni-kov, Yu.A., Drachev, L.A., Kaulen, A.D., Khitrina, L.V., Skulachev, V.P. (1978). FEBS Lett. 90, 190-194.

Ovchinnikov, Yu.A. (1984). Abstracts of 16th FEBS Meeting, Moscow, p. 65.

London, E., Khorana H.G. (1982). J. Biol. Chem. 257, 7003-7011.

Huang, K.S., Bayley, H., Liao, M.J., London, E., Khora-na, H.G. (1981). J. Biol. Chem. 256, 3802-3809.

Liao, M.-J., London, E., Khorana, H.G. (1983). J. Biol. Chem. 258, 9949-9955.

Nathans, J., Hoggnes, D. (1984). Cell, 34, 807-814.

Stryer, L., Hurley, J.B., Fung, K.-K. (1981). Trends in Biochem. Sci. 6, 245-247.

THE ELECTROGENIC Na$^+$, D-GLUCOSE COTRANSPORTER: ISOLATION AND FIRST INSIGHT IN ITS MODE OF FUNCTION:

GIORGIO SEMENZA
Laboratorium für Biochemie der Eidgenössischen Technischen Hochschule, ETH-Zentrum, Universitätstr. 16, CH 8092 Zürich/Switzerland.

Our ideas on the mode of functioning of membrane carriers have undergone a sizeable change since the "carrier" concept was originally introduced. The generally accepted (but never demonstrated) "diffusive" or "rotative" mode of operation at one time derived support from the work on some model compounds, particularly on valinomycin. Now, only a few years later, however, it becomes clear that, since the carriers of natural membranes are intrinsic proteins, they are to be expected to insert vectorially into the membranes at the time of (or immediately after) their synthesis. As they must have both hydrophilic and hydrophobic areas on their surface, they can hardly be expected to tumble over (to "rotate") at any appreciable rate.

This does not mean, however, that within the membrane protein operating as "carrier" a portion should not move concomitantly with, and related to, substrate transport (we will define operationally this portion as the "gate"). Only the existence of this kind of movement can adequately account for the well known features of carrier kinetics, in particular of counterflow - and it is only fair to say that, whatever the mechanical models used, the definition of "carrier" has always been functional, i.e. kinetic in nature. Perhaps the best definition of "carrier" is that of a transport agency which can expose its substrate binding site(s) to both sides of the membrane alternatively, but never simultaneously; "carrier" being thus a special type of (gated) "channel" or "pore" (1).

Proceedings of the 16th FEBS Congress
Part B, pp. 279-289
© 1985 VNU Science Press

The small-intestinal Na^+-D-glucose cotransporter is asymmetric with respect to the plane of the membrane in both its chemical (2-4) and functional (5) properties. This stable asymmetry thus effectively rules out "diffusive" or "rotative" modes of operration in the case of this transporter also, and makes an asymmetric channel (or pore) most likely. Its binding sites for Na^+ and for the sugar are more easily accessible from the cytosolic side than from the luminal side (5,6).

Since the Na^+, D-glucose cotransporter has the kinetic properties of a "carrier" notably that of showing the counterflow phenomenon, it must have a mobile portion (a "gate", see above). Some knowledge of some property of this gate is necessary, if a plausible model of the mode of operation of this "asymmetric gated channel" is to be constructed.

THE "GATE" BEARS A NEGATIVE CHARGE OF 1 OR 2 ($z=-1$ or $z=-2$).

This conclusion is based on the following experimental observations:
(i) $\Delta\psi$-dependence of transinhibition. It can be shown that in an electrogenic cation-dependent cotransport system the extent of transinhibition by the "substrate$_{in}$" or by Na^+_{in} is affected by $\Delta\psi$ (negative at the trans side). One can conclude that independently of the degree of asymmetry of the cotransporter and of the Na^+:substrate stoichiometric ratio, a negative $\Delta\psi$ leads to a decreased trans-inhibition, if the mobile part of the (unloaded) cotransporter carries one or two negative charges, but to an increased transinhibition of this mobile part is electrically neutral. In actual fact, the transinhibition by D-glucose$_{in}$ follows the prediction of the models with $z=-1$ or $z=-2$, and is not compatible with model with $z=0$. We conclude that the "gate" of the translocator bears, in the substrate-

free form at least one negative charge (5).

(ii) Lack of effect of $\Delta\psi \ll 0$ on the rate of dissociation of phlorizin from the cotransporter. If the gate carries a negative charge of 1 and the Na^+: phlorizin stoichiometry of binding is one (which is made likely by the $\bar{n}$ coefficient being equal to one, for the intestinal (6) and for the renal cotransporter (7)) the ternary complex (phlorizin-Na^+-cotransporter$^-$) is electrically neutral and the rate of phlorizin dissociation should not be affected by $\Delta\psi \ll 0$. This is indeed the case for both the intestinal(6) and the renal (7) cotransporter. (Fig. 1).

Furthermore, the apparent K_m-values for D-glucose uptake are independent of the pH in the 6.5-9.5 range; at lower pH the apparent K_m increases sharply (8). It is quite possible, therefore, that the negative charge in the "gate" or elsewhere in one of the sites binding either substrates is a carboxylate group. This conclusion would also agree with recent observations by Weber and Semenza (1984 unpublished) that D-glucose transport is inhibited irreversibly by dicyclohexenylcarbodiimide.

Summing up the considerations above, a negatively charged gated channel (or pore) with substrate binding sites more easily accessible (at $\Delta\psi \sim 0$) from the cytosolic than from the extracellular side is the most likely model for the small-intestinal Na^+, glucose cotransporter. In addition, kinetic analysis shows that the only partially occupied forms of the cotransporter (say, only loaded with either Na^+ or D-glucose) have very small translocation probabilities as compared with those of the empty or the fully occupied cotransporter. Also, (Iso) Ping Pong mechanisms can be ruled out (5).

A PLAUSIBLE MECHANISTIC MODEL (Ref. 5).

The large quantitative difference in the kinetic

properties of the Na^+,glucose cotransporter at $\Delta\psi \sim 0$ as compared at $\Delta\psi <<0$ show that it exists in two forms (or families of forms), the one prevailing at $\Delta\psi \sim 0$ (i.e., Form I, Fig. 2) and the other one (the "energized" form) prevailing at $\Delta\psi <<0$ (Forms II through IV, Fig. 2).

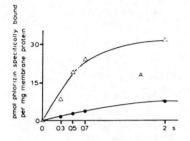 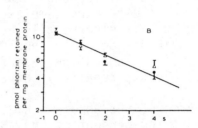

Fig. 1 Time course of phlorizin binding (A) and release (B) in the presence of an initial (out>in) gradient of NaSCN (Δ) or sodium cyclamate (●). In A, specific phlorizin binding (phlorizin 10µM, pH 6.5; a 100 mM out, 0 in gradient of either NaSCN or sodium cyclamate) was obtained as the difference in binding in the presence of 25 mM D-fructose minus that in the presence of 25 mM D-glucose. In B, the vesicles were first pre-equilibrated in 100 mM sodium cyclamate, pH 6.5. At time -1s phlorizin (10µM) was added and a choline SCN gradient (100 out, 0 in) was established. At time zero the vesicle suspension was diluted 50 times in either 100 mM NaSCN (Δ) or 100 mM sodium cyclamate (●). (From ref. 6).

Each of the two (families of) forms operate as a "mobile carrier" in Läuger's (1) sense, but with different energetic profiles (and thus with at least some of the individual rate constants different) in the "translocation" events. Thermodynamically, the difference between "nonenergized" and "energized" forms is apparent in the capability of the latter (but absent in the former) of producing accumulation of substrates starting from inital $(Na^+)_{in} = (Na^+)_{out}$ and $(Glc)_{in} = (Glc)_{out}$.

Even at the cost of stating the obvious we want to emphasize that the displacement of the substrate binding sites depicted in Fig. 2 need not imply their actual movement. Indeed a change in their

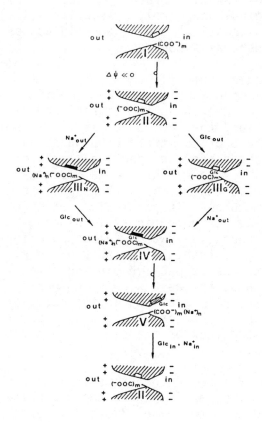

Fig. 2: A likely mode of operation of the small-intestinal Na^+, D-glucose cotransporter(s): an asymmetric gated channel (or pore) responsive to $\Delta\Psi$. The D-glucose (and phlorizin) binding site is indicated white (low affinity), or black (high affinity), or shaded (indefinite affinity). Subscript m: it is not known whether m is 1 or 2; subscript n: it is not known whether the Na^+: D-glucose flux ratio is 1 or 2. For details, see text under the original paper (5).

accessibility from either side of the membrane (which could be related with protein fluctuation) is a perfectly logical and likely possibility (1).) Accordingly, "translocation" and "change in accessibility" are used here as synonymes.

We will also assume that: (i) the "gate" is (a part of) the Na^+ binding site (the alkali cations vastly prefer O over N or S as the ligand) and, (ii) the "orientation" (or "accessibility"), as well as the affinity state of substrate binding sites must change in a concerted and identical fashion. The "gated channel (or pore)" of the Na^+, D-glucose cotransporter is asymmetric with respect to the plane of the membrane. In particular, at $\Delta\psi \sim 0$ and at low substrate concentrations all binding sites have a spontaneously inwardly directed orientation (5). In Form I, then, Na^+_{in} and D-glucose$_{in}$ each have access to the respective binding site$_{in}$ and trap the cotransporter as a slowly (or non-) translocating binary complex. This is the basis of the transinhibitions by Na^+ or by D-glucose from the "in" side and for the lack of transinhibitions from the "out"-side (5).

In the presence of a $\Delta\psi << 0$ (negative inside) the "gate" (and with it, by an ill-understood mechnism, the D-glucose binding sites also) "moves" towards the outside or is made otherwise accessible from the "out"-side (Form II).

Na^+_{out} can now bind to the gate (Form III N), which increases the affinity of the sugar binding site. The mechanism whereby the binding of Na^+ to its site affects the affinity (or, rather, the K_m) of the sugar binding site for its own substrate is still a matter of speculation. However, the drastic change in the coulombic field near the COO^--gate upon Na^+ binding and the (even if minute) reorientation of the "gate" under $\Delta\psi$ provide ample possibilities.

284

Alternatively (but less likely with poor sugar substrates), D-glucose as the first may bind to its outwardly exposed binding site (Form II), leading to Form III G. Neither Form III N nor Form III G crosses fast the membrane (or, rather, expose and liberate the lone bound substrate to the in-side).

From either Form III N or III G the "fully occu-pied" Form IV is generated, in which the gate is neutralized by Na^+, or even made positive (if the gate carries a charge of -1 and can bind 2 Na^+). This makes the gate snap back (Form V) in the "spontaneous" inwardly directed positioning (as in Form I), the more so if it is now positively charged. In Form V the binding sites (and thus the substrates) are exposed towards the inside, where they are libe-rated (we do not know in which order). Reappearance of the negative charge in the gate makes it again respond to $\Delta\psi$ and snap towards the outside (Form II). The combined effect of Na^+ would thus be that of modu-lating the function of the sugar binding site and of changing the energy profile of the channel so as to favor the exposure of the sugar binding site towards one or the other side of the membrane. An important condition for this "shoveling" mechanism to operate is that, as suggested above, the translocations (or changes in accessibility) of all substrate bin-ding sites must take place in a concerted, identi-cal fashion.

The model provides a unifying and realistic basis to at least three of the major characteristics of the small-intestinal Na^+D-glucose cotransporter: the Na^+, ($\Delta\psi$)-dependent phlorizin binding (Form III only binds phlorizin optimally, as discussed in detail by Toggenburger et al. (6)), the flux coupling between $Na^+$and D-glucose (mainly Form IV, the fully occupied complex, liberates the subs-trates at the trans side), and perhaps, most impor-tant of all, the accumulation of an unloaded com-pound (D-glucose) being driven by $\Delta\psi$, with the proviso that Na^+ is also present. It is an attempt to explain in molecular terms the phenomenon of flux coupling in secondary active transport which was put forward for the first time by Crane, Miller and Bihler in 1961 (8).

It seems likely that the mechanism depicted in Fig. 2 be common to the kindred kidney cortex Na^+, D-glucose cotransporter(s), the mobile part of which also probably bears in the free form, a negative charge of 1 (7). Also a recent, independent observation of Hilden and Sacktor (9) on the kidney cotransporter(s) fits beautifully in the mechanistic model of Fig. 2. In cortex membrane vesicles in the total absence of Na^+, $\Delta\psi$ (negative inside) promotes phlorizin binding and a (slow) uptake of D-glucose, the K_d- and K_m-values being large. This is exactly what the transition between Form I and Form II (Fig. 2) predicts: a $\Delta\psi$ (negative inside) leads to exposure of the substrates' binding sites towards the outside, leaving them, however, in the low-affinity form. In addition, Form II (when combined with D-glucose) must have a small, but detectable out-in translocation probability.

TOWARDS THE ISOLATION AND IDENTIFICATION OF THE COTRANSPORTER.

Much work and a variety of approaches have been directed towards this goal (for a review see ref. 10). Our own group using monoclonal antibodies has recently isolated and identified a 72 kDa from small-intestinal membranes (11).

A number of criteria indicate that this polypeptide is one part or a whole of the cotransporter, i.e.: (i) it interacts with monoclonal anti body directed against this membrane component:it is retained by immunoadsorbents prepared from them, (ii) it is eluted therefrom by moderate concentrations of D-glucose, (iii) it is eluted therefrom by moderate concentrations of phlorizin, (iv) it is the only band retained and eluted when digitonin-solubilizates of deoxycholate-extracted membranes are used, (v) the 72 kDa apparent molecular weight corresponds to that of a band previously shown to be specifically photolabeled by 4-azido-phlorizin (12), (vi) the 72 kDa apparent molecular weight corresponds to that previously suggested on the basis of semi-selective labeling with $HgCl_2$, or of partial negative purification (13), (vii) the low density of the 72 kDa component is compatible with the low density of the Na^+, glucose cotransporter; (viii) it is the only band showing protection by D-glucose + Na^+ against labeling by fluorescein-isothiocyanate (14).

Whether these criteria are sufficient, and whether the 72 kDa band is the sole component of the (a) cotransporter, future work will demonstrate.

ACKNOWLEDGEMENTS: The financial support of the SNSF, Berne and of Nestlé Alimentana, Vevey, is gratefully acknowledged.

REFERENCES:

1. Läuger, P. (1980) Kinetic properties of ion carriers and channels. J. Membrane Biol. 57, 163-178.

2. Klip, A., Grinstein, S. and Semenza, G. (1979). Transmembrane disposition of the phlorizin binding protein of intestinal brush borders. FEBS Lett. 99, 91-96.

3. Klip, A., Grinstein, S. and Semenza, G. (1979). Distribution of the sulfhydryl groups in in-

testinal brush border membranes. Localization
of side-chains essential for glucose transport
and phlorizin binding. Biochim. Biophys. Acta
558, 233-245.

4. Klip, A., Grinstein, S., Biber, J. and Semenza,
(1980). Interaction of the sugar carrier of
intestinal brush border membranes with $HgCl_2$.
Biochim. Biophys. Acta 598, 100-114.

5. Kessler, M. and Şemenza, G. (1983). The small-
intestinal Na^+D-glucose cotransporter: an
asymmetric gated channel (or pore) responsive
to $\Delta\psi$. J. Membr. Biol. 76, 27-56.

6. Toggenburger,. G., Kessler, M. and Semenza, G.
(1982) Phlorizin as a probe of the small-
intestinal Na^+,D-glucose cotransporter. A
model. Biochim. Biophys. Acta 688, 557-571.

7. Aronson, P.S. (1978) Energy-dependence of phlorizin binding to isolated renal microvillus
membranes. J. Membrane Biol. 42, 81-98.

8. Crane, R.K., Miller, D. and Bihler, I. (1961) The
restriction on possible mechanism of intesti-
nal active transport of sugars. In: Membrane
Transport and Metabolism. A. Kleinzeller and
A. Kotyk, eds., pp.439-449. Czech. Acad. Sci.
Press, (Prague).

9. Hilden, S. and Sacktor, B. (1982) Potential-
dependent D-glucose uptake by renal brush border membrane vesicles in the absence of sodium. Am. J. Physiol. 242, F340-F345.

10. Semenza, G., Kessler, M., Hosang, M., Weber, J.
and Schmidt, U. (1984). Biochemistry of the
Na^+, D-glucose cotransporter of the small-
intestinal brush-border membrane: the state
of art in 1984. Biochim.Biophys.Acta (in press).

11. Schmidt, U., Eddy, B., Fraser, C.M., Venter, J.C. and Semenza, G. (1983). Isolation of (a subunit of) the Na^+ D-glucose cotransporter(s) of rabbit intestinal brush border membranes using monoclonal antibodies. FEBS Lett. 161, 279-283.

12. Hosang, M., Gibbs, E.M., Diedrich, D.F. and Semenza, G. (1981). Photoaffinity labeling and identification of (a component of) the small intestinal Na^+, D-glucose transporter using 4-azidophlorizin. FEBS Lett. 130, 244-248.

13. Klip, A., Grinstein, S. and Semenza, G. (1979). Partial purification of the sugar carrier of intestinal brush border membranes. Enrichment of the phlorizin binding component by selective extractions. J. Membrane Biol. 51, 47-73.

14. Peerce, B.E. and Wright, E.M. (1984) Conformational changes in the intestinal brush border sodium-glucose cotransporter labeled with fluorescein isothiocyanate. Proc. Natl. Acad. Sci. USA 81, 2223-2226.

KINETICS OF ATP SYNTHESIS/HYDROLYSIS BY THE MITOCHONDRIAL ATP-SYNTHASE COMPLEX

A.D. VINOGRADOV, E.A. VASILYEVA, O.A. EVTUSHENKO
Department of Biochemistry, School of Biology, Moscow
State University, Moscow 117234, U.S.S.R.

Most of the available information on the mechanism of oxidative phosphorylation is based on the studies of ATPase reaction catalyzed by the mitochondrial preparations of different degree of resolution. Being itself extremely useful this information would become somehow ambiguous if one assumes that the sequence of the reaction steps during ATP hydrolysis is not the same as that during ATP synthesis. The purpose of this report is to summarize our previous data (1-7,9) and to present some new results which indicate that the ATPase reaction catalyzed by the submitochondrial particles (coupled or uncoupled) is not the simple reversal of ATP-synthase reaction.

The participation of the coupling factor F_1 in ATP synthesis and hydrolysis in the mitochondrial membrane can be described in a very general form as follows:

1. $\qquad ATP \longleftarrow F_1 \longrightarrow ADP + P_i + n\bar{H}^+$

2. $\qquad ATP \longrightarrow F_1^H \longrightarrow ADP + P_i$

$\qquad\qquad\qquad\qquad \Big\uparrow \text{ fast}$

$\quad ADP + P_i + n\bar{H}^+ \longleftarrow F_1^S \longrightarrow ATP$

3. $\qquad ATP \longrightarrow F_1^H \longrightarrow ADP + P_i$

$\quad ADP + P_i + n\bar{H}^+ - F_1^S \longrightarrow ATP$

Proceedings of the 16th FEBS Congress
Part B, pp. 291–299
© 1985 VNU Science Press

4. $$\text{ATP} \longrightarrow F_1^H \longrightarrow \text{ADP} + P_i$$

$\Big\downarrow$ slow

$$\text{ADP} + P_i + n\bar{H}^+ \xleftarrow{} F_1^S \longrightarrow \text{ATP}$$

Model 1 describes the simplest mechanism where F_1 operates as the reversible H^+-ATPase and catalyzes synthesis or hydrolysis of ATP depending on $\Delta \mu_{H^+}$ magnitude. The kinetic properties of F_1 in this case are determined by $\Delta \mu_{H^+}$ and free energy of ATP hydrolysis through the Haldane relation.

Model 2 describes the existence of two reaction pathways for ATP synthesis and hydrolysis with rapid equilibrium between some intermediates of "uncoupled" ATPase and $\Delta \mu_{H^+}$-dependent ATP-synthase. In this model the hydrolysis of ATP is not tightly coupled with the vectorial proton translocation and a leakage of ATP energy occurs depending on equilibrium and rate constants for an interconversion between the intermediates of ATPase (F_1^H) and ATP-synthase (F_1^S) reactions.

Model 3, which is highly unprobable and considered here for the sake of completeness, describes the synthesis or hydrolysis of ATP as being catalyzed by two different enzymes. It is clear that the mechanisms of synthesis and hydrolysis in such a model may be quite different and no Haldane relation exists for the net reactions in both directions.

Model 4 which has been proposed in our previous publications (1,2) describes the existence of two slowly (compare to the turnover numbers) interconvertible states of F_1 - hydrolase and synthase originally designated as F_1^H and F_1^S, respectively. An important consequence of this model is that the net ATP hydrolysis can not be described as the reversal of net ATP synthesis and at any given relatively short time models 3 and 4 are kinetically equivalent. In other words F_1^S and F_1^H can be considered as the "kinetically formed isoenzymes". It should be emphasized that we have proposed a hypothesis on different reaction pathways for ATP synthesis and hydrolysis (1-3) in a strict sense: it may include different binding sites for the substrates (products)

on the enzyme molecule during its operation in both directions, or it may be due to the different intramolecular transformation of the same enzyme-substrate (product) complexes when ATP synthesis or hydrolysis occur.

INTERACTION OF ADP AND P_i WITH THE MEMBRANE-BOUND F_1

The membrane-bound or soluble F_1 specifically binds ADP
at the high affinity site which is kinetically distinct
from that where ADP is released during ATP hydrolysis
($K_i \sim 10^{-8}$M, $k_{off} \approx 0.2$ min^{-1}) (4-7). The saturation of
this site with ADP completely inhibits ATPase activity.
The slow ATP-dependent activation of ADP-inhibited ATPase
apparently occurs through the formation of ADP$\cdot F_1 \cdot$ATP
complex where ATP is bound at the ATPase catalytic site
(6). P_i has no effect on the affinities of ATP and ADP
to the catalytic site of ATPase whereas it strongly decreases the affinity of "slow" ADP-specific site to
ADP (2,3). The factor of negative cooperativity for
ADP and P_i binding measured as inhibition and activation
of ATPase in the presence of both modulators is about
equal to 100; thus in the presence of saturating P_i the
affinity of ADP-specific inhibitory site to ADP is in
the same order of magnitude as K_m for ADP in oxidative
phosphorylation (3). These and some other findings
allow to suggest that ADP-specific ATPase inhibitory
site in F_1 molecule serves as the substrate binding
site during oxidative phosphorylation. In harmony with
this proposal it has been found that under certain
conditions ADP is the "unidirectional" inhibitor of
ATPase reaction catalyzed by the coupled submitochondrial particles (1). This result can hardly be explained
by any model of the reversible F_1 operation except for
model 4 (see above).

WHETHER INHIBITORY ADP IS BOUND AT THE CATALYTIC SITE
OF ATPase?

Although several lines of evidence suggest that ADP
binds with F_1 at the site different from that where
ADP is released during overall ATP hydrolysis, it has
beeb argued that inhibitory effect of ADP is due to

293

the formation of a dead-end complex as the result of
"incorrect" P_i release before ADP during ordered ATP
hydrolysis (8). Thus, it seemed of interest to check
this possibility. Fig. 1 shows that both ADP and ATP
used in a very low concentrations are able to inhibit
ATPase activity of submitochondrial particles and the
treatment of nucleotide-inhibited enzyme with ATP-regenerating system completely restores the original activity. An important point illustrated by Fig. 1 is
that if ATP-regenerating system is added before ATP it
prevents an inhibitory effect of the latter. This result
clearly shows that ADP formed from ATP at ATPase catalytic site must appear in the surrounding medium in

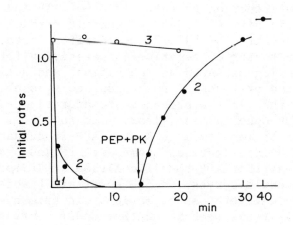

Fig. 1. Inactivation of ATPase by ATP.
        AS - submitochondrial particles (1 mg/ml) were
        incubated at 25°C in the mixture containing
        (final concentrations): KCl - 0.1M, MOPS - 10 mM,
        EDTA - 50 µM, $MgCl_2$ - 2 mM (pH 7.0). 1 - 0.8 µM
        ADP was added at zero time; 2 - 0.8 µM ATP was
        added at zero time, incubation was continued
        and phosphoenol pyruvate (3 mM) and pyruvate
        kinase (20 units/ml) were added where indicated;

294

3 - phosphoenol pyruvate and pyruvate kinase
were added before ATP. The initial rates of
ATPase were measured at 25°C in the assay mixture comprising (final concentrations): KCl -
0.1 M, MOPS - 10 mM, EDTA - 50 μM, MgCl$_2$ - 2 mM,
phosphoenol pyruvate - 2 mM, NAD·H - 0.25 mM,
rotenone - 5 μM, FCCP - 1 μM, pyruvate kinase -
3.3 units/ml, lactate dehydrogenase - 5 units/ml,
ATP - 75 μM. The reaction was started by the
addition of submitochondrial particles to the
assay mixture.

order to inhibit ATPase activity. In other words, the
sequence of the events during ATP-induced inactivation
of ATPase should be described as:

$$\cdot F_1 \cdot \underset{+ATP}{\longleftrightarrow} \cdot F_1 \cdot ATP \underset{-P_i}{\longleftrightarrow} \cdot F_1 \cdot ADP \underset{-ADP}{\longleftrightarrow} \cdot F_1 \cdot \underset{+ADP}{\longleftrightarrow} ADP \cdot F_1 \cdot$$

active   inactive

and not as:

$$F_1 \cdot \underset{+ATP}{\longleftrightarrow} F_1 \cdot ATP \underset{-P_i}{\longleftrightarrow} F_1 \cdot ADP.$$

active   inactive

DOES ADP-INHIBITED F$_1$ ARISE DURING ATP HYDROLYSIS
COUPLED WITH PROTON TRANSLOCATION?

Unidirectional inhibition of ATPase by ADP (1) qualitatively shows that the mechanisms of a direct and reverse
reactions of ATP hydrolysis/synthesis are not the same.
This interpretation, however, meets some difficulties
when applied quantitatively. An ATPase activity of the
coupled particles is evidently the sum of the activity
coupled with the vectorial proton translocation and
that which is due to an operation of F$_1'$s bound to the
particles with the membrane permeable to protons. The
possibility thus exists that "slow" F$_1$·ADP complex
arises as a dead-end intermediate only during operation
of the proton permeable particles. To find out whether
ADP-inhibited F$_1$ is formed when the membrane potential

exists, we studied the effects of azide and sulphite
on ATP-dependent reduction of NAD^+ by succinate, i.e.
on coupled ATPase. As we have shown earlier azide stabilizes $F_1 \cdot ADP$ complex whereas sulphite prevents its formation (9). As shown in Fig. 2, the patterns of inhibition by azide are the same for net ATP hydrolysis and
for ATPase coupled with the vectorial proton translocation (ATP supported reverse electron transfer).

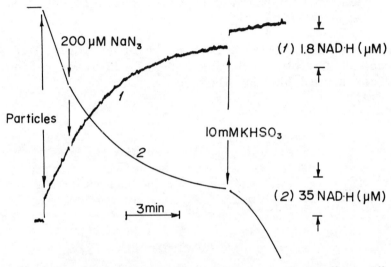

Fig. 2. Effects of azide and sulphite on the "total"
and "coupled" ATPase.
AS - submitochondrial particles (11 mg/ml)
were preincubated at 25°C for 40 min in the
mixture containing (final concentrations):
HEPES-KOH (pH 8.0) - 10 mM, sucrose - 0.25 M,
EDTA - 50 µM, potassium succinate - 10 mM,
bovine serum albumin - 1 mg/ml, KCN - 1 mM,
phosphoenol pyruvate - 1 mM, pyruvate kinase -
3 units/ml, $MgCl_2$ - 1 mM, oligomycin - 0.2
µg/mg of protein. After incubation the particles were stored in ice during the experiments (about 1 h). The reverse electron transfer (curve 1) was assayed at 25°C by the addition of 160 µg of the preincubated particles
to 2 ml assay cuvette containing (final con-

centrations): the same components as for pre-incubation except for oligomycin and ATP-regenerating system, Mg–ATP – 1 mM, NAD^+ – 1 mM. The total ATPase (curve 2) was assayed in the mixture containing the same components as for curve 1 and NAD·H – 0.45 mM, phosphoenol pyruvate – 5 mM, pyruvate kinase – 10 units/ml, lactate dehydrogenase – 7 units/ml. The rates of both processes without further additions were constant during the registration time.

Remarkably, when sulphite is added after inhibition by azide has been completed an activation of net ATPase up to the initial level occurs, whereas no "coupled" ATPase is now operating. It was shown in the separate experiments (not shown) that sulphite inhibits ATP-supported reverse electron transfer. Therefore these results suggest that F_1·ADP complex is formed during coupled ATPase reaction and moreover the formation of such a complex is apparently a prerequisite of $\Delta\mu_{H^+}$-dependent reversible H^+-ATPase. The special experiments show that neither azide nor sulphite influence respiratory control ratio measured for the particles under the conditions as in Fig. 2 (2.8 and 1.7 with NAD·H and succinate as the substrates, respectively). It may thus be concluded that the hydrolysis of ATP in the presence of sulphite is uncoupled at the level of F_1 operation.

THE MODEL OF PSEUDOREVERSIBLE MITOCHONDRIAL ATPase

The scheme which accounts for our data published previously and reported here is depicted below. According to the scheme the ratio between slowly interconvertible synthase (left part) and hydrolase (right part) states of F_1 is under control of ADP/ATP ratio; from this point of view ADP-specific high affinity inhibitory site should be considered as the regulatory site for ATPase activity of the enzyme. However, this site serves as the substrate binding site during the catalytic cycle of phosphorylation. On the other hand, ATP-specific binding site responsible for the forma-

297

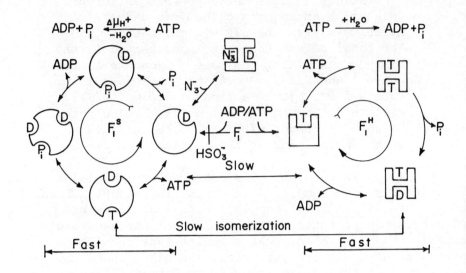

tion of a hydrolase state may be considered as the regulatory site for ATP-synthase activity and as the catalytic one for ATPase. The coordinated functioning of
only two nucleotide binding sites is shown for the sake
of simplicity; the model can be further developed taking
into account three subunit symmetry   (10) and the total
number of nucleotide binding sites in F_1 (11).

REFERENCES

1. Minkov, I.B., Fitin, A.F., Vasilyeva, E.A., Vinogra-
     dov, A.D. (1980). Differential effects of ADP on
     ATPase and oxidative phosphorylation in submito-
     chondrial particles. Biochem. Int. 1, 478–485.
2. Vinogradov, A.D., Vasilyeva, E.A., Yalamova, M.V.
     (1982). Pseudoreversibility of ATP hydrolysis/syn-
     thesis as revealed by the effects of ADP and P_i
     on mitochondrial adenosine triphosphatase. In:
     Second European Bioenergetics Conference Short
     Reports, LBTM-CNRS Edition, Lyon, 113–114.
3. Yalamova, M.V., Vasilyeva, E.A., Vinogradov, A.D.
     (1982). Mutually dependent influence of ADP and
     P_i on the activity of mitochondrial adenosine

triphosphatase. Biochem. Int. 4, 334-344.

4. Fitin, A.F., Vasilyeva, E.A., Vinogradov, A.D.
   (1979). An inhibitory high affinity binding site
   for ADP in the oligomycin-sensitive ATPase of
   beef-heart submitochondrial particles. Biochem.
   Biophys. Res. Communs. 86, 434-439.

5. Minkov, I.B., Fitin, A.F., Vasilyeva, E.A., Vinogradov, A.D. (1979). Mg^{2+}-induced ADP-dependent inhibition of the ATPase activity of beef-heart mitochondrial coupling factor F_1. Biochem. Biophys.
   Res. Communs. 89, 1300-1306.

6. Vasilyeva, E.A., Fitin, A.F., Minkov, I.B., Vinogradov, A.D. (1980). Kinetics of interaction of
   adenosine diphosphate and adenosine triphosphate
   with ATPase of bovine heart submitochondrial particles. Biochem. J. 188, 807-815.

7. Vasilyeva, E.A., Minkov, I.B., Fitin, A.F., Vinogradov, A.D. (1982). Kinetic mechanism of mitochondrial adenosine triphosphatase. ADP-specific inhibition as revealed by the steady-state kinetics.
   Biochem. J., 202, 9-14.

8. Boyer, P.D., Kohlbrenner, W.E., Smith, L.T., Feldman, R.E. (1982). A unifying hypothesis for ADP
   participation in catalysis and control of F_1
   ATPases. In: Second European Bioenergetics Con-
   ference Short Reports, LBTM-CNRS Edition, Lyon,
   p. 23-24.

9. Vasilyeva, E.A., Minkov, I.B., Fitin, A.F., Vinogradov, A.D. (1982). Kinetic mechanism of mitochondrial adenosine triphosphatase. Inhibition by
   azide and activation by sulphite. Biochem. J.,
   202, 15-23.

10. Ioshida, M., Sone, N., Hirata, H., Kagawa, J. (1979).
    Reconstitution of adenosine triphosphatase. Com-
    parison of the structure in thermophilic bacte-
    rium PS3 with those in mitochondria, chloroplasts
    and Escherichia coli. J. Biol. Chem., 254, 9525-
    9533.

11. Cross, R.L., Nalin, C.M. (1982). Adenine nucleotide
    binding sites on beef heart F_1-ATPase. Evidence
    for three exchangable sites that are distinct from
    three noncatalytic sites. J.Biol.Chem. 257,2874-2881.

CONTROLLING MECHANISMS IN MITOCHONDRIAL RESPIRATION

L. WOJTCZAK, K. BOGUCKA, J. DUSZYŃSKI, M. PUKA
and A. ŻÓŁKIEWSKA
Nencki Institute of Experimental Biology,
Pasteura 3, 02-093 Warsaw, Poland

In pioneering studies of Chance and Williams [1] a particular role in controlling the rate of mitochondrial respiration was attributed to the availability of external ADP. Later on, however, the importance of the ATP/ADP ratio and, consequently, of the adenine nucleotide translocator as the controlling factors has been stressed. It is suggested [2] that this translocator operates under disequilibrium conditions, although a view has also been presented [3] that the respiratory chain from NADH up to cytochrome c operates close to equilibrium with ATP synthetase and that cytochrome oxidase is the only controlling site. This controversy can be reconciled by assuming a multisite control mechanism. By introducing the concept of the control strength, it has been shown [4,5] that the rate of mitochondrial respiration may be simultaneously regulated by the adenine nucleotide translocator, cytochrome oxidase, the substrate carrier and the respective dehydrogenase.

According to the chemiosmotic theory of energy coupling [6], the electrochemical proton potential (the protonmotive force, $\Delta\tilde{\mu}_{H^+}$) can be regarded formally as the intermediate of oxidative phosphorylation. Therefore, it was of particular interest to see how this potential is controlled by mitochondrial respiration and ATP synthesis and, on the other hand, how its magnitude influences the overall flux through the energy coupling system. By

Proceedings of the 16th FEBS Congress
Part B, pp. 301–306
© 1985 VNU Science Press

modulating the rates of respiration and ATP
synthesis with specific inhibitors we have
shown [7] that $\Delta\tilde{\mu}_{H^+}$ and its major component,
the membrane potential ($\Delta\psi$) vary only slightly, whereas the respiration is changed considerably (Fig. 1). This points to a high degree
of homeostasis of the mitochondrial protonmotive force or, in other words, to a high sensitivity of fluxes through the respiratory chain
and ATP synthetase to small changes of $\Delta\tilde{\mu}_{H^+}$.
The relationship between the two fluxes and
$\Delta\tilde{\mu}_{H^+}$ is schematically illustrated in Fig. 2.

Homeostasis of the protonmotive force is
probably an important feature of mitochondrial
metabolism. It also allows to explain coupling
phenomena entirely in terms of the "classical"
chemiosmosis without the necessity of introducing the concept of localized proton gradients.

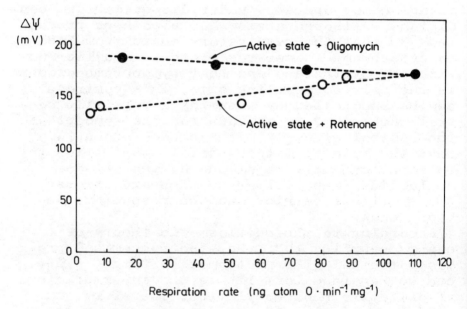

Fig. 1. Dependence of the membrane potential
($\Delta\psi$) on the rate of respiration in rat liver
mitochondria oxidizing glutamate + malate under
active state conditions. From [7].

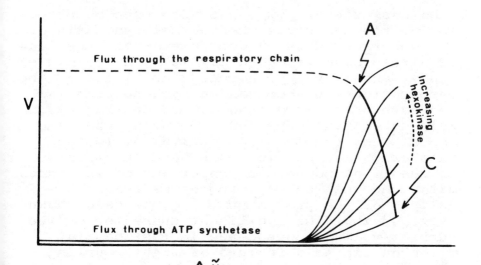

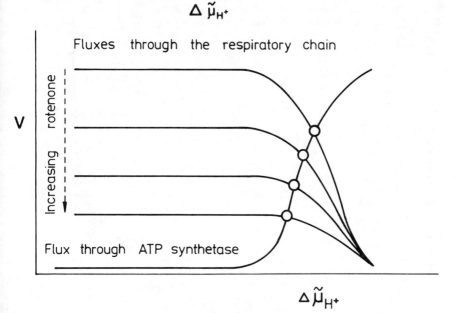

Fig. 2. Relationships between the protonmotive force ($\Delta\tilde{\mu}_{H^+}$) and fluxes (V) through the respiratory chain and ATP synthetase. Indications: A, active state; C, resting state. From [7].

Homeostasis of $\triangle\tilde{\mu}_{H^+}$ has also been observed in the resting state when no net synthesis of ATP occurred. Here, a decrease of the respiration rate also produced little or no change of $\triangle\tilde{\mu}_{H^+}$, and only a pronounced inhibition of the respiration was accompanied by a substantial decrease of the protonmotive force (Fig. 3). This non-linear dependence between $\triangle\tilde{\mu}_{H^+}$ and the rate of respiration (equivalent to the rate of proton pumping) has been interpreted as result of non-ohmic properties of the inner mitochondrial membrane [8] or as result of "slips" of the proton pump [9]. We have shown (Fig. 4) that the non-linear character of the current/voltage dependence in resting state mitochondria is a feature of tight coupling.

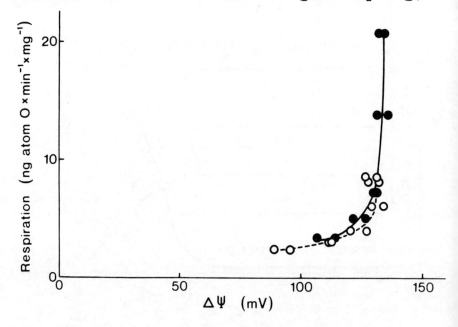

Fig. 3. Dependence between the membrane potential and the rate of respiration in the resting state. Mitochondria oxidizing succinate (●) and glutamate + malate (O) were titrated with malonate and rotenone, respectively.

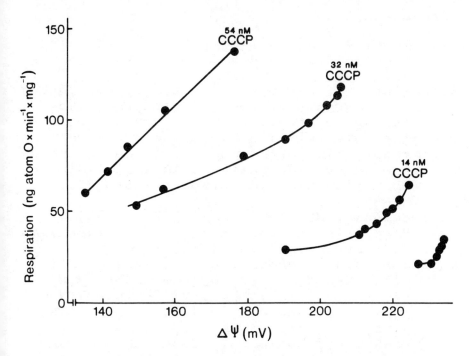

Fig. 4. Effect of partial uncoupling on the dependence between $\triangle \psi$ and the respiration rate. Mitochondria respiring with succinate were titrated with malonate in the presence of various concentrations of carbonylcyanide m-chlorophenylhydrazone (CCCP).

By gradually uncoupling the particles the curve becomes less steep at its initial part, and finally an almost linear dependence is obtained. It is difficult to explain this in terms of slips of proton pumps. The non-ohmic property of the membrane can also hardly account for this result, as the non-linearity appears at various values of $\triangle \psi$. We are now developing an approach in which the non-linear relation between $\triangle \tilde{\mu}_{H^+}$ and the respiration is related to the heterogeneity of isolated mitochondria.

References:

1. Chance, B. and Williams, G.R. (1956). The respiratory chain and oxidative phosphorylation. Adv. Enzymol. 17, 65-134.
2. Küster, U., Letko, G., Kunz, W., Duszyński, J., Bogucka, K. and Wojtczak, L. (1981). Influence of different energy drains on the interrelationship between the rate of respiration, protonmotive force and adenine nucleotide patterns in isolated mitochondria. Biochim. Biophys. Acta 636, 32-38.
3. Erecińska, M. and Wilson, D.F. (1982). Regulation of cellular energy metabolism. J. Membr. Biol. 70, 1-14.
4. Groen, A.K., Wanders, R.J.A., Westerhoff, H.V., Van der Meer, R. and Tager, J.M. (1982). J. Biol. Chem. 257, 2754-2757.
5. Tager, J.M., Wanders, R.J.A., Groen, A.K., Kunz, W., Bohnensack, R., Küster, U., Letko, G., Böhme, G., Duszyński, J. and Wojtczak, L. (1983). Control of mitochondrial respiration. FEBS Lett. 151, 1-9.
6. Mitchell, P. (1966). Chemiosmotic coupling in oxidative and photosynthetic phosphorylation. Biol. Rev. 41, 445-502.
7. Duszyński, J., Bogucka, K. and Wojtczak, L. (1984). Homeostasis of the protonmotive force in phosphorylating mitochondria. Biochim. Biophys. Acta, in press.
8. Nicholls, D.G. (1974). The influence of respiration and ATP hydrolysis on the proton-electrochemical gradient across the inner membrane of rat-liver mitochondria as determined by ion distribution. Eur. J. Biochem. 50, 305-315.
9. Pietrobon, D., Azzone, G.F. and Walz, D. (1981). Effect of funiculosin and antimycin A on the redox-driven H^+-pumps in mitochondria: On the nature of "leaks". Eur. J. Biochem. 117, 389-394.

THE SODIUM TRANSPORT DECARBOXYLASES

PETER DIMROTH
Institut für Physiologische Chemie der TU
München Biedersteiner Straße 29, 8000 München
40, FRG

INTRODUCTION

Energy conversion into the biologically useful
form of ATP generally involves two distinct
steps. Chemical or light energy is first converted into an intermediate of high energy
which provides the immediate driving force for
ATP synthesis in the second energy conversion
step. In substrate level phosphorylation the
energy-rich intermediate is a phosphoryl compound with high group transfer potential from
which ATP is synthesized by phosphate transfer
to ADP in the soluble compartment of the cell.
Generally, the energy-rich phosphoryl compounds
are formed by catabolic redox processes and
only in rare cases are catabolic non-redox
processes accompanied by ATP synthesis. All the
other energy conversion mechanisms involve
vectorial membrane reactions. The intermediate
of high energy from which ATP synthesis is
accomplished in most cases is an electrochemical gradient of protons ($\Delta\mu H^+$) generated by
proton pumps from the primary energy sources.
The latter energy conversion mechanisms involve
mostly either photosynthetic electron transfer
or chemical redox processes. A novel type of
energy conversion mechanism has been detected
with the sodium transport decarboxylases. The
primary energy conversion is the transduction
of decarboxylation energy into an electrochemical gradient of Na^+ ions ($\Delta\mu Na^+$). Subsequently, the $\Delta\mu Na^+$ is used as an energy source for
active transport or ATP synthesis.
    The enzymes acting as sodium transport decar-

Proceedings of the 16th FEBS Congress
Part B, pp. 307–313
© 1985 VNU Science Press

boxylases are oxaloacetate decarboxylase of
Klebsiella aerogenes (1-3), methylmalonyl-CoA
decarboxylase of Veillonella alcalescens (4,5)
or Propionigenium modestum (6) and glutaconyl-
CoA decarboxylase of Acidaminococcus fermen-
tans (7). As far as we know is the occurence of
these energy converting enzymes restricted to
anaerobic bacteria. The enzymes are induced by
the substrate of the respective fermentation
pathway and besides their function in energy
conservation they are essential catalysts for
the degradation of the fermentation substrate.
The large negative free energy change (6-7
kcal/mol) of the decarboxylation reactions
provides the driving force for the active
transport of Na^+ ions.

Table 1: Subunit composition of the sodium
transport decarboxylases

Enzyme	Subunit	Approximate M_r
	α	65 000 (b)
Oxaloacetate	ß	34 000
decarboxylase	ɣ	12 000
Methylmalonyl-CoA	α	60 000
decarboxylase	ß	33 000
	ɣ	18 500 (b)
	δ	14 000
b=biotin-containing subunit		

Molecular properties
All three sodium transport decarboxylases are
tightly bound to the membranes, specifically
activated by Na^+ ions ($K_M \sim 1$ mM) and contain
biotin as a prosthetic group. This biotin content has greatly facilitated the purification
of these enzymes which is achieved by affinity
chromatography on monomeric avidin-Sepharose
columns (5,6,8). The subunit compositions of

the decarboxylases are summarized in Table 1
and indicate that there are several weight
homologous subunits in these decarboxylases.
These could thus perform a similar function in
the catalytic cycle.

Decarboxylation mechanism. The decarboxylation
mechanism involves three distinct steps as
shown below. The first step is a carboxyl
transfer from the substrate to the biotin
prosthetic group of the enzyme (eqn 1). This is
followed by the decarboxylation of the carboxy-
biotin enzyme intermediate (eqn 2) and Na^+ ions
are transported during the overall reaction
from the interior of the bacterial membrane to
the exterior (eqn 3).

$$R-COO^- + E\text{-biotin} \rightleftharpoons R\text{-H} + E\text{-biotin-}CO_2^- \qquad (1)$$

$$E\text{-biotin-}CO_2^- + H^+ \longrightarrow E\text{-biotin} + CO_2 \qquad (2)$$

$$2\ Na^+_{in} \longrightarrow 2\ Na^+_{out} \qquad (3)$$

$$R-COO^- + H^+ + 2\ Na^+_{in} \longrightarrow R\text{-H} + CO_2 + 2\ Na^+_{out}$$

The carboxyltransferase activity (eqn 1) of
oxaloacetate decarboxylase has been demonstrated
by the isotopic exchange between $[1\text{-}^{14}C]$
pyruvate and oxaloacetate (9). The reaction was
completely independent from the presence of
Na^+ ions and was catalyzed by the α-subunit of
the decarboxylase (10). The ß and the ɣ-subunit
apparently take part in the other reactions of
the catalytic cycle. These are integral membrane
proteins which are only released by detergents
whereas the α-chain is loosely attached to the
membrane and behaves like a soluble protein
after dissociation from the membrane by freezing

and thawing in presence of 1 M LiCl (10).

Reconstitution of Na$^+$ transport. The Na$^+$ transport activity of the sodium transport decarboxylases was reconstituted by incorporating the
purified enzymes into phospholipid vesicles
using the detergent dilution method with octyl-
glucoside as the detergent (3,7,11). These
proteoliposomes upon substrate decarboxylation
performed an electrogenic uptake of Na$^+$ ions
creating a Na$^+$ concentration gradient equivalent
to about 50 mV and a membrane potential of
around 60 mV. The total sodium motive force
generated was thus 110 mV which is equivalent to
a free energy change of 2.5 kcal/mol of transported ion. Since the free energy of the decarboxylation reactions is about 6-7 kcal/mol, this
is sufficient to pump two mol Na$^+$ ions against
the concentration gradient. When direct measurements of the stoichiometry were performed it was
found that close to two mol Na$^+$ ions were taken
up by the vesicles per mol substrate decarboxylation in the initial phase of the transport.
Later, after a Na$^+$ concentration gradient had
developed over the proteoliposomal membrane, the
stoichiometry changed since decarboxylation
proceeded at a high rate even after reaching the
steady state internal Na$^+$ concentration. Nevertheless, partial coupling remained since the
decarboxylation rate increased about twofold by
adding monensin which immediately destroyed the
Na$^+$ concentration gradient. This coupling
results from an energy requiring exchange of
internal and external Na$^+$ ions as catalyzed by
the Na$^+$ transport decarboxylases.
  One of the fundamental features of coupled
vectorial transport systems is reversibility.
It was therefore expected that the sodium transport decarboxylases were reversible systems, as
well, if the same principles of vectorial energy

coupling were valid. Substrate decarboxylations by the soluble enzymes are completely irreversible. Under the conditions of vectorial energy coupling, however, with oxaloacetate decarboxylase or methylmalonyl-CoA decarboxylase incorporated into proteoliposomes the decarboxylation reactions were reversed if a Na^+ ion gradient of proper direction and magnitude was applied (12). The best system to study this reversibility are proteoliposomes reconstituted with oxaloacetate decarboxylase and methylmalonyl-CoA decarboxylase. One of the decarboxylases served in generating an electrochemical Na^+ gradient upon decarboxylation of its substrate and the other decarboxylase performed the carboxylation reaction under consumption of the energy of the electrochemical Na^+ gradient. This is the first example of an unfavorable carboxylation reaction which is energized by an electrochemical Na^+ gradient and not by ATP hydrolysis.

The reconstituted transcarboxylase system also provides a model for physiologically more relevant processes, e.g. ATP synthesis mediated by a Na^+ circuit. The anaerobic bacterium Propionigenium modestum grows from the fermentation of succinate to propionate and CO_2. The degradation proceeds via succinyl-CoA, methylmalonyl-CoA and propionyl-CoA with neither substrate nor electron transport phosphorylations. Rather, all biologically useful energy stems from the decarboxylation of methylmalonyl-CoA to propionyl-CoA which is converted into an electrochemical Na^+ gradient by methylmalonyl-CoA decarboxylase. A novel type of Na^+-dependent ATPase in the bacterial membrane synthesizes ATP from ADP and inorganic phosphate under consumption of the Na^+ ion gradient. This is the first example of ATP synthesis energized by a Na^+ gradient and also the first example where the chemical energy of a decarboxylation reaction provides all of the energy for life (6).

Methylmalonyl-CoA decarboxylase pumps 2 mol Na^+ ions through the membrane generating a sodium motive force of 110 mV, equivalent to 5 kcal/2 mol Na^+ ions. This amount of energy is not sufficient to support ATP synthesis. However, if 3 or 4 mol Na^+ ions were traversing the membrane at the given $\Delta\mu Na^+$, the energy would increase to 7.5 and 10 kcal, respectively, which could energetically balance the synthesis of ATP from ADP and inorganic phosphate. ATP synthesis in this organism therefore requires that the Na^+/ATP stoichiometry is higher than that of Na^+/methylmalonyl-CoA. Less than 1 mol ATP is therefore synthesized per fermentation cycle. This is accomplished by accumulating the energy of more than one decarboxylation reaction in the form of $\Delta\mu Na^+$. The smallest quantum of biologically useful energy is therefore not that of ATP hydrolysis but that of an ion forming a gradient over a membrane. Other microorganisms growing from an energy span which is insufficient for the synthesis of a total mol of ATP per fermentation cycle probably depend on analogous energy conservation mechanisms.

References

1. Dimroth, P. (1980) A new sodium transport system energized by the decarboxylation of oxaloacetate. FEBS Lett. 122, 234-236.
2. Dimroth, P. (1982) The generation of an electrochemical gradient of sodium ions upon decarboxylation of oxaloacetate by the membrane-bound and Na^+-activated oxaloacetate decarboxylase from Klebsiella aerogenes. Eur. J. Biochem. 121, 443-449.
3. Dimroth, P. (1981) Reconstitution of sodium transport from purified oxaloacetate decarboxylase and phospholipid vesicles. J. Biol.

Chem. 256, 11974-11976.
4. Hilpert, W. & Dimroth, P. (1982) Conversion of the chemical energy of methylmalonyl-CoA decarboxylation into a Na^+ gradient. Nature (Lond.) 296, 584-585.
5. Hilpert, W. & Dimroth, P. (1983) Purification and characterization of a new sodium transport decarboxylase. Methylmalonyl-CoA decarboxylase from Veillonella alcalescens. Eur. J. Biochem. 132, 579-587.
6. Hilpert, W. Schink, B. & Dimroth, P. (1984) Life by a new decarboxylation-dependent energy conservation mechanism with Na^+ as coupling ion. EMBO J. 3, in press.
7. Buckel, W. & Semmler, R. (1983) Purification characterization and reconstitution of glutaconyl-CoA decarboxylase, a biotin-dependent sodium pump from anaerobic bacteria. Eur. J. Biochem. 136, 427-434.
8. Dimroth, P. (1982) Purification of the sodium transport enzyme oxaloacetate decarboxylase by affinity chromatography on avidin Sepharose. FEBS Lett. 141, 59-62.
9. Dimroth, P. (1982) The role of biotin and sodium in the decarboxylation of oxaloacetate by the membrane-bound oxaloacetate decarboxylase from Klebsiella aerogenes. Eur. J. Biochem. 121, 435-441.
10. Dimroth, P. & Thomer, A. (1983) Subunit composition of oxaloacetate decarboxylase and characterization of the α-chain as carboxyltransferase. Eur. J. Biochem. 137, 107-112.
11. Hilpert, W. & Dimroth, P. (1984) Reconstitution of Na^+ transport from purified methylmalonyl-CoA decarboxylase and phospholipid vesicles. Eur. J. Biochem. 138, 579-583.
12. Dimroth, P. & Hilpert, W. (1984) Carboxylation of pyruvate and acetyl-CoA by reversal of the Na^+ pumps oxaloacetate decarboxylase and methylmalonyl-CoA decarboxylase. Biochemistry, in press.

DIRECT AND INDIRECT INTERACTION BETWEEN PRIMARY AND SECONDARY TRANSPORT IN BACTERIA

MARIEKE G.L. ELFERINK, JAN M. VAN DIJL, KLAAS J. HELLINGWERF AND WIL N. KONINGS
Department of Microbiology, University of Groningen. Kerklaan 30, 9751 NN HAREN. The Netherlands

The chemiosmotic hypothesis of Mitchell predicts that the proton motive force is the driving force for energy requiring processes like solute transport and ATP synthesis. However, in our experiments we showed that in the phototrophic bacterium Rhodopseudomonas sphaeroides the existence of a proton motive force alone is not sufficient for solute uptake but also turnover of the cyclic electron transfer chain is necessary (1). This led us to investigate in detail the role of the electron transfer chain in solute transport in both Rps. sphaeroides and in cells and cytoplasmic membrane vesicles of Escherichia coli. For this aim a thermostated vessel was constructed in which we can measure continuously the $\Delta\psi$ (with an ion selective TPP^+ electrode) and the respiration rate (with an oxygen electrode). From this vessel simultaneously samples are taken and filtrated to measure the uptake of radioactive compounds. Furthermore, all experimental conditions were such that the proton motive force is composed out of a $\Delta\psi$ only, because the ΔpH is abolished with nigericin. For the calculation of the $\Delta\psi$ a proper correction for aspecific TPP^+ binding was applied (2).

The direct interaction between the primary proton pump and secondary transport systems was initially observed in Rps. sphaeroides. When the initial rate of uptake of the amino acid alanine is measured at a constant light intensity (= constant rate of cyclic electron transfer), the rate of transport depends exponentially on the size of the proton motive force. However, at constant proton motive force values the rate of transport is a linear function of the light intensity and is not constant as would be expected from the chemiosmotic hypothesis. At low light intensities there is no uptake of alanine, even when the proton motive force is high (Fig. 1).

Proceedings of the 16th FEBS Congress
Part B, pp. 315–321
© 1985 VNU Science Press

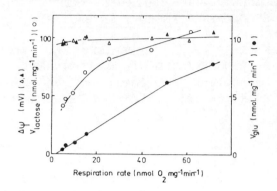

Fig. 1. The relation between V_{ala} and $\Delta\psi$ at constant light intensity and between V_{ala} and light intensity at constant $\Delta\psi$ in cells of <u>Rps. sphaeroides</u>.

Alanine uptake and $\Delta\psi$ were measured simultaneously in cells treated with EDTA and nigericin at different light intensities. The incubation medium contained: 50 mM potassium phosphate pH 8, 5 mM $MgSO_4$, 50 µM ^{14}C alanine, 4 µM tetraphenylphosphonium, cells at 0.64 mg protein/ml and various concentrations of valinomycin. Upper pannel: the alanine uptake rate (V_{ala}) as a function of $\Delta\psi$ at constant light intensity. Lower pannel: V_{ala} as a function of light intensity at constant $\Delta\psi$ values. Data from the upper pannel were replotted.

Fig. 2. The inital rate of lactose and glutamate uptake and the magnitude of $\Delta\psi$ as a function of the respiration rate in cells of <u>E. coli</u>.

Cells of <u>E. coli</u> were pretreated with EDTA and nigericin. Lactose resp. glutamate uptake, $\Delta\psi$ and respiration were measured simultaneously at increasing KCN concentrations. The incubation medium contained: 50 mM potassium phosphate pH 8, 5 mM $MgSO_4$, 200 µM ^{14}C-lactose or 50 µM ^{14}C Na-glutamate, 4 µM TPP^+, cells at 1.1 mg protein/ml. The KCN concentration was varied between 0 and 5 mM. o initial rate of lactose uptake; o initial rate of glu uptake; Δ membrane potential measured simultaneously with lactose uptake; Δ membrane potential measured simultaneously with glu uptake.

Such an interaction between the electron transfer system and solute transport carriers is not specific for Rps. sphaeroides. In a strain of Rps. sphaeroides in which the E. coli transport protein for lactose was incorporated via genetic transformation a similar relation between the rate of cyclic electron transfer and lactose transport was observed (3). Kinetic analysis of the changes in the initial rate of both alanine and lactose uptake indicates that the regulation is due to a light dependent change in the number of active carrier molecules in the membrane.

Recent studies in our laboratory demonstrated that similar interactions between the transport carrier proteins and the linear electron transfer chain exist in Rps. sphaeroides and also in E. coli (4), however, in the latter organism differences between the various transport systems are observed. The initial uptake rate of glutamate and lactose were measured in E. coli cells as a function of the respiration rate (Fig. 2). Respiration was progressively inhibited by the addition of increasing amounts of potassium cyanide. The proton motive force ($\Delta\psi$) under these conditions remained approximately constant. The initial rate of uptake of glutamate decreased proportionally with the rate of respiration and at low respiration rates no uptake occurs. For glutamate uptake in addition to a proton motive force respiration is obligatory, like for solute transport in Rps. sphaeroides. On the other hand the rate of transport of lactose decreased with the respiration rate, but is not completely abolished in the absence of electron transport. At very low respiration rates there is still a significant rate of accumulation of lactose.

To investigate the difference between glutamate and lactose uptake in more detail the uptake of both solutes was measured with a proton motive force imposed with a potassium diffusion potential under anaerobic and aerobic conditions (Fig. 3). Glutamate is not transported under anaerobic conditions, even when the $\Delta\psi$ is high. But a much more striking observation is that under aerobic conditions both glutamate and lactose are transported even when the $\Delta\psi$ is zero. It should be noted that in E. coli cells electrons are transferred to oxygen, from endogenous substrates, when this acceptor is available.

317

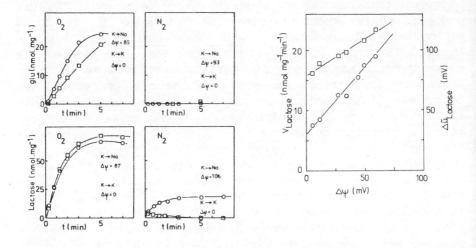

Fig. 3. Glutamate and lactose transport driven by a potassium diffusion potential under aerobic and anaerobic conditions in E. coli cells.

E. coli cells were pretreated with EDTA and suspended in 100 mM potassiumphosphate pH 8, 5 mM $MgSO_4$, 40 µM valinomycin at a protein concentration of 75 mg/ml. The uptake experiment was started by a dilution of the cell suspension 1:100 in 100 mM sodium phosphate pH 8. 5 mM $MgSO_4$, 4 µM TPP[+], 200 µM ^{14}C lactose or 50 µM ^{14}C Na-glutamate, respectively. For the control experiments cells were diluted in potassium phosphate buffer with the same additions.

Fig. 4. The initial rate of lactose uptake and steady state accumulation level as a function of the $\Delta\psi$, titrated with valinomycin in E. coli membrane vesicles.

Lactose uptake, $\Delta\psi$ and respiration rate were measured simultaneously at 30°C and at increasing valimomycin concentrations. The incubation medium contained: 50 mM potassium phosphate pH 7.0, 5 mM $MgSO_4$, 3 µM TPP[+] and the vesicles suspension in a protein concentration of 0.3 mg/ml. A nigericin containing vesicles-suspension was pretreated with 0-2 µM valinomycin. The uptake experiment was started by adding 200 µM ^{14}C lactose to the vesicles suspension.

318

Lactose transport does occur, with a potassium diffusion potential under anaerobic conditions but the initial rate of uptake and steady state accumulation level is much lower than in the presence of oxygen. Lactose uptake could only be abolished when both a $\Delta\psi$ and electron transfer are absent. These results indicate that both a proton motive force and electron transfer can - independently - provide energy for lactose transport in E. coli. This suggestion is confirmed by the observation that under anaerobic conditions, where the proton motive force is the only driving force for lactose uptake, the steady state accumulation level of lactose is in equilibrium with the artificially imposed $\Delta\psi$ with a stoichiometry of H^+/lactose of 1, the same stoichiometry as observed in oxygen-pulse experiments (5). If one assumes that lactose is transported with one proton under all conditions, the extra energy provided by turnover of the electron transfer chain allows the cells larger steady state accumulation levels of lactose than the extant $\Delta\psi$.

The interaction between the electron transfer chains and transport carriers is not restricted to H^+/symport systems but also occurs in Na^+/methyl ß-D-thiogalactopyranoside (TMG) symport via the melibiose transport carrier of E. coli. This is a strong argument against the involvement of local proton pools or local proton pathways in the direct interaction.

In order to obtain more information about the mechanism that is the basis for the direct interaction the lactose transport system has been studied in more detail in cytoplasmic membrane vesicles of E. coli. In these vesicles linear electron transfer is initiated with D-lactate as electron donor. The initial rate of lactose accumulation decreased with decreasing respiration rate when electron transfer is inhibited with increasing amounts of the lactate dehydrogenase (LDH) inhibitor oxamate, but the steady state accumulation level of lactose correlated more with the $\Delta\psi$. However, when the respiratory chain is titrated with increasing amounts of KCN both the initial uptake rate and steady state accumulation level of lactose decreased with the respiration rate. The proton motive force under these conditions decreased slightly.

When the respiratory chain is inhibited with oxamate at

the level of LDH the components of the electron transfer chain will become oxidized. On the other hand, when the respiratory chain is inhibited with KCN at the level of the terminal oxidase, the components of the electron transfer chain will become in a reduced form.

In parallel experiments the $\Delta\psi$ was titrated with valinomycin and the rate of lactose uptake was measured as a function of the $\Delta\psi$ (or: the proton motive force, Fig. 4). Under these conditions the respiration rate remained approximately constant. It was clear that the slight decrease in proton motive force observed with the electron transfer chain inhibitors could not account for the observed decrease in uptake rate.

The decrease in uptake rate and steady state accumulation level obtained with both electron transfer chain inhibitors was corrected for the expected decrease in both parameters due to the decrease in proton motive force under these circumstances. From this correction it is clear that there is no difference in uptake rate of lactose between an oxidized or reduced electron transfer chain. The turnover rate determines the rate of uptake, when the $\Delta\psi$ is the same. However, there is a difference in the steady state accumulation level of lactose between an (partially) oxidized and a reduced electron transfer chain. This leads to the conclusion that efflux of lactose is inhibited when electron transfer chain components come in the oxidized form.

That oxamate inhibits efflux of lactose in membrane vesicles of E. coli was shown already ten years ago by Kaback et al. (6). Here this observation is independently confirmed and in addition it is shown that the $\Delta\psi$ is unchanged under these conditions.

An alternative explanation by Westerhoff and van Dam (7) that oxamate translocation inhibits efflux can be excluded, since the same results are obtained when lactose uptake is driven by PQQ dependent glucose dehydrogenase (GDH) in membrane vesicles of E. coli. In E. coli an apo-GDH is present, which is converted into the active holo-enzyme upon addition of its prosthetic group pyrrolo-quinolinequinone (PQQ). This system is ideal for transport studies, because the rate of electron transfer can be increased by adding increasing amounts of PQQ to glucose containing vesicles. Therefore, in that case the use of ill-defined respiratory chain inhibitors can be avoided. For the redox state of the components of the electron transfer chain addition of decreasing amounts of PQQ is comparable to the inhibition with oxamate. When the respiratory chain is titrated with glucose/PQQ lactose efflux is also inhibited.

In membrane vesicles there is a significant initial uptake rate and steady state accumulation level of lactose at $\Delta\psi$ is zero (Fig. 4). The remaining uptake activity could only be abolished with electron transfer chain inhibitors or with anaerobic conditions.

SUMMARIZING CONCLUSIONS

1 Evidence is provided for a redox linked attenuation of carrier activity.
2 For some carriers turnover of the electron transfer chain is obligatory, for others a proton motive force or electron transfer is sufficient.
3 Both a proton motive force and electron transfer can – independently – provide energy for solute transport in bacteria.
4 The experimental observations cannot be explained by postulation of a local proton diffusion pathway.

REFERENCES

1 M.G.L. Elferink, I. Friedberg, K.J. Hellingwerf, W.N. Konings (1983) Eur.J.Biochem. 129: 583–587
2 J.S. Lolkema, K.J. Hellingwerf, W.N. Konings (1982) Biochim.Biophys.Acta 681: 85–94
3 M.G.L. Elferink, K.J. Hellingwerf, F.E. Nano, S. Kaplan, W.N. Konings (1983) FEBS Lett. 164: 198–190
4 M.G.L. Elferink, K.J. Hellingwerf, M.J. van Belkum, B. Poolman, W.N. Konings (1984) FEMS Microbiol.Lett. 21: 293–298
5 I.R. Booth, W.J. Mitchell, W.A. Hamilton (1979) Biochem.J. 182: 687–696
6 H.R. Kaback, E.M. Barnes (1971) J.Biol.Chem. 246: 5523–5531
7 H.V. Westerhoff, K. van Dam (1979) Current Topics in Bioenergetics 9: 1–62

THE PROTONMOTIVE ACTIVITY OF THE CYTOCHROME SYSTEM: VECTORIALITY AND CO-OPERATIVITY

SERGIO PAPA, MICHELE LORUSSO, FERRUCCIO GUERRIERI, DOMENICO GATTI AND DOMENICO BOFFOLI

Institute of Biological Chemistry, Faculty of Medicine and Centre for the Study of Mitochondria and Energy Metabolism, University of Bari, Italy

According to Mitchell the protonmotive activity of the cytochrome system of mitochondria is a direct consequence of vectorial arrangement in the membrane of primary redox reactions (1,2).

Papa et al., on the other hand, proposed that H^+ can be transported, across the membrane, on protolytic groups co-operatively linked to e^- transfer at the metal centers (3,4).

In the quinone cycle of Mitchell (2) $4H^+$ are effectively translocated from the matrix (N) to the cytosolic (P) phase per $2e^-$ flowing from quinol to oxygen, as consequence of hydrogen conduction from the N to the P side of the membrane by quinones, acting in a cycle on both sides of b cytochromes, and vectorial e^- conduction from the P to the N side by hemes b_{566} and b_{562} (2,4,5), and the redox centers of cytochrome oxidase, with H^+ consumption for oxygen reduction to H_2O from the N aqueous phase.

It is agreed that aerobic oxidation of cytochrome c generates $\Delta\mu H^+$ and that this is, first all, due to asymmetry of O_2 reduction to H_2O (1,2,4-6).

According to Wikström co-operative proton transfer would confer to the oxidase also a proton pumping capacity (6). Observations from Mitchell's (7) and our group (8,9) cast, however, doubts on cytochrome oxidase functioning

Proceedings of the 16th FEBS Congress
Part B, pp. 323–330

in the native membrane, under steady-state conditions, as a proton pump.

Besides the Q cycle (2) a cytochrome b cycle has also been proposed for proton translocation in cytochrome c reductase (6). Difficulties to explain the observations available, purely in terms of direct ligand conduction or, alternatively, by co-operative H^+ transfer, have led us to consider the possibility that H^+ translocation derives from combination of these two types of mechanisms (8,9).

We developed a model (Fig.1) where ubiquinol of the pool delivers 1 e^- to protein-bound semiquinone, through an antimycin-insensitive reaction, at a site in protonic equilibrium with the N space. The anionic ring of the semiquinone is attracted at the P side of the membrane and is oxidized by cytochrome b_{566}, which then transfers e^- to cytochrome b_{562}, at the N side, and from this to bound semiquinone through an antimycin sensitive reaction. Protonation of the UQ°/UQH_2 couple from the N side upon reduction and H^+ release at the P side, upon oxidation, both provided by specific proton conduction path-

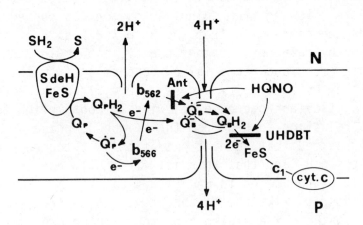

Fig.1. Q-gated pump mechanism for H^+ translocation in cytochrome c reductase (8).

ways in the proteins, would result in transmembrane H^+ translocation. Since the semiquinone has pK around 5-6 this can transfer $4H^+$ per $2e^-$ at physiological pH's.

$\Delta\mu H^+$ exerts a back pressure on internal e^- transfer within the b-c_1 complex (10). b-c_1 vesicles were supplemented with traces of cytochrome c and cytochrome oxidase. Duroquinol gave a steady-state e^- flow to oxygen and reduction of cytochromes b_{566}, b_{562} and c_1 (Fig.2). Valinomycin caused oxidation of cytochromes b_{566} and transition of c cytochromes towards reduction. Cytochrome b_{562} underwent an oxidation which was smaller than the redox changes of the other two components.

Addition of nigericin per se had small effect on the redox level of b and c cytochromes. Addition of valinomycin to the particles supplemented with nigericin caused marked oxidation of b_{566} and reduction of c cytochromes but only small oxidation of b_{562}.

According to the Q cycle, $\Delta\psi$ collapse should accelerate e^- flow from b_{566} at the P side to b_{562} at the N side of the membrane, but not further e^- flow from b_{562} to cytochrome c_1, which is mediated by electroneutral transmembrane hydrogen conduction by QH_2. The present observations can, on the other hand, be explained by electrogenic H^+ translocation associated to e^- flow from b_{562} to c_1, as envisaged in our model.

Fig. 3 shows that when the soluble reductase was treated with ^{14}C-DCCD, a major binding of the reagent to the 8 kDa band was observed, with attenuation of this band and decrease of its migration. The 12 kDa band and the Fe-S protein band were also reduced after treatment with DCCD and a new band with a weight of 40 kDa appeared, which did not exhibit radioactivity (11).

It is likely that polypeptide(s) in the 8 kDa band, after reaction with ^{14}C-DCCD get cross-linked with the Fe-S protein in a reaction leading to release of urea derivative of ^{14}C-DCCD.

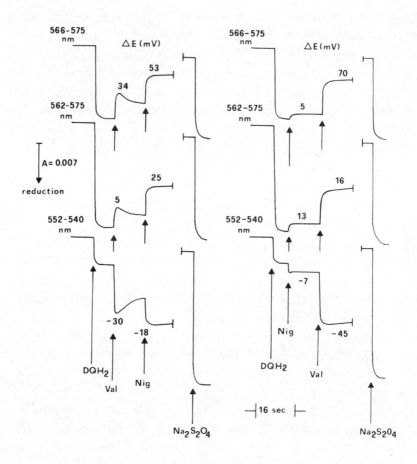

Fig.2. Effect of valinomycin and nigericin on steady-
        state redox level of b and c_1 cytochromes in
        b-c_1 vesicles.

b-c_1 vesicles (0.2 mg protein/ml) in 125 mM choline-chlo-
ride, 10 mM K-chloride, 0.5 mM K-phosphate (pH 7.2) and
50 μM EDTA were supplemented with 1 μM ferricytochrome c
and 0.37 μM purified cytochrome oxidase. The reaction was
started by the addition of 300 μM duroquinol. Where indicated, 1 μg/ml valinomycin and 1 μg/ml nigericin were added. The figures on the traces represent the steady-state
redox transitions.(For details see ref.10).

326

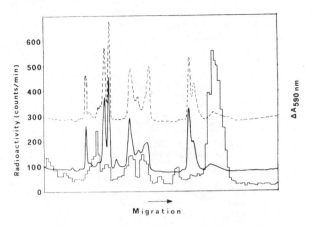

Fig.3. Densitometric profiles and ^{14}C-DCCD distribution
of Coomassie Blue stained gels of b-c$_1$ complex
treated with ^{14}C-DCCD.
For details see ref.11. Symbols: (---), control; (——),
plus ^{14}C-DCCD.

Modification of the b-c$_1$ complex with DCCD inhibited H$^+$
release elicited by the addition of duroquinol to cytochrome c supplemented b-c$_1$ vesicles, but had no significant effect on cytochrome c reduction (11).

The 8 and 12 kDa bands and possibly also the Fe-S protein, modified and cross-linked by DCCD, seem, therefore,
to be involved in the coupling between electron flow and
vectorial proton translocation.

Fig. 4 shows that treatment of the isolated cytochrome
c reductase with papain resulted in enhanced migration of
core protein II and of the 15 kDa subunit, indicative of
their partial cleavage. There was also decrease of the
band corresponding to the Fe-S protein and appearance of
two new bands which may represent cleavage products of
the Fe-S protein.

Papain digestion of the soluble enzyme, before incorporation in liposomes, resulted in inhibition of e$^-$ flow
and suppression of vectorial H$^+$ translocation (Table I).

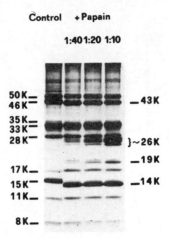

Fig.4. SDS-PAGE (12-20% acrylamide gradient gel in 6 M
urea) of b-c$_1$ complex; effect of increasing concentrations of papain (w:w).

The residual release of 1 H^+/e^- derives, in fact, from
the scalar oxidation of quinol by cytochrome c.

TABLE I. PROTON TRANSLOCATION AND ELECTRON TRANSFER BY
b-c$_1$ COMPLEX TREATED WITH PAPAIN.
b-c$_1$ complex was treated with papain (1:20, w:w) for 30
min at 25°C in Tris-sucrose-hystidine buffer (pH 8.0)
containing 5 mM cysteine and 2 mM EDTA.Aliquots were treated with 10% T.C.A. for SDS-PAGE.The enzyme was reconstituted into liposomes by cholate dialysis.

	Rate of H^+ release	Rate of cyt.c reduction	H^+/e^-
	($nmol \cdot min^{-1} \cdot mg$ protein^{-1})		
Control	660	342	1.93
Papain treated	328	276	1.19

It was apparent from the results that whilst the inhibition of e$^-$ flow was correlated with the digestion of
the Fe-S protein, the suppression of vectorial H$^+$ translocation was correlated with digestion of core protein II
and the 15 kDa protein.

What presented support the concept that vectorial organization of protolytic redox reactions represents a central step in the coupling between e$^-$ flow and H$^+$ transport
in the quinone-cyt.c segment of the chain. The possibility
that the anisotropy derives simply from vectorial e$^-$ flow
and diffusion of quinone molecules (2) appears, however,
to be unsufficient to explain the observation available.

Polypeptides of the cytochrome c reductase may provide
H$^+$ conducting pathways. Asymmetric H$^+$ conduction along
specific sequences may be promoted by redox-linked pK
shifts of basic and acid residues engaged in salt bridges (9).

REFERENCES

1. Mitchell, P. (1966). Chemiosmotic coupling in oxidative
    and photosynthetic phosphorylation. Glynn Research,
    Bodmin.

2. Mitchell, P. (1976). Possible molecular mechanism of
    the protonmotive function of cytochrome systems.
    J. Theor. Biol. 62, 327-367.

3. Papa, S., Guerrieri, F., Lorusso, M. and Simone, S.
    (1973). Proton translocation and energy transduction
    in mitochondria. Biochimie 55, 703-716.

4. Papa, S. (1976). Proton translocation reaction in the
    respiratory chain. Biochim.Biophy. Acta 456, 39-84.

5. Papa, S., Lorusso, M., Izzo, G. and Capuano, F. (1981).
    Control of electron transfer in the cytochrome system

of mitochondria by pH, transmembrane pH gradient and electrical potential. Biochem. J. 194, 395-406.

6.Wikström, M., Krab, K. and Saraste, M. (1981). Proton-translocating cytochrome complexes. Ann. Rev. Biochem. 50, 623-655.

7.Mitchell, P. (1980). Protonmotive cytochrome system of mitochondria. Ann. N.Y. Acad. Sci. 341, 564-584.

8.Papa, S., Lorusso, M. and Guerrieri, F. (1982). Energy transfer by redox proteins in mitochondria. In: Cell Function and Differentiation, G. Akoyunoglou et al. (eds). Alan R. Liss, Inc., New York, pp. 423-437.

9.Papa, S. (1982). Molecular mechanism of proton transloe-cation by the cytochrome system and the ATPase of mi-tochondria. Role of proteins. J. Bioenerg. Biomembr. 14, 69-86.

10.Papa, S., Lorusso, M., Boffoli, D. and Bellomo, E.(1983). Redox-linked proton translocation in the $b-c_1$ complex from beef-heart mitochondria reconstituted into pho-spholipid vesicles. General characteristics and con-trol of electron flow by $\Delta\mu H^+$. Eur. J. Biochem. 137, 405-412.

11. Lorusso, M., Gatti, D., Boffoli, D., Bellomo, E. and Papa, S. (1983). Redox-linked proton translocation in the $b-c_1$ complex from beef-heart mitochondria recon-stituted into phospholipid vesicles. Studies with chemical modifiers of aminoacid residues. Eur. J. Biochem. 137, 413-420.

THE RESPIRATION-COUPLED Na$^+$ PUMP IN VIBRIO ALGINOLYTICUS: Na$^+$ TRANSLOCATION AT NADH-QUINONE OXIDOREDUCTASE SEGMENT

HAJIME TOKUDA
Research Institute for Chemobiodynamics, Chiba University, 1-8-1 Inohana, Chiba 280, Japan

INTRODUCTION

As proposed by the chemiosmotic theory of P. Mitchell (1, 2), the vectorial translocation of H$^+$ by respiratory chain or H$^+$-motive ATPase leads to the generation of an electrochemical potential of proton (proton motive force) across the membrane. The proton motive force (Δp) is composed of an electrical component $\Delta\psi$ (negative inside) and chemical component ΔpH (alkaline inside) in the following relatinship:

$$\Delta p = \Delta\psi - Z\Delta pH \qquad (\text{in mV}) \qquad (1)$$

where Z is equal to 59 at room temperature. It is well established that Δp drives various energy-dependent reactions. Many active transport sytems are coupled to the inwardly directed proton movement. Generation of the electrochemical potential of sodium (sodium motive force) is performed by a Δp-driven Na$^+$/H$^+$ antiport system (3) and, hence, secondary to the generation of the proton motive force. This type of bioenergetics is common to most of non-halophilic bacteria in which energy-generating reactions and energy-consuming reactions are performed by proton circulation across the membrane.

On the other hand, recent studies on the energy coupling mechanisms in the marine bacterium _Vibrio alginolyticus_, that requires Na$^+$ for growth, revealed that bioenergetics of this strain is performed by sodium circulation across the membrane. The sodium motive force was found to be an immediate driving force for amino acids and sucrose transports (4). It was also reported that the flagella motility of this strain is driven by the sodium motive force (5). Above all, the presence of

Proceedings of the 16th FEBS Congress
Part B, pp. 331–339
© 1985 VNU Science Press

a Na^+-motive respiratory chain (6, 7) is astonishing. This system generates the sodium motive force as a direct result of respiration and seems to play an important role in the energetics of this strain. Furthermore, the mechanism of the Na^+-motive respiratory chain is of great interest since this system is expected to give important informations concerning the controversial mechanism for cation extrusion by respiration (8, 9).

THE RESPIRATION-COUPLED Na^+ PUMP IN VIBRIO ALGINOLYTICUS

Effects of CCCP on the generation of the sodium motive force

The activity of the Na^+-motive respiratory chain (Na^+ pump) is maximum at alkaline pH but minimum at acidic pH (7). In contrast, the extrusion of H^+ by respiration occurs over the pH range of 6 to 9. Therefore, bioenergetics of V. alginolyticus shows striking differences in the sensitivity to a proton conductor, carbonyl-cyanide m-chlorophenylhydrazone (CCCP), depending on external pH. At acidic pH, the immediate result of respiration is the generation of the proton motive force. Since CCCP short-circuits the extrusion of H^+, neither $\Delta\psi$ nor ΔpH is generated in the presence of CCCP (10). The generation of the sodium motive force at acidic pH is performed only by the Na^+/H^+ antiport system. Therefore, collapse of the proton motive force by CCCP leads to the inhibition of Na^+ extrusion and active transports (6). On the other hand, at alkaline pH, the Na^+ pump generates $\Delta\psi$ by the electrogenic extrusion of Na^+. Influx of H^+ induced by CCCP does not short-circuit this Na^+ extrusion and continues until a steady-state is reached. At the steady-state, $\Delta\psi$ (negative inside) and ΔpH (acidic inside) of similar magnitude but in opposite polarity are generated, resulting in the collapse of Δp. Generation of the ΔpH is driven by CCCP resistant $\Delta\psi$, therefore, the magnitude of the ΔpH never exceeds the magnitude of CCCP resistant $\Delta\psi$. This means that no net influx of H^+ occurs at the steady-state. Thus, the $\Delta\psi$ at alkaline pH is resistant to CCCP unless the generation of ΔpH (inside acidic) is suppressed (7). Since the generation of the sodium motive force occurs in the presence of CCCP, active uptake of solutes (6) and flagella motility (5) are resistant to CCCP when the Na^+ pump functions.

Isolation of the Na^+ pump-defective mutants

The growth of V. alginolyticus became remarkably resistant to CCCP when the Na^+ pump functions (11). Minimal inhibitory concentration for CCCP was 4 μM at pH 6.5 whereas that at pH 8.5 was higher than 80 μM (12). These findings clearly indicate that the proton motive force is not essential for growth when the Na^+ pump functions and that the sodium motive force is able to play a central role in the energetics of V. alginolyticus. Taking advantage of these findings, an attempt was made to isolate the Na^+ pump-defective mutants. The strains unable to grow in the presence of CCCP were selected at pH 8.5 (12). In contrast to the wild type cells, the isolated mutants, Nap 1 and Nap 2, were unable to extrude Na^+ in the presence of CCCP. On the other hand, the activity of H^+ extrusion by respiration was similar in all the strains examined. These results indicate that the mutants are specifically defective in the Na^+-motive respiratory chain. It became also clear that Na^+ extrusion by the mutants is performed only by the Na^+/H^+ antiport system.

Coupling site of the Na^+ pump

Respiratory activities were examined (13) in membranes prepared from osmotically lysed cells of the wild type, Na^+ pump-defective mutants and a spontaneous revertant, Nap 2R. It may be important to point out that the membranes used in these experiments are not closed vesicles and permeable to dextran (14). NADH oxidase activity in these membranes was examined at pH 7.5 as a function of salt concentration (Fig. 1). The NADH oxidase of the wild type and revertant required Na^+ for maximum activity. About 0.2 M NaCl gave an maximum activity, whereas stimulation by KCl was slight. On the other hand, the NADH oxidase of the mutants did not show any specific requirement for Na^+. The activities determined in NaCl and KCl were essentially the same. From these results, it became clear that the Na^+ requirement of NADH oxidase, which has been found before

333

(14), is due to the Na$^+$ pump.

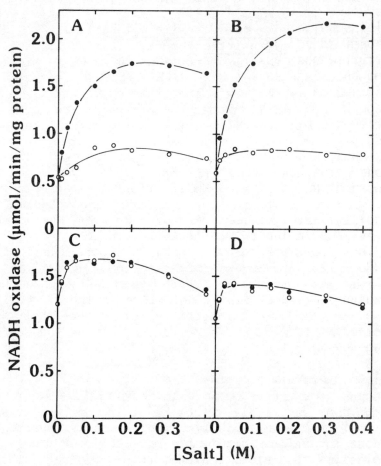

Fig. 1 Effect of salt on the NADH oxidase of <u>V.</u> <u>alginolyticus</u> membranes (13). NADH oxidase activity was determined in various concentrations of KCl (O) or NaCl (●). Membranes were prepared from the wild type (A), Nap 2R (B), Nap 1 (C), and Nap 2 (D).

The activity of NADH oxidase was determined as a function of pH in KCl and NaCl. In NaCl, the activities of the wild type and revertant were dependent on pH with an optimum at pH about 8. In KCl, however, the activities of both membranes were less dependent on pH and always lower than those determined in NaCl. As a result, the difference between activities determined in KCl and NaCl, or the Na^+-dependent activity, was maximum at pH about 8 and minimum at pH 6. These results are in good agreement with the pH dependence of the Na^+ pump determined in whole cells (7). On the other hand, the NADH oxidase of mutant membranes showed no specific requirement for Na^+ over the whole pH range tested.

In order to determine the Na^+-dependent site of NADH oxidase, the effects of cations and electron donors on ubiquinol formation by membranes were examined (Table 1).

Table 1 Effects of salt and electron donor on QH_2 formation (13).

Membrane	Salt (0.2 M)	Activity (μmol/min/mg protein)	
		NADH	G3P
wild type	KCl	0.37	0.48
	NaCl	0.99	0.46
Nap 1	KCl	0.43	0.43
	NaCl	0.42	0.43
Nap 2	KCl	0.51	0.78
	NaCl	0.54	0.83
Nap 2R	KCl	0.29	0.59
	NaCl	0.82	0.65

The assays were performed in the presence of 5 μM ubiquinone-1 (Q-1) and 10 mM KCN which was added to inhibit the re-oxidation of ubiquinol-1 (QH_2). In the presence of NADH as an electron donor, QH_2 formation by the wild type and revertant was dependent on Na^+, whereas the activity of mutant membranes was not affected by species of cation. When glycerol-3-phosphate (G3P) was used as an electron donor, however, all the membranes showed Na^+-independent QH_2 formation. These results clearly indicate that the Na^+-dependent site of NADH oxidase is localized in NADH:quinone oxidoreductase segment.

Inhibition of NADH oxidase and QH_2 formation by a respiratory inhibitor, 2-heptyl-4-hydroxyquinoline-N-oxide (HQNO), was exmained (Fig. 2). HQNO specifically

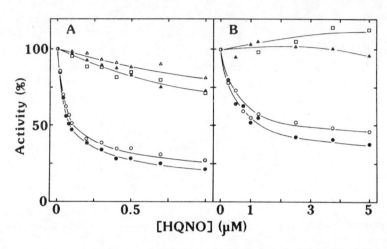

Fig. 2. Inhibition of NADH oxidase and QH_2 formation by HQNO (13). NADH oxidase (A) and NADH-linked QH_2 formation (B) were assayed in 0.2 M NaCl with membranes prepared from the wild type (O), Nap 1 (△), Nap 2 (▲), and Nap 2R (●). A symbol (□) represents Na^+-independent NADH oxidase (A) and G3P-linked QH_2 formation (B) of the wild type.

inhibited the Na^+-dependent NADH oxidase of the wild type and revertant membranes, whereas the Na^+-independent NADH oxidase of the mutants was little affected by the inhibitor. It should be noted that the Na^+-independent activity of the wild type membranes observed in the absence of Na^+ was also insensitive to HQNO. Similarly, the Na^+-dependent QH_2 formation by the wild type and revertant membranes observed in the presence of NADH was sensitive to HQNO. In contrast, G3P-linked QH_2 formation by the wild type and NADH-linked QH_2 formation by the mutant were neither dependent on Na^+ (Table 1) nor sensitive to HQNO (Fig. 2). From these results, it is evident that HQNO specifically inhibits the Na^+-dependent NADH:quinone oxidoreductase, that is, the coupling site of the Na$^+$ pump. It has been reported (7) that the inactivation of the Na$^+$ pump by HQNO in whole cells was overcome by the addition of an artificial electron donor, N,N,N',N'-tetramethyl-p-phenylenediamine (TMPD). However, the TMPD-dependent energization of the Na$^+$ pump was found to be dependent on oxidized, but not reduced, TMPD (13).

CONCLUSION

The scheme given in Fig. 3 summarizes the conclusion on the coupling site of the Na$^+$-motive respiratory chain of V. alginolyticus. The Na$^+$ requirement of NADH oxidase was found to be due to the Na$^+$ pump. Inhibition by HQNO

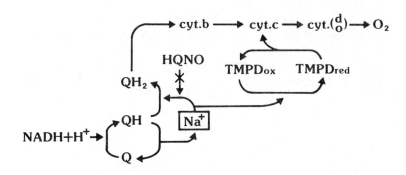

Fig. 3. Schematic representation of the Na$^+$-motive respiratory chain (13). The translocation site of Na$^+$ is shown as $\boxed{\text{Na}^+}$. Q, QH, and QH$_2$ indicate quinone, semiquinone radical, and quinol, respectively. ox, oxidized; red, reduced.

was specific to this Na$^+$-dependent NADH oxidase. Moreover, the NADH:quinone oxidoreductase was characterized as a Na$^+$-dependent, HQNO-sensitive site of NADH oxidase. Therefore, the translocation of Na$^+$ by respiration seems to occur at the NADH:quinone oxidoreductase segment. It was recently found that the ubiquinol formation takes place via semiquinone radicals. Interestingly, this radical formation is neither dependent on Na$^+$ nor sensitive to HQNO. On the contrary, the

337

subsequent formation of ubiquinol, presumably by the dismutation of semiquinone radicals, is dependent on Na^+ and sensitive to HQNO. Therefore, it seems likely that the Na^+ translocation is coupled to the formation of quinol from semiquinone radical. HQNO presumably inhibits the Na^+ pump by preventing this reaction. It seems also likely that the oxidized TMPD, which is a radical, accepts electrons from the coupling site and, thus, is able to energize the Na^+ pump.

REFERENCES

1. Mitchell, P. (1968). Chemiosmotic coupling and energy transduction. Glynn Research, Bodmin, Cornwall, England.
2. Mitchell, P. (1973). Performance and conservation of osmotic work by proton-coupled solute porter systems. J. Bioenerg. 4, 63-91.
3. West, I. C. and Mitchell, P. (1974). Proton/sodium ion antiport in Escherichia coli. Biochem. J. 144, 87-90.
4. Tokuda, H., Sugasawa, M. and Unemoto, T. (1982). Roles of Na^+ and K^+ in α-aminoisobutyric acid transport by the marine bacterium Vibrio alginolyticus. J. Biol. Chem. 257, 788-794.
5. Chernyak, B. V., Dibrov, P. A., Glagolev, A. N., Sherman, M. Yu. and Skulachev, V. P. (1983). A novel type of energetics in a marine alkali-tolerant bacterium (ΔμNa-driven motility and sodium cycle). FEBS Lett. 164, 38-42.
6. Tokuda, H. and Unemoto, T. (1981). A respiration-dependent primary sodium extrusion system functioning at alkaline pH in the marine bacterium Vibrio alginolyticus. Biochem. Biophys. Res. Commun. 102, 265-271.
7. Tokuda, H. and Unemoto, T. (1982). Characterization of the respiration-dependent Na^+ pump in the marine bacterium Vibrio alginolyticus. J. Biol. Chem. 257, 10007-10014.
8. Mitchell, P. (1979). Compartmentation and communication in living systems. Ligand conduction: a general catalytic principle in chemical, osmotic and chemi-

osmotic reaction systems. Eur. J. Biochem. 95, 1–20.

9. Wikström, M. and Krab, K. (1980). Respiration–linked H$^+$ translocation in mitochondria:stoichiometry and mechanism. Curr. Top. Bioenerg. 10, 51–101.

10. Tokuda, H., Nakamura, T. and Unemoto, T. (1981). Potassium ion is required for the generation of pH–dependent membrane potential and ΔpH by the marine bacterium Vibrio alginolyticus. Biochemistry 20, 4198–4203.

11. Tokuda, H. and Unemoto, T. (1983). Growth of a marine Vibrio alginolyticus and moderately halophilic V. costicola becomes uncoupler resistant when the respiration–dependent Na$^+$ pump functions. J. Bacteriol. 156, 636–643.

12. Tokuda, H. (1983). Isolation of Vibrio alginolyticus mutants defective in the respiration–coupled Na$^+$ pump. Biochem. Biophys. Res. Commun. 114, 113–118.

13. Tokuda, H. and Unemoto, T. (1984). Na$^+$ is translocated at NADH:quinone oxidoreductase segment in the respiratory chain of Vibrio alginolyticus. J. Biol. Chem. 259, 7785–7790.

14. Unemoto, T., Hayashi, M. and Hayashi, M. (1977). Na$^+$–dependent activation of NADH oxidase in membrane fractions from halophilic Vibrio alginolyticus and V. costicolus. J. Biochem. (Tokyo) 82, 1389–1395.

MOLECULAR AND ENZYMATIC BASIS OF CARCINOGENESIS

PROTO-ONCOGENE RELATED AND RETROVIRAL RELATED SEQUENCES IN A HUMAN GENOME

Lev L. KISSELEV
Institute of Molecular Biology, the USSR Academy of
Sciences, 117984 Moscow

This paper briefly summarizes the data obtained recently
by I. M. Chumakov, E. R. Zabarovsky, V. S. Prassolov,
V. L. Mett, F. B. Berditchevsky and L. O. Tretyakov
at the author's laboratory. The aim of this work was
to examine in a more detail the proto-oncogenese of
a human genome in terms of its number, diversity and
possible mechanisms of inactivation taking as a model
human counterparts of well known retroviral oncogene
mos present in the Moloney strain of murine sarcoma
virus (MSV), a derivative of a murine leukemia virus
(MLV) which acquired a piece of cellular genome after
long cultivation. The problem of cellular proto-oncogenes and respective retroviral onc genes has been
reviewed many times, most recently by several authors
(1-4).

In 1979 we observed that $cDNA_{MSV}$ hybridizes with two
EcoRI-fragments of a total human placental DNA (5,6).
In parallel, in mouse genome a unique mos-positive
14-15 kb-fragment generated by EcoRI has been revealed,
cloned and mapped (7-9). In rat a similar unique EcoRI-
-fragment was detected, too (5,6).

To proceed further in evaluation of structure and
mapping of the MSV-related regions in human genome,
we prepared a mos-specific probe (10,11) by cloning
a fragment of a double-stranded DNA_{MSV} synthesized in
disrupted virions and used it for screening a human
gene library in phage λ Charon 4A strain (11,12).
It turned out that human DNA inserts in recombinant
phages as follows from molecular hybridization data
with mos-specific and retroviral specific probes and
physical mapping might be subdivided into two types:
(i) related to portions of MLV genome that may be con-

Proceedings of the 16th FEBS Congress
Part B, pp. 343–351

sidered as endogenous proretrovirus or its fragment(s) related to or similar with MLV, (ii) related to both mos-specific and retroviral-specific nucleotide sequences resembling in certain sence a sarcoma-like provirus.

Obviously, the better insight into understanding of this phenomenon might be achieved with more thorough studies of these DNA regions and such investigation has been undertaken (13). Several cloned fragments of human DNA contain sequences resembling mos. The physical maps of them are different and they belong to different regions of human genome being nonallelic to each other (with one exception of gp7 and gp8 phages). The family of mos-related sequences is characterized also by the presence of retroviral-like sequences neighbouring or overlapping with the mos-related regions. Moreover, the same DNA fragment contains also Alu element typical for human genome and widely spread within it. The observed mosaic is not a consequence of redistribution of these structural elements due to repeated molecular cloning since genomic DNA restriction fragments generate the same sizes hybridizable with appropriate probes at least for one of the DNA inserts in λ gp5.

A detailed mapping with a set of restriction enzymes of one of these clones, λ gp5, fully confirmed the mosaic distribution of the mos-, retro- and Alu-elements within human DNA insert (13,14). Next step consisted of sequencing a part of the λ gp5 insert by means of chemical degradation technique of Maxam and Gilbert and by dideoxy method of Sanger.

Firstly, we sequenced a NV-1 region (HindII fragment of λ gp5), 841 bp long (15) which hybridizes both with mos and Alu probes. Analysis of the sequence showed the presence of two Alu elements. The first one maps at position 59-339 and is flanked by 8-bp direct repeats. The second Alu is located at positions 449-756 and is flanked by 9-bp repeats. Both Alu elements have the same orientation and display a considerable homology (84% and 86%) to the consensus structure but less homology (80%) to each other.

These two Alu repeats interrupt the stretch of nucleotides that is homologous to a part of the proto-mos

344

coding region. Three homologous domains can be deduced
from the sequence. The first one at position 1-58 is
homologous to 868-924 bp of hu-mos or to 784-840 bp
of the murine counterpart. To optimize the allignment
of homologous regions we assumed that a few short (less
then 3 bp) deletions and insertions are not shared by
the λ gp5 insert and proto-mos. The second domain begins just after the short direct repeat flanking the
first Alu element at position 347 and continues to
the beginning of the second Alu element at position
448. The homologysis to 918-1022 bp of hu-mos and to
834-938 bp of the murine counterpart. The last domain
starts at the end of 9-bp repeat flanking the second
Alu element at position 767 and continues to the end
of the sequenced region. This domain is homologous to
985-1058 bp of the human and to 901-974 bp of the murine
proto-mos genes. The unique feature of this homology
is the partial overlapping of the regions homologous
to proto-mos. We have calculated the statistical probability of finding such homology between 250-bp random
sequences and found it improbable (10^{-20}).

The DNA region homologous to proto-mos cannot code
for any polypeptide larger than 28 amino acids because
of the dense distribution of termination codons. This
finding substantiated our suspicion that we were probably dealing with a pseudogene of proto-mos. Moreover,
we were unable to find anything resembling concensus
sequences for splicing signals in the vicinity of the
Alu elements, therefore these repeats cannot be excised
from the transcripts.

One could propose that inactivation of the duplicated
copy of proto-mos was attained by duplications in the
coding region of this gene. Such aberrations are located
in the regions flanking Alu elements and have rather
peculiar structures, indicating that duplication occurred in more than one step. More recent duplication
is evident from the existence of short perfect direct
repeats immediately flanking each Alu element. Moreover,
even longer stretches of nucleotides flanking Alu repeats are homologous to the one and the same region
of proto-mos as illustrated in the case of sequences
around the site of the second Alu element. The same

38-bp stretch of proto-mos is homologous not only to
34 bp (including the left 9-bp-direct repeat) immediately before this element, but also to 40 bp following
the direct repeat on the right side of the Alu. The
relation to proto-mos can reflect the common origin
of these regions, although now they do not possess a
significant degree of homology to each other. The higher
rate of changes accumulated between two pseudogenes
than between a pseudogene and an active one can explain
this fact. The probable cause of this old duplication
could be the transposition of the ancient form of Alu
element to the amplified proto-mos. The nucleotide
changes accumulated during this time could have erased
the homology between the duplicated regions although
the relatedness to a more conserved, active proto-mos
can still be seen. More recently, 9 bp derived from
the proximal region of the left side repeat were duplicated and transposed to the right side of the Alu element. The possible reason for this duplication could
be the process of conversion of the Alu element into
its present form. The same model based on the postulated two steps in the process of repeat formation also
explains the aberrations at the sides adjacent to the
first Alu element. The ancient duplication was 7-bp
long and some resemblence is still preserved. The second
step resulted in duplication of the left repeat and
its translocation to the right side of the Alu element.
This fact argues against the probability that the association of Alu elements with the duplication is the
result of mere coincidence.

Without regard to the possible role of Alu elements
in the inactivation of potentially oncogenic copies
of proto-mos our results represents one of the first
proofs of the mobile nature of Alu repeats.

The other mos-related region, designated CL-1 has
been also sequenced (16). Starting from 273 nucleotide
the sequence is homologous to mu-mos gene after 74
nucleotide counting from ATG initiation codon. The
homology is around 55% and stops at position 453. It
is remarkable that homology of CL-1 region with mos
starts approximately at the same site where a recombination between proto-mos and retroviral genome of

MoMuLV has taken place (17) and where IAP integrates in plasmacytomas (18). The right part of the CL-1 is 50% homologous to the 3'-end of viral mos beginning at position 773 of the latter up to the end of the sequenced region.

The homology between NV-1 and CL-1 is around 50% i.e. of the same order as between these regions, hu- and mu-mos genes. Thus it is reasonable to assume that the NV-1 and CL-1 regions diverged very early fromeach other and from the progenitor of human proto-mos gene.

When comparisons have been made, it turned out that CL-1 is closer to mu-mos than to hu-mos in its sequence. This unusual situation might be explained by the fact that initial screening of the library has been undertaken with viral mos (nearly identical with mu-mos), not with hu-mos probe (11).

The main difference between mu-mos and hu-mos, on one hand, and CL-1, on the other consists in existence of a long stretch of nucleotides present inside the gene in the first two cases and absent in the latter. Two explanations might be suggested. Either due to homologous recombination an internal part of the gene was excised (this is probable since the deleted part is flanked by short homologous regions) or if the de-leted part represented an exon of the progenitor intron--containing mos gene, CL-1 had appeared in the past as a result of an alternative splicing.

Since mos-related regions of CL-1 contain termination codons in all frames one may tentatively assign the CL-1 region to a pseudogene, too. However, in pseudo-genes the degree of homology to the initial gene should be roughly the same along the polynucleotide chain. This is not the case for CL-1, for example, between positions 392-453 and 442-532 the homology is high (60-65%) whereas between positions 533-601 and 636-685 it is low (~ 36%). Furthermore, molecular hybridiza-tion of a part of CL-1 region with DNA from various species proved high conservation of its structure being inconsistant with pseudogene nature of this region.

Therefore the CL-1 region belonging structurally to mos-related sequences may be functionally different. Obviously, this question remains open till more infor-

mation become available on the function and structure
of mos-related domains in human genome.

The mos-related region of CL-1 is flanked downstream
by a sequence resembling the leader non-translatable
sequence of MLV-Mo RNA. Moreover, next to it a sequence
was recognized which is partially complementary to
mammalian initiator tRNA^{Met}. Finally, tRNA binding site
neighboured with a sequence resembling a U5 region of
retroviral long terminal repeats (19). This pattern
strongly suggests that part of the CL-1 region represents a fragment of proretroviral genome including
three features of it - non-translatable region, tRNA
binding site and U5 region of LTR.

These sequence data are in full agreement with the
previous results mentioned above which showed the presence of retroviral like elements in the ORAgp5 and
other loci of human genome.

A homology between the U5 like sequence of CL-1 and
U5 regions of LTRs lies within 50-55% irrespectively
of the retroviruses taken into comparison. Among them
are retroviruses of C, B and A types and VL-30 retroviral like elements. The highest degree of homology
(58%) is with the U5 region of Mo-MuLV. Although the
homology between CL-1 and U5 seems to be not very high
it should be stressed that the same holds true if to
compare the U5 regions of various known LTRs of different proviruses. Furthermore, if to combine various
regions of U5 from different viruses into a composite
U5, its homology raises up to 80% with respect to CL-1.

The sequence organization of the whole CL-1 region
and molecular hybridization data led us to conclude
that ORAgp5 locus contains a part of endogeneous human
proretrovirus. This conclusion is strengthened by the
observation that the U5 like region is reiterated about
10 times in a human genome (a value close for other
mammalian and avian endogenous retroviruses), and is
present at 5'end of polyA containing RNAs of normal
and malignant human cells 21-35S in size (19).

The tight linkage between mos like sequences and proviral like sequences strongly supports the hypothesis
proposed by us earlier which postulates the involvement of proretroviruses in amplification of proto-

-oncogenes. This proposal is also consistent with a different chrosomal location of hu-mos and ORAgp5 loci in a human genome (20).

Summarizing, we assume (21) that (a) proto-oncogenes are diverged and amplified mostly by a non-tandem duplication; (b) proretroviruses are involved in proto-oncogene amplification; (c) proto-oncogenes might be inactivated by mobile genetic elements and other types of genetic rearrangements; (d) new reiterated expressable proretroviral like element is discovered in mammalian genome.

Those conclusions are based on our experience with mos gene and human genome, however they can be probably extrapolated to other proto-oncogenes and to genomes of other higher eukaryotes.

Dedicated to the memory od Professor V. A. Engelhart, the organizer of the FEBS Meeting Symposium on molecular oncology.

REFERENCES

1. Aaronson, S. A. (1983). Unique aspects of the interactions of retroviruses with vertebrate cells. Cancer Res. 43, 1-5.
2. Bishop, J. M. (1983). Cellular oncogenes and retroviruses. Ann. Rev. Biochem. 52, 301-354.
3. Duesberg, P. H. (1983). Retroviral transforming genes in normal cells? Nature 304, 219-226.
4. Willecke, K. and Schäfer, R. (1984). Human oncogenes. Hum. Genet. 66, 132-142.
5. Chumakov, I. M., Prassolov, V. S. and Kisselev, L. L. (1979). Mammalian DNA sequences homologous to the src gene of Moloney murine sarcoma virus Hoppe Zeoler's. Z. Physiol. Chem. 360, 1023.
6. Chumakov, I. M., Prassolov, V. S. and Kisselev, L. L. (1980). Mammalian nucleotide sequences related to the src gene of Moloney sarcoma virus and their mapping. Dokl. AN SSSR (Moscow) 252, 232-235.
7. Tronick, S. K., Robbins, K. C., Canaani, E., Devare, S. G., Andersen, P. R. and Aaronson, S. A. (1979). Molecular cloning of Moloney murine sarcoma virus: arrangement of virus related sequences

within the normal mouse genome. Proc. Natl. Acad. Sci. USA, 76, 6314-6318.

8. Jones, M., Bosselman, R. A., Van den Hoorn, F. A., Berns, A., Fan, H. and Verma, I. M. (1980). Identification and molecular cloning of Moloney mouse sarcoma virus specific sequences from uninfected mouse cells. Proc. Natl. Acad. Sci. USA 77, 2651-2655.

9. Oscarsson, M., McClements, W. L., Blair, D. G., Maizel, J. V. and Van de Woude, G. F. (1980). Properties of a normal mouse cell DNA sequence (sarc) homologous to the src sequence of Moloney sarcoma virus. Science 207, 1222-1224.

10. Chumakov, I. M., Zabarovsky, E. R., Mett, V. L., Prassolov, V. S. and Kisselev, L. L. (1981). Cloning of fragment of Moloney murine sarcoma virus containing its oncogene. Dokl. AN SSSR (moscow) 259, 219-222.

11. Chumakov, I. M., Zabarovsky, E. R., Mett, V. L., Prassolov, V. S. and Kisselev, L. L. (1982). Human nucleotide sequences related to the transforming gene of a murine sarcoma virus: studies with cloned viral and cellular DNAs. Gene 17, 19-26.

12. Zabarovsky, E. R., Chumakov, I. M., Prassolov, V. S. and Kisselev, L. L. (1980). Construction of human gene library and cloning of nucleotide sequences homologous to genomes of murine sarcoma and leukemia viruses. Dokl. AN SSSR 255, 1275-1277.

13. Zabarovsky, E. R., Chumakov, I. M., Prassolov, V. S. and Kisselev, L. L. (1984). Human genomic regions containing homologs of oncogenes and retroviral genes. Proto-mos gene family and an unusual structure of the ORAgp5 locus. Mol. Biol. (Moscow) 18, 60-82.

14. Zabarovsky, E. R., Chumakov, I. M. and Kisselev, L. L. (1983). Tight linkage of retroviral-like sequences to a variant human c-mos gene in the human genome. Gene 23, 379-384.

15. Zabarovsky, E. R., Chumakov, I. M., Prassolov, V. S. and Kisselev, L. L. (1984). The coding region of the human c-mos pseudogene contains Alu repeat insertions. Gene, in press.

16. Zabarovsky, E. R., Prassolov, V. S., Tretyakov, L. O., Chumakov, I. M. and Kisselev, L. L. (1984). Bioorg. Chem. (Moscow) 10, in press.
17. Van Beveren, C., Van Straaten, F., Galleshaw, J. A. and Verma, I. M. (1981). Nucleotide sequence of the genome of a murine sarcoma virus. Cell 27, 97-108.
18. Cohen, J. B., Unger, T., Rechavi, G., Canaani, E. and Givol, D. (1983). Rearrangement of the oncogene c-mos in mouse myeloma NSI and hybridomas. Nature 306, 797-799.
19. Chumakov, I. M., Zabarovsky, E. R., Prassolov, V. S., Mett, V. L. and Kisselev, L. L. (1985). Human genomic regions containing homologs of oncogenes and retroviral genes. 2. New class of retroviral elements. Mol. Biol. (Moscow) 19, in press.
20. Berditchevsly, F. B. and Chumakov, I. M. 81985). Chromosomal segregation of the two genes from the human mos family. Dokl. Akad. Nauk SSSR (Moscow), in press.
21. kisselev, L. L., Chumakov, I. M., Zabarovsky, E. R., Prassolov, V. S., Mett, V. L., Berditchevsky, F. B. and Tretyakov, L. O. (1985). Human genome: proto-oncogenes and proretroviruses. Folia biol. (Praha), in press.

ALTERED AND CRYPTIC PROVIRAL SEQUENCES IN MAMMALIAN TUMOUR CELL LINES AND CHARACTERIZATION OF RESCUED ASVs

J. SVOBODA, J. GERYK, V. LHOTÁK, J. PICHRTOVÁ
Institute of Molecular Genetics, Czechoslovak Academy of
Sciences, 166 37 Prague, Czechoslovakia.

Avian sarcoma viruses (ASV), a prototype of which is Rous
sarcoma virus (RSV), provide one of the best elaborated
models for study of retrovirus-mediated oncogenesis.

RSV has been studied extensively for many years, and
various approaches to its analysis have been developed.
One of them is the use of mammalian hosts, which was
disoovered by Zilber and Kryukova and Svet-Moldavsky and
Skorikova (1).

We established and characterized the first virogenic
mammalian tumour cell line XC containing an unexpressed
RSV genome. The non-infectious viral genome persisted
indefinitely in this line and in all cell clones as a
stable genetic marker, which allowed us to postulate
already in the early sixties that the viral genome is
integrated in XC cells as a provirus (2). We suggested
and showed that infectious transforming virus can be rescued from virogenic cells by their fusion with indicator
chicken fibroblasts. Finally, XC cells were successfully
emplyed to prove for the first time the DNA nature of
retroviral provirus by transfection procedure.

XC cells have a complicated arrangement of proviral
structures. Restriction enzymes, which digest provirus
only twice, such as SacI, also yield a number of junction
fragments, demonstrating that proviruses had been integrated at different sites of the cell genome. (3). In XC
cells one to two microchromosomes were also found (4).

Our previous, long-term karyological study of RSV
transformed mouse cells showed that variable numbers of
double-minute chromatin bodies (dms) are present, with a
high frequency, in such lines. After repeated passages l
the dms became replaced by stable microchromosomes (5).
These and additional observations suggested that the provirus may have been amplified in the XC cell line via dms

Proceedings of the 16th FEBS Congress
Part B, pp. 353–359
© 1985 VNU Science Press

knowm to be involved in cell gene amplification. This possibility is now being tested.

XC cells harbour two types of provirus. Type I provirus has the same EcoRI restriction pattern as has PR RSV, but is not rescuable by fusion with chicken fibroblasts. Type II provirus is rescuable and contains anadditional EcoRI site responsible for the generation of a 0.9 Md fragment (3,6).

To study the character and degree of possible modification of type II provirus, we produced a series of hamster cell lines using cloned virus obtained by transfection of chicken cells with XC DNA. A number of such tumours were first examined for provirus expression and virus rescue (7).

In collaboration with D. Stéhelin's laboratory we constructed the genetic maps of proviral structures integrated in several hamster tumour cell lines (6). The most deleted proviral structure was found in cryptovirogenic H-19 cells. It is represented by the v-src gene flanked by LTR's, and is accomodated on a 1.6 Md EcoRI fragment. Employing cell fusion with chicken cells infected with transformation-defective PR-C virus, we were not successful in rescuing transforming virus from this cell line. However the cryptic proviral structure present in H-19 cells is clearly expressed and it codes for src mRNA. Recently it was established that H-19 cells also synthesize pp60^{v-src} (8). Cryptic proviral structure may have arisen by reverse transcription of src mRNA. It can be revealed on unique DNA restriction fragments, as on one 3.4 Md HindIII fragment. Structural analysis of cloned 3.4 Md fragment will clarify the genesis of cryptic provirus.

Recently we returned to the problem of transforming virus rescue from H-19 cells ans employed RAV-1, a naturally occurring avian leukosis virus. When H-19 cells were fused with RAV-1-infected chicken fibroblasts, abou 2 foci per dish appeared, and several individual foci were isolated and grown. They produced very little transforming virus, but about two-three logs of focus forming units were obtained during further subcultures.

Individual focus progeny viruses were used for mass transformation of japanese quail cells. The DNA was iso-

354

lated from fully transformed cultures and used for
EcoRI and BglII restriction mapping, as shown schematically in Fig. 1. In the first step, EcoRI-digested and
blotted DNAs were hybridized with the src probe. Three
focus isolates (F6, G8, E7) contained the viral src gene
sequences on a 1.6 Md fragment, which comigrates exactly
with the src fragment.present in H-19 cells. Only in the
case of focus progeny virus E6 was the src fragment
localized on an unusual 2.2 fragment. Using the pol
probe we established that this fragment also contains
pol gene sequences. This finding showed that the src
gene was accomodated together with the pol sequences.
on one fragment. Fig. 2 illustrates hybridization with
the pATV-8 probe, which detects all ASV sequences. Only
in the track of E6 did three new EcoRI fragments
(1.0, 1.8, and 2.2 Md) appear, which were absent in
control RAV-1-infected quail cells. Further hybridization
experiments clearly revealed that all three anomalous
EcoRI E6 fragments contain LTRs. For hybridization,
nick-translated plasmid containing two LTRs was used,
which was constructed by Dr. Tatosyan.

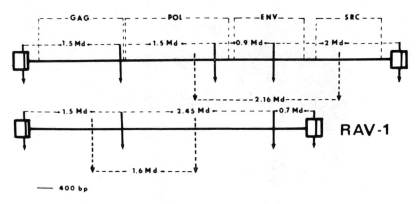

Figure 1. Schenatic drawing of the structure of type II
provirus (upper part) and RAV-1 (lower part). EcoRI sites
are indicated by solid arrows, BglII sites by dashed
arrows. LTRs are boxed.

Finally, we employed BglII and hybridized the blot
with the src probe. In E6 and F6, the v-src-containing
bands were absent. In G8, there were two bands (1.25 and
1.8 Md), and one 2-Md fragment in E7. H-19 cells, a
cell clone, produced two src-containing junction
fragments distinguishable from others. Double digestion

pATV 8

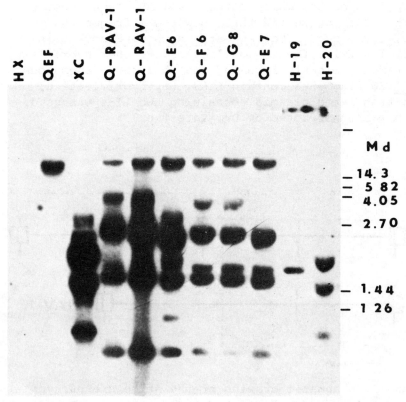

Figure 2. EcoRI restriction pattern of proviral DNAs from
quail cells (Q) transformed with viruses (E6, F6, G8, E7)
rescued from H-19 cells. HX - normal hamster DNA.

with EcoRI and BglII again revealed anomalous proviral
bands only in the E6 DNA.

Based on these data, we may propose tentatively the
structural features of rescued ASVs (Fig. 3). In E6,
the cryptic v-src may have become recombined in the
middle of the RAV-1 genome, outside BglII sites, which
resulted in the loss of these RAV-1 BglII sites and,
in addition, probably also in acquisition of some pol
sequences in the cryptic src structure. EcoRI cleavage
will then produce three anomalous proviral LTR-equipped
fragments and BglII digestion will result in the formation of only junction src containing fragments of
different sizes in the DNA from at random virus-trans-
formed permissive cells, which do not produce distinct
bands, and this fits with our experimental data.

In F6, a similar situation may be presumed, because no
src containing BglII bands were found. However, no anomalous EcoRI fragments were seen. It is therefore more
likely that a cryptic provirus alone may have become
integrated at different sites in the cell genome.

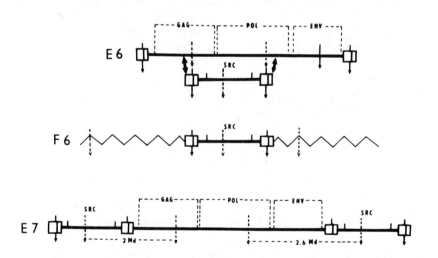

Figure 3. Schemes of proviral structures of three transforming viruses (E6, F6, E7) rescued from H-19 cells.
Double arrows indicate the tentative site of recombination. Broken line indicates cell DNA.

357

In the case of E7, one 2-Md BglII src fragment was
found but, after EcoRI digestion, no rearrangements
of proviral structure were again noted. This would be
in agreement with the model in which cryptic provirus
became joint by recombination in LTR with the left
(5') end of the RAV-1 genome. Such a structure would
generate a 2-Md BglII src-containing fragment. Additional
viral probes and restriction enzymes will be employed
to draw complete genetic maps of rescued viruses.

The results from our analysis of viruses rescued from
cryptovirugenic cells indicate that this model will be
useful for study of recombination activity of v-src and
the ways in which it can be transferred by other retroviruses. Finally, it makes it possible to explore the
ways in which transforming ASV is reformed from v-src
and a helper virus.

REFERENCES

1. Zilber, L. A. (1965). Pathogenicity and oncogenicity
   of Rous sarcoma virus for mammals. Progr. Exp.
   Tumor Res. 7, 1-48 (Karger, Basel-New York).
2. Svoboda, J. and Hlozánek, I. (1970). Role of cell
   association in virus infection and virus rescue.
   Adv. Cancer Res. 13, 217-269.
3. Mitsialis, A., Katz, R. A., Svoboda, J. and Guntaka,
   R. V. (1983). Studies on the structure and organization of avian sarcoma proviruses in the rat XC
   cell line. J. Gen. Virol. 64, 1885-1893.
4. Tantravahi, U., Erlanger, B. F. and Miller O. J.
   (1982). The rat XC sarcoma cell line: ribosomal
   RNA gene amplification and banded karyotype.
   Cancer Genet. Cytogenet. 5, 63-73.
5. Sainerová, H. and Svoboda, J. (1981). Stability
   of C-banded and C-bandless microchromosomes in
   clonal sublines of the RVP_3 mouse tumor grown
   serially in vivo. Cancer Genet. Cytogenet. 3, 93-99.
6. Svoboda, J., Lhoták V., Geryk, J. Saule, S., Raes,
   M. B. and Stehelin, D. (1983). Characterization
   of exogenous proviral sequences in hamster tumor
   cell lines transformed by Rous sarcoma virus rescued
   from XC cells. Virology 128, 195-209.

7. Geryk, J., Sainerová, H., Sovová, V. and Svoboda,
   J. (1984). Characterization of cryptovirogenic,
   virus-productive and helper-dependent virogenic
   hamster tumour cell lines. Folia biol. (Praha) 30,
   152-164.
8. Grofová, M. Bízik, J., Blahová, S., Geryk, J. and
   Svoboda, J. Identification of transformation-specific
   proteins synthesized in cryptovirogenic cells.
   Folia biol. (Praha) in press.

STRUCTURAL BASIS OF INTERRELATION OF MOLECULAR MECHANISMS OF CANCEROGENESIS AND IMMUNITY

V.P.ZAV'YALOV
All-Union Research Institute of Applied Microbiology,142200 Serpukhov,Moscow Region,USSR

At present there is a great deal of data indicating a homology of protein products of oncoviruses and oncogenes with normal proteins of
host cells.In some cases an extent of homology
of amino acid sequences is so wide that it is
evident even for a non-specialist.A most characteristic example is the homology between a
transforming protein of simian sarcoma virus
p28^{sis} (sis protein) and platelet-derived
growth factor (PDGF) /1/.But in most cases the
homology is not so evident,and special approaches are required to reveal and prove it.My
investigations were aimed at developing such
an approach to elucidate one of the most important problems of cancerogenesis- the mechanism of slipping of oncoviruses and the cells
transformed by them out of control of immune
system.
   The approach supposed is based on the experimental data indicating that spatial structure of functionally and evolutionarily related
proteins has a signicantly higher similarity
that their primary structure.Thus,the conclusion of a common evolutionary precursor for
the proteins compared should be based on the
similarity of their conformations.At present,
direct experimental data on the three-dimensional structure of proteins may be obtained
only by the X-ray analysis.However,the protein
conformation is coded by the amino acid se-
quence.The decoding of this code will allow a
theoretical estimation of spatial structures
of proteins without the employment of the ex-

Proceedings of the 16th FEBS Congress
Part B, pp. 361–370
© 1985 VNU Science Press

perimental methods.Although the problem has not
been solved in general,at present it is possible to predict,with high degree of probability,
a spatial arrangement of globular proteins with
high content either of α-helices or β-struc-
tures.Occasionally,many proteins of immune system belong to the one of these types.It should
be noted that the bilayer β-sheet structure
of immunoglobulin (Ig) domains and the α-heli-
cal conformation of interferons (IFNs) were
successfully predicted by us with the help of
our methods /2,3/,and subsequently confirmed
experimentally by the X-ray analysis /4/ and
circular dichroism /5/.A general scheme for
prediction of secondary structure was as fol-
lows.At first,the main type of secondary structure of the protein under study was determined
by the nomograms /3/ from amino acid composi-
tion.In case of high content of α-helices,a
double α-helical net /3/ was used to localize α-helical sites capable of forming a hydrophobic core.Further, α-helical segments were folded into a globule according to the method described in /3/.In case of high content
of β-structures,the β-folded sites were localized with the help of the method reported
in /4/.Then fitting of β-folded sites was
used to seek for a homology with highly β-
folded proteins of immune system.At first,we
employed these methods for the analysis of the
spatial structure of the sis protein highly
homologous to PDGF.It was found that the main
type of secondary structure of the protein
should be α-helix,its content was estimated
to be 50%.In the polypeptide chain of the sis
protein one can identify five α-helical sites
capable of forming a hydrophobic core.As the
number of α-helical sites and their length
were found to be the same as those of IFNs,we
decided to pack α-helical segments into the
three-dimensional structure previously suggest-

ed for IFNs /6/.Fig.1 shows a schematic representation of the predicted three-dimensional structures of IFNs,interleukins (ILs) and sis protein.The comparison of the hydrophobic cores of the sis protein and IFN-β revealed an identity in 9 of 27 positions,above 30% of homology.Analogous similarity was observed by comparing the structures of IFNs and T-cell growth factor (TCGF or IL-2) and of IL-3 and IFN-α .

The analysis of the alignment of these proteins allows one to conclude that IFNs,ILs and growth factors (GFs) studied form a superfamily of hormones united by a structural and evolutionary similarity.Recently,the experimental data have been obtained indicating a functional interaction of GFs,IFNs and ILs /7,8/.These hormones (we suggest to name them "intercellons") seem to be important components of the united system of regulation of proliferation and differentiation of cells.ILs represent a part of the system directly related to immune cells. It is natural that an uncontrolled interference of products of oncoviruses and oncogenes in the system of regulation of proliferation and differentiation of cells should be one ofthe most significant causes of tumor growth.In fact,in case of simian sarcoma,a cause of tumor growth is an uncontrolled production of a PDGF-like sis protein by the transformed cells /1/,and in case of T-cell leukemia – an uncontrolled expression of receptors for TCGF on the surface of the transformed T-lymphocytes /9/.

As has been mentioned at the beginning of the present report,a very important problem in the mechanism of cancerogenesis is the elucidation of molecular causes of slipping of oncoviruses and the cells transformed by them out of control of immune system.

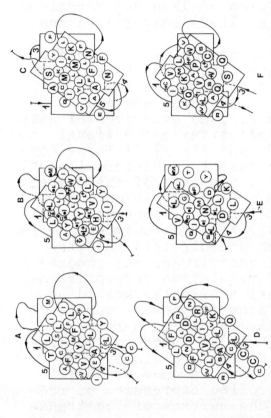

Fig.1 The schematic representation of the expected tertiary structures of IFNs-α(A),-β(B),-ℓ(C),IL-3 (D),IL-2 (E),p28sis(F).
Boxes and numbers indicate α-helical segments.The amino acid residues forming the hydrophobic core are given in one-letter symbols.
Large letters indicate side-chains in the upper α-helical layer.
Small letters denote the side-chains in the lower α-helical layer.
The amino acid residues coinciding in IL-3 and IFN-α, IL-2 and IFN-
β,p28sis and IFN-β are indicated by open circles,shaded circles
and crosses,respectively.The direction of the polypeptide chain is
indicated by arrows going from the N-terminus to C-terminus.

Mimicry of the proteins,oncovirus products,under host proteins can be one of the causes of a similar effect.A phenomenon of mimicry of the sis protein under PDGF is really obvious. Besides,the experimental data were obtained speaking for mimicry of envelope (env) oncovirus proteins.According to Baird et al. /10/, the env protein of Moloney murine leukemia virus (MoMuLV) displays reactivity with antibodies to murine IgM.In view of these data, we decided to analyse the structure of the env protein of human adult T-cell leukemia virus (ATLV) /11/.It turned out that as well as for Ig's the β -structure is predicted as the main secondary structure for the env protein of ATLV.The fitting of β -folded sites and cysteines in the env protein with the corresponding sites and cysteines in Ig domains allows the polypeptide chain of this protein to be packed into four Ig-like domains.The C-terminal domain of the env protein of ATLV is highly homologous with the C-terminal part of the env protein p15E MoMuLV /12/ (Fig.2).At the same time this part of p15E of MoMuLV has a statistically reliable homology with the second constant domain of the heavy chain of murine IgM /13/,the homology being higher than that observed by comparing the second and third constant domains of the same IgM.The homology in primary structure of the env proteins of leukemia viruses and of Ig domains forming an Fc-subunit can reflect their common functional activity,for instance,the interaction with the Fc-receptors of cells.The experimental investigations show that p15E of oncogenic retroviruses actively suppress immune response due to the interaction with T-lymphocytes and the suppression of IL-2 production /14/.

A statistically significant homology is found by us between the structure of the hypo-

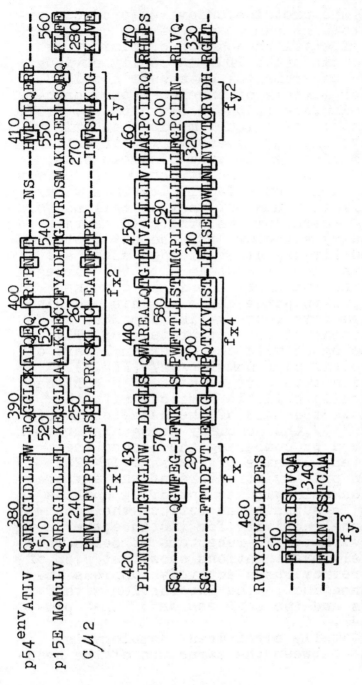

Fig.2 The alignment of amino acid sequences of the env proteins of ATLV /11/, MoMuLV /12/ and C 2 domain of murine IgM /13/. Designations are the same as in Fig.3.

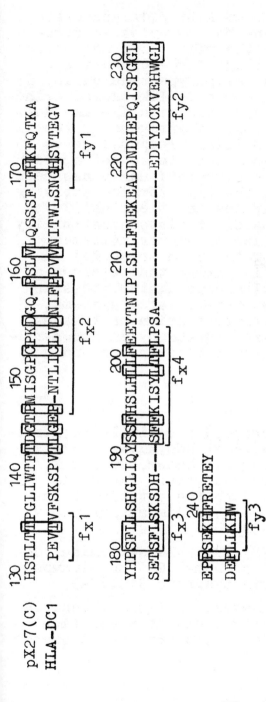

```
              130          140        150           160            170
pX27(C)  HSTLT PGLIWTF DGTF MISGP CPKD GQ- PSLM LQSSSFIF FKFQTKA
HLA-DC1        PEV VFSKSPV LGE - NTLI CLVD NIF PVN ITWLSNG SVTEGV
                  └─fx1─┘        └──────fx2──────┘    └───fy1───┘

              180       190        200           210         220           230
         YHPSFL LSHGLIQY SS FHSLH FEEYTNIPISLLFNEKEADDNDHEPQISPGL
         SETSFL SKSDH - SF EKISYL TE LPSA- - - - - - - - - - EDIYDCKVEHW GL
         └──fx3──┘         └──fx4──┘                          └──fy2──┘

         EPPSEKH FRETEY
         DEPLIKHW
          └fy3┘
            240
```

Fig.3 The alignment of primary structures of the predicted C-terminal domain of pX27 ATLV /11/ and HLA-DC1 /16/.Amino acid residues
are given in one-letter symbols.Numbers indicate positions of the
residues in the sequence of pX27 ATLV,translated from the nucleotide sequence of the ATLV genome /11/.Identical residues are boxed.
Deletions are designated by dashes.Brackets indicate segments of
β-pleated structure.

thetical protein pX27 of ATLV /11/ and histocompatibility antigens. The β -pleated structure is predicted as the main conformation for
this protein. The fitting of β -folded sites
and cysteines allows the polypeptide chain of
pX27 to be packed into two Ig-like domains. The
highest homology is observed with Ig-like domains of histocompatibility antigens of the II
class, the products of immune response genes
(Fig.3). This fact can appear to be not acciden-
tal as recently a direct relationship has been
demonstrated between the transforming activity
of oncogenic adenoviruses and their ability
to reduce the expression of histocompatibility
antigens on the surface of the transformed
cells /15/. In view of the data presented in
the report, the idea is formed that a cause of
tumor growth is simultaneous disturbances in
the regulation of two interrelated systems,
proliferation and differentiation of tissues
and immunity, which are induced by an uncontrolled action of products of oncoviruses and oncogenes.

Reference list

1. Waterfield, M.D., Scrace, G.T., Whittle, N., Stroo-
   bant, P., Johnsson, A., Wasteson, A., Westermark,
   B., Heldin, C.-H., Jung San Huang, Deull, T.F.
   (1983). Platelet-derived growth factor is
   structurally related to the putative transforming protein p28^{sis} of simian sarcoma virus. Nature 304, 35-39

2. Zav'yalov, V.P. (1973). Probable N-terminal domains conformation of human G1 (Eu) immunoglobulin. Biochim. Biophys. Acta 310, 70-75

3. Zav'yalov, V.P., Denesyuk, A.I. (1982). Possible
   conformation of interferons: a prediction
   based on amino acid composition and sequence.
   Immunol. Lett. 4, 7-14

4. Poljak,R.J.,Amzel,L.M.,Chen,B.L.,Phizacker-
ley,R.P.,Saul,F.(1974).The three-dimensional
structure of the Fab' fragment$_o$of a human
myeloma immunoglobulin at 2.0 Å resolution.
Proc.Natl.Acad.Sci.USA 71,3440-3444

5. Bewley,T.A.,Levine,H.L.,Wetzel,R.(1982)
Structural features of human leucocyte interferon A as determined by circular dichroism spectroscopy.Int.J.Peptide Prot.Res.
20,93-96

6. Zav'yalov,V.P.,Denesyuk,A.I.(1984).Evolu-
tionary,conformational and functional interrelationship of α -, β - and γ - in-
terferons.Doklady Akademii Nauk SSSR (in
Russian) 275,242-246

7. Inglot,A.D.,Albin,M.(1983).Interaction of
mouse interferon and platelet-derived growth
factor during multiplication of BALB/c 3T3
cells.J.Interferon Res.3,75-81

8. Kawase,I.,Brooks,C.G.,Kuribayashi,K.,Ola-
buenaga,S.,Newman,W.,Gillis,S.,Henney,C.S.
(1983).Interleukin 2 induces γ -interfe-
ron production:participation of macrophages
and NK-like cells.J.Immunol.131,288-292

9. Lando,Z.,Sarin,P.,Megson,M.,Greene,W.C.,
Waldman,T.A.,Gallo,R.C.,Broder,S.(1983).
Association of human T-cell leukemia virus
with the Tac antigen marker for the human
T-cell growth factor receptor.Nature 305,
733-736

10. Baird,S.,Lesley,J.,Raschke,W.(1983).Mono-
clonal antibodies to murine leukemia virus
gp 70 recognize the same T lymphoma cell
surface molecules as anti-immunoglobulin.
J.Immunol.131,1576-1581

11. Seiki,M.,Hattori,S.,Hirayama,Y.,Yoshida,M.
(1983).Human adult T-cell leukemia virus:
Complete nucleotide sequence of the provirus genome integrated in leukemia cell DNA.
Proc.Natl.Acad.Sci.USA 80,3618-3622

12. Shinnick,T.M.,Lerner,R.A.,Sutcliffe,S.G. (1981).Nucleotide sequence of Moloney murine leukaemia virus.Nature 293,543-548
13. Kehry,M.R.,Fuhrman,J.S.,Schilling,J.W.,Rogers,J.,Sibley,C.H.,Hood,L.E.(1982).Amino acid sequence of a mouse μ chain: Homology among heavy chain constant region domains. Biochemistry 21,5415-5424
14. Copelan,E.A.,Rinehart,J.J.,Levis,M.,Mathes, L.,Olsen,R.,Sagone,A.(1983).The mechanism of retrovirus suppression of human T-cell proliferation in vitro.J.Immunol.131,2017-2020
15. Schrier,P.I.,Bernards,R.,Vaessen,R.T.M.J., Houweling,A.,van der Eb,A.J.(1983) Expression of class I major histocompatibility antigens switched off by highly oncogenic adenovirus 12 in transformed rat cells.Na ture 305,771-775
16. Auffray,Ch.,Korman,A.J.,Roux-Dosseto,M., Bono,R.,Strominger,J.L.(1982).c-DNA clone for the heavy chain of the human B-cell alloantigen DC1: Strong sequence homology to the HLA-DR heavy chain.Proc.Natl.Acad. Sci.USA 79,6337-6341

IONIC CHANNELS AND CELLULAR METABOLISM

INTRACELLULAR REGULATION OF IONIC CURRENTS THROUGH CHEMOEXCITABLE NEURONE MEMBRANE

CHEMERIS N.K., ILJIN V.I.
Lab. of Nerve Cell Biophysics, Inst. of Biological Physics, USSR Acad. Sci., Pushchino, Moscow Reg., 142292, USSR

In this paper we present the data on regulation of chloride currents controlled by nicotinic-like acetylcholine receptors (AChR) in identified giant neurones of pond-snail *Limnaea stagnalis*. We succeeded to show that functioning of the acetylcholine (ACh)-activated chloride channels is regulated by both intracellular ionized Ca and cyclic AMP.
In 1974 in our lab Drs Kislov and Kazachenko found a rather sharp decrease in the slope of the voltage-current relationship of ACh-induced current at depolarization of *Limnaea* neurone soma membrane. In their subsequent study these authors had shown that the effect of membrane depolarization on ACh-induced conductance could not result from a voltage-clamp artifact or from rectification of Cl^--channels, alteration of ionic equilibrium potential, ionophoresis of ACh away from the membrane, speeding up a densitization of the AChR's /1/. On the other hand some data were obtained that the phenomenon observed is related somehow to activation of electroexcitable Ca-channels at membrane depolarization. So the conductance of the cholinoreceptive membrane fell and the maximal electroexcitable Ca-current developed in one and the same region of membrane voltages. Bath-applied Mn^{2+} (10 mM), a known Ca-channel blocker, led to elimination of depolarization-dependent inactivation of the AChR's and linearization of the voltage-current curve of the ACh-induced current. And conversely, at elevation of external Ca^{2+} the inactivation streng-

Proceedings of the 16th FEBS Congress
Part B, pp. 373–378

thened /2/.

But the decisive experiments testifying the direct participation of intracellular ionized Ca in AChR inactivation were carried out by Dr Chemeris. In his experiments on dialysed neurones /3/ Dr Chemeris found that the effects of membrane depolarization on the ACh-induced currents are imitated by direct introduction of Ca^{2+} into the cell interior. The effects of both membrane depolarization and inward Ca-current were eliminated by intracellular application of 5 mM EGTA. The dependence of the degree of inactivation of responses to ACh on intracellular concentration of ionized Ca appears to be of the simple Langmuir-like form /4/. The maximal inhibition is achieved at Ca^{2+} concentration of about 0.1 mM. The apparent dissociation constant is close to 2.1 µM.

Thus, the conductance of excited cholinoreceptive membrane is controlled by the level of free Ca inside a cell. Elevation of intracellular Ca^{2+} leads to decrease in neurone responses to ACh no matter whether it is due to the Ca-influx through electroexcitable Ca-channels at membrane depolarization, or release from mitochondria upon their poisoning by dinitrophenole, or due to direct introduction of Ca-enriched solution into the cell interior.

Intracellular Ca-dependent inactivation of the AChR's develops quickly /4/: at excitation of the inward Ca-current it reaches the maximum within several hundreds of milliseconds. The recovery of the receptors from inactivation proceeds also rapidly with the rate very close to that of binding of excess of free Ca inside molluscan nervous cells (e.g. /5, 6/).

We found that the Ca-dependent inactivation is not the only way of regulation of AChR functioning in soma membrane of *Limnaea* neurones. In collaboration with Drs Akopyan and Bocharova we showed that functioning of the receptors is also modulated by intracellular cyclic AMP.

The original observation made in 1979 was the
decrease in ACh-induced conductance by 20-40%
at application of serotonin (5HT) or dopamine
(DA). We studied the origin of the inhibitory
effect of biogenous amines and came to conclusion that it is mediated by intracellular cyclic
AMP on the basis of the following data /7/. Intracellular application of GTP, a cofactor of
mediator-sensitive adenylate cyclase, enhances
the effect of DA on ACh responses. Activation of
membrane adenylate cyclase by NaF imitates the
inhibitory effect of biogenous amines. Activation of cellular phosphodiesterase by Ca^{2+} weakens
the inhibition and papaverine prevents this effect. And at last, intracellular application of
cyclic AMP imitates completely the inhibitory
effect of biogenous amines.
Although both intracellular regulators, ionized
Ca and cyclic AMP, inhibit ACh-induced currents,
their actions differ in several respects. First,
there are differences in kinetics. Ca-dependent
inactivation develops within few seconds, per-
sists during that period of time when free Ca
concentration is increased and recovers completely within several seconds. In the case of cyclic AMP-dependent inhibition the maximal effect
is reached within 2-3 min. The lowered responses
to ACh persist over the whole period of time,
when biogenous amines are applied externally or
cyclic AMP internally. Complete recovery of the
responses to ACh is not observed even after
washing out of biogenous amines or cyclic AMP
for an hour (residual inactivation is of about
15-20%). In contrast, the degree of inhibition
of the AChR's by free Ca is determined only by
the effective concentration of ionized Ca. The
maximal inhibition of ACh-induced current (of
about 80%) can be easily achieved at intensive
excitation of Ca-channels and this inhibition
recovers completely following the binding of
free Ca to intracellular structures.
The discrepances in kinetics may determine the

differences in possible physiological significance of these two ways of regulation of the
same neuronal response. Elevation of intracellular free Ca at Ca-action potential generation
might influence the cholinergic postsynaptic potential only in the case when these two membrane
events follow each other within 1-2 s. This regulation is rapid and short-term. At activation
of neuronal adenylate cyclase, $e.g.$ by mediators
of monoamine group, the modulation of the AChR
functioning is slower in time and long-term.
This may be one of the real mechanisms of plas-
tic changes in efficiency of synaptic transmission at the level of postsynaptic membrane.
The Ca-dependent inactivation and cyclic AMP-dependent inhibition seem also to differ in their
mechanisms. In a number of biochemical studies
cyclic AMP-dependent phosphorylation of nicotinic ACh receptors was found without any indications to possible consequences of such phosphorylation for receptor functioning ($e.g.$ /8/). In
our case the effect of biogenous amines seems
also to be mediated by cyclic AMP-dependent
phosphorylation since the inhibitor of phosphorylation, talbutamide, weakens the inhibitory
effect of both 5HT and cyclic AMP by twofold.
Thus, phosphorylation of the AChR's may result
in decrease of cholinergic membrane conductance.
There exist some evidence that calmodulin-depen-
dent phosphorylation of the AChR's may also occur /9/. But in our case, Ca-dependent inactivation of the AChR is not affected by trifluopera-
zine, a known inhibitor of calmodulin. Moreover,
we think that Ca-dependent inactivation is associated with no biochemical process at all. In
fact, 5HT-induced inhibition which seems to be
coupled with the synthesis of cyclic AMP and
phosphorylation, disappears completely at temperature lowering to $2^{o}C$; by contrast, for Ca effect the temperature coefficient Q_{10} is rather
small (close to 1.8 /4/). Moreover, we found
that Sr^{2+} is half as effective as Ca^{2+} in de-

creasing the ACh-induced conductance, while cal-
modulin-dependent processes are highly selective
towards Ca^{2+}. And at last, Ca-dependent inactivation of the AChR's fits the simple Langmuir
isoterm which is compatible with monomolecular
reaction, whereas activation of calmodulin requires 2-4 Ca ions to be bound. These data altogether allow us to assume that Ca-dependent
inactivation is related to some physical process.
Thus although both free Ca and cyclic AMP decrease the ACh-induced membrane conductance,
this seems to be in one case the result of some
physical process and in another case - of biochemical modification of the AChR.
What is changed in AChR functioning at modulation? We compared the "concentration-response"
curves for ACh in control and at "injection" of
Ca ions into cell interior through activated Ca-
channels and found that Ca decreases the affinity of the AChR's (by ~ 1.5) without any effect
on the maximal response. These data are qualitatively similar to the findings of Chang and Neumann on the purified AChR's /10/ and compatible
with the idea that activation of the AChR requires one bound Ca ion to be released. At high
concentration of intracellular Ca^{2+} the release
of bound Ca is limited because of lowered affinity of the receptor to ACh.
Thus intracellular free Ca seems to modulate the
affinity of the AChR. But there is nothing to
say at present what is changed in receptor functioning upon cyclic AMP modulation. This question requires further investigations.

1. Kazachenko, V.N., Kislov, A.N., Veprintsev,
    B.N. (1979). Cholino-receptive membrane
    inactivation caused by depolarization of
    Limnaea stagnalis neurones. Comp. Biochem.
    Physiol. 63C, 61-66.
2. Kazachenko, V.N., Kislov, A.N., Kurchikov
    A.L., Chemeris, N.K. (1981). Intracellular

calcium initiates acetylcholine receptor inactivation. Biofizika.26, 1052-1056 (in Russian).

3. Kostyuk,P.G., Kryshtal,O.A., Pidoplichko,V.I. (1978). Estimation of conductance of a single calcium-channel according to current fluctuations using the effect of EGTA.Dokl. Akad.Nauk SSSR.238, 478-485 (in Russian).

4. Chemeris,N.K., Kazachenko,V.N., Kislov,A.N., Kurchikov,A.L. (1982). Inhibition of acetylcholine responses by intracellular calcium in *Limnaea stagnalis* neurones. J.Physiol. (Lond.). 323, 1-19.

5. Ahmed,Z., Connor,J.A.(1979). Measurement of calcium influx under voltage clamp in molluscan neurones using the metallochrome dye Arsenazo III. J.Physiol.(Lond.) 286, 61-82.

6. Smith,S.J., Zucker,R.S.(1980). Aequorin response facilitation and intracellular calcium concentration in molluscan neurones. J.Physiol.(Lond.). 300, 167-196.

7. Akopyan,A.R., Chemeris,N.K.,Iljin,V.I., Veprintsev,B.N.(1980).Serotonin,dopamine and intracellular cyclic AMP inhibit the responses of nicotinic cholinergic membrane in snail neurones. Brain Res. 201, 480-484.

8. Huganir,R.L., Greengard,P.(1983). cAMP-dependent protein kinase phosphorylates the nicotinic acetylcholine receptor. PNAS USA. 80, 1130-1134.

9. Smilowitz,H., Hadjian,R.A., Dwyer,I., Feinstein,M.B.(1981). Regulation of acetylcholine receptor phosphorylation by calcium and calmodulin. PNAS USA.78, 4708-4712.

10.Chang,H.W., Neumann,E.(1976). Dynamic properties of isolated acetylcholine receptor proteins: release of calcium ions caused by acetylcholine binding. PNAS USA.73, 3364-3368.

THE BOVINE CARDIAC MUSCLE BINDING SITES FOR CALCIUM-ANTAGONISTS:

P.RUTH, V.FLOCKERZI, E.v.NETTELBLADT, F.HOFMANN
Pharmakologisches Institut der Universität, Im Neuenheimer Feld 366, D-6900 Heidelberg, Germany.

Opening and closing of the Ca^{2+} channel controls the intracellular $[Ca^{2+}]$ of many cells(1). In cardiac muscle opening of these channels is facilitated by phosphorylation of a membrane component by cAMP-dependent protein kinase(2,3). The Ca^{2+} channels are blocked by a heterogenous group of compounds refered to as "Calciumantagonist"(4). Among these compounds are the phenylalkylamines verapamil and its desmethoxyderivative (-)D888, the benzothiazepine diltiazem and the dihydropyridines nitrendipine and nimodipine. Recently, tritiated congeners of these compounds have been used to identify calcium channels in broken cell preparations(5-8). Specific high affinity sites for these compounds have been found in different tissues including skeletal muscle, heart, smooth muscle and brain(9). So far the physiological significance of these binding sites has not been established beyond doubt. Four different Ca^{2+} antagonists have been used to identify in cardiac muscle membranes the physiological sites for these compounds.

METHODS

Crude membranes were prepared from the middle portion of fresh bovine cardiac muscle at 4°C. Finely minced muscle (400g) was washed twice with buffer A(10 mM histidine, 750 mM NaCl, pH7.5). The muscle was disrupted for 2 min in 4 volumes of buffer A with an Ultra Turrax Tissuemizer. The pellet obtained after low speed centrifugation(9000xg) was rinsed with buffer A and rehomogenized in the original buffer volume for 15 sec. The crude membranes were immediately stored at -80°C. Sarcolemma and membranes sedimenting at higher density were prepared as described in (10). The binding of dihydropyridines was determined at 20°C in 0.25 ml of 50 mM TRIS-HCl, pH7.4, containing 1 mM $CaCl_2$ and 1 nM (^{3}H)-nimodipine or 1 nM (^{3}H)-nitrendipine. Non-

Proceedings of the 16th FEBS Congress
Part B, pp. 379–384
© 1985 VNU Science Press

specific binding was determined in the presence of 5 and
2 µM nitrendipine and nimodipine, respectively. The binding of phenylalkylamines was determined at 20°C in 0.25ml
of 50 mM TRIS-HCl, pH7.4, containing 1 mM EDTA, 0.1 mg/ml
bovine serum albumine and 3-5 nM (^3H)-verapamil or (^3H)-
(-)D888. Nonspecific binding was determined in the presence of 10 µM unlabelled ligand. After 20 min incubation,
0.2 ml were spotted on a GF/C filter which was washed with
4x2 ml ice cold 50 mM TRIS-HCl buffer, pH7.4.

RESULTS

The proportion of specific to total binding did not differ
significantly between the four ligands when crude membranes were used and was between 20% and 30%. Specific
binding to sarcolemma varied considerably among the ligands being 30% for verapamil, 41% for (-)D888 and 70-90%
for the dihydropyridines. Specific binding of the Calciumantagonists depended on the amount of membrane protein
added and was optimal between 0.1 to 0.4 mg/ml. Specific
binding did not increase when the incubation time was extended over 30 min at 20°C. Pretreatement of the membranes
for 30 min at 30°C with trypsin(30µg/mg protein) destroyed
completely specific binding of each antagonist. Specific
binding was modulated by different metal ions(Fig.1).
Verapamil binding was maximal in the presence of 1 mM
EDTA and was inhibited halfmaximally by 0.3 mM Co^{2+},
0.6 mM Ni^{2+}, 1.5 mM Ba^{2+}, 3 mM Ca^{2+}, 3.4 mM Mn^{2+} and 5.1 mM
Mg^{2+}. In contrast, binding of nitrendipine was inhibited
by 70% in the presence of 1 mM EDTA.
Specificity of binding sites
Variation of the concentration of (^3H)-nitrendipine between 0.01 and 2.0 nM resulted in an apparent hyperbolic
saturation curve (Fig.2), which yielded a K_D value of
0.23 $\pm$ .09 nM and an apparent density of 0.7 $\pm$ .06 pmol/mg
in five different sarcolemma preparations. A second site
was detected at higher ligand concentrations. The K_D value
was confirmed by following rate constants: k_{+1} .23 $\pm$ .007
(n=3) 1/nmolxmin; k_{-1} .023 $\pm$ .002 (n=3) 1/min yielding a
K_D value of 0.1 $\pm$ .002 nM. A site with a similar K_D value
was detected by nimodipine which ligand allowed also the

Fig. 1: Metal requirement of specific calcium-antagonist binding.
Crude membranes (100 μg) were incubated in the presence of 1 mM EDTA and the indicated concentrations of free Ca²⁺. (●) verapamil; (o) nitrendipine.

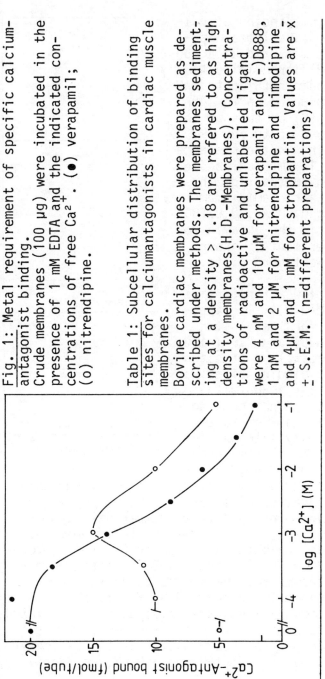

Table 1: Subcellular distribution of binding sites for calciumantagonists in cardiac muscle membranes.
Bovine cardiac membranes were prepared as described under methods. The membranes sedimenting at a density > 1.18 are refered to as high density membranes(H.D.-Membranes). Concentrations of radioactive and unlabelled ligand were 4 nM and 10 μM for verapamil and (-)D888, 1 nM and 2 μM for nitrendipine and nimodipine and 4μM and 1 mM for strophantin. Values are x̄ ± S.E.M. (n=different preparations).

Fraction	Verapamil	(-)D888	Nitrendipine	Nimodipine	Strophantin
Homogenate	.14+.02(19)	.09+.01 (6)	.10+.02(20)	.06+.01(10)	2.9+ .4 (6)
Sarcolemma	.26+.03 (9)	.25+.03(16)	.65+.05(11)	.62+.19 (4)	56.3+5.3(14)
H.D.-Membran.	.20+.04 (6)	.41+.04 (6)	.36+.06 (6)	.28+.03 (6)	4.4+ .5 (6)

Fig. 2: Equilibrium binding of calciumantagonist to sarcolemma. Specific binding was measured at a con·
centration of (^3H)nitrendipine(A)up
to 2 nM,(^3H)-nimodipine(B)up to 2nM
and unlabelled compound up to 100nM
and (^3H)-(-)D888 (C) up to 4 nM and
unlabelled compound up to 300 nM.
Nonspecific binding in the presence
of 2 µM(A,B) and 10 µM(C)unlabelled
compound has been subtracted. The
concentration of sarcolemmal membrane protein was 0.08(A), 0.07(B)
and 0.2(C) mg/ml in the assay.A representative experiment is shown.
The insets show Scatchard plots.

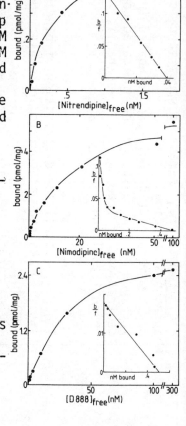

measurement of a low affinity site
(K_D=23.8 $\pm$ 2.5 nM(n=5)). The apparent B_{max} values for these sites
were .23 $\pm$ .03 (n=5) and 7.8 $\pm$ 1.0
(n=5)pmol/mg protein.In most cases
a single class of binding sites was
detected with (^3H)-(-)D888 with an
apparent K_D of 25 $\pm$ 6 nM and a density of 1.8 $\pm$ .36 pmol/mg protein
(n=6).A high affinity site was observed (app.K_D=1 nM) in some preparations.(^3H)-nimodipine was rea-
dily displaced by unlabelled nimodipine and nitrendipine
with apparent IC_{50} values of 14 and 22 nM, respectively.
The dihydropyridine binding site had apparently a hundred fold lower affinity for the phenylalkylamines. Nimodipine binding was inhibited at 10 µM by (+) and (-)vera-
pamil 55% and 30% and by (-) and (+) D600 (methoxyvera-
pamil) 30%. Diltiazem at 10 µM showed no effect. (^3H)-
(-)D888 was halfmaximally displaced by 18 and 90 nM unlabelled (-)D888 and (-) verapamil, respectively. (-)D600
displaced it halfmaximally at 70 nM. The (+) isomers of
verapamil and D600 had lower affinities as the (-)isomers
with apparent IC_{50} values of 180 and 600 nM, respectively.

Binding of $(^3H)-(-)D888$ was only marginally affected by nimodipine and nifedipine. Binding of nimodipine or $(-)$ D888 was not affected by prazosin, yohimbine, tetrodotoxin, atropin and atenolol added at 10 µM.

Subcellular distribution of the binding sites

Homogenates of bovine cardiac muscle had apparent binding densities of .14, .09, .1, .06, and 2.9 pmol/mg protein for verapamil, $(-)D888$, nitrendipine, nimodipine and strophantin, respectively (Table 1). The apparent densities of these sites increased in the crude membranes suggesting that the majority of them was of particulate nature. The binding sites for strophantin, dihydropyridines and phenylalkylamines were enriched 20, 7-8 and 2-3 fold in sarcolemma and 2, 3-4 and 2-4 fold in high density membranes. Although these values were obtained under conditions which saturated only the high affinity binding sites they represent probably a correct distribution of the binding sites. The affinities of the binding sites did not change with purification as tested in single preparations. Further experiments showed that the binding sites for phenylalkylamines copurify with free sarcoplasmic reticulum.

DISCUSSION

The present study demonstrates that bovine cardiac muscle contains at least two separate binding sites for the phenylalkylamines and the dihydropyridines. These sites are not identical with the α and β adrenoreceptor, the muscarinic receptor and the sodium channel. They are probably distinct entities as revealed by their different requirement for divalent metal ions, their copurification with different membrane fractions and their inability to bind compounds of the other group with high affinity. The existence of two distinct binding sites for dihydropyridines and phenylalkylamines in cardiac muscle has been predicted previously from non-competitive inhibition curves of (^3H)-nitrendipine binding by verapamil(11). The K_D value of the low affinity site for dihydropyridines (24 nM) is very similar to the concentration needed to inhibit halfmaximally contraction in cardiac muscle (33 nM)(12).

The apparent IC_{50} value for verapamil and D600 (70-90 nM) to inhibit $(^3H)-(-)$D888 binding and contraction of cardiac muscle (70-100 nM)(13,14) are also almost identical. This suggests that at least the low affinity sites detected in these studies may be identical with part of the cardiac Ca^{2+} channel.

Aknowledgement: We thank Dr.Hoffmeister from Bayer AG, Dr.Hollmann and Dr.Kretschmar from Knoll AG for providing the organic calciumantagonists. This work was supported by a grant from DFG.

REFERENCES

1. Reuter,H. (1984) Ann.Rev.Physiol.46, 473-484.
2. Osterrieder,W.,Brum,G.,Hescheler,J.,Trautwein,W., Flockerzi,V.and Hofmann,F. (1982) Nature 298, 576-578.
3. Brum,G.,Flockerzi,V.,Hofmann,F.,Osterrieder,W. (1983) Pflügers Arch.398, 147-154.
4. Fleckenstein,A. (1977) A.Rev.Pharmac.Toxic. 17,149-166.
5. Bellemann,P.,Ferry,D.,Lübbecke,F.and Glossmann,H. (1981) Arzneimittel-Forsch. 31, 2064-2067.
6. Hulthén,V.L.,Landmann,R.,Bürgisser,E.,Bühler,F.R. (1982) J.Cardiovasc.Pharmacol. 4, S291-SS293.
7. Glossmann,H.,Ferry,D.,Lübbecke,F.,Mewes,R.,Hofmann,F. (1982) TrendsPharmacol.Sci. 3, 431-437.
8. Holck,M.,Thorens,S.,Haeusler,G. (1982) Eur.J.Pharmacol. 85, 305-315.
9. Snyder,S.H. (1984) Science 224, 22-31.
10. Flockerzi,V.,Mewes,R.,Ruth,P.,Hofmann,F. (1983) Eur.J. Biochem. 135, 131-142.
11. Ehlert,F.J.,Itoga,E.,Roeske,W.R.,Yamamura,H.I., (1982) Biochem.Biophys.Res.Commun.104, 937-943.
12. DePover,A.,Lee,S.,Matlib,M.A.,Whitmer,K.,Davis,B.A., Powell,T.,Schwartz,A. (1983) Biochem.Biophys.Res. Commun. 113, 185-191.
13. Millard,R.W.,Grupp,G.,Grupp,I.L.,DiSalvo,J.,DePover,A., Schwartz,A. (1983) Circ.Res. 52, (Suppl.I), 29-39.
14. Pelzer,D.,Trautwein,W.,McDonald,T.F. (1982) Pflüger's Archs. 394, 97-105.

EFFECTS OF cAMP OR CATALYTIC SUBUNIT OF PROTEIN KINASE ON CARDIAC CALCIUM CHANNELS.

W. TRAUTWEIN, G. BRUM and W. OSTERRIEDER
Physiology 2, Univ. Saarland, 6650 Homburg/Saar, F.R.G.

In ventricular myocytes,isolated from the adult guinea pig heart by enzymatic digestion with collagenase,pressure injection through a glass pipette of a small volume of 1 mM cAMP dissolved in 150 mM KCl into the cell prolongs the action potential (AP) and shifts its plateau in positive direction. Simultaneously the amplitude of the Ca current is greatly increased. Bath perfusion with adrenaline or theophylline produced similar effects. Pressure injection of catalytic subunit of the cAMP-dependent protein kinase (C) produced cAMP-like effects: The AP was prolonged and the plateau was shifted in positive direction (Fig. 1A). In contrast to cAMP injection the changes lasted for a long time. Simultaneously with the alterations in the AP, in the voltage-clamp experiments, the Ca current was drastically increased (Fig. 1B).

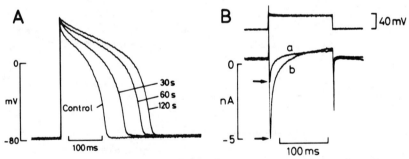

Fig. 1A: Superimposed AP's, control and after 30 s, 60 s & 120 s (steady state) of injection of catalytic subunit (From ref.[1]). B superimposed currents in response to step depolarizations from -40 mV to zero mV (top), a control, b after injection of C (From ref.[2]).

Proceedings of the 16th FEBS Congress
Part B, pp. 385–390
© 1985 VNU Science Press

The effects of C were seen in less than 3 s after beginning of injection but the delay could not be reliably resolved. C was prepared by Dr. Hofmann (Heidelberg) from fresh bovine hearts [3]. The injections increased C by about 1-10 µM/l, a value which is 1-10 times higher than the total concentration of the protein kinase in the heart.

When the AP was prolonged by injection of C, perfusion with adrenaline did not produce further prolongation. Obviously the Ca permeability was saturated and adrenaline could not produce an additional increase. The result suggests that there is only on type of Ca channels, activated by either adrenaline or C.

To study the question whether under physiological conditions C is involved in the modulation of the Ca current, the regulatory subunit, R, was injected. As far as it is known the only function of R is to bind C and thereby inhibit its phosphotransferease activity [4]. Injection of R lowered the plateau of the AP and, in most

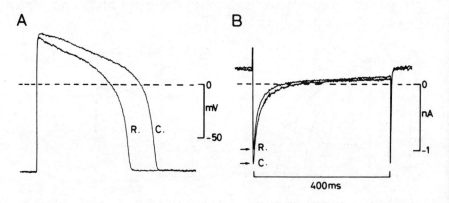

Fig. 2: Injection of R on AP (A superimposed control, C, and R effect) and membrane current (B superimposed C and R, for peaks see arrows). The currents were on step depolarization from -40 to zero mV (unpublished experiment from Kameyama and Trautwein).

experiments, shortened its duration. Simultaneously the amplitude of the Ca current was reduced. The reduction varied between 10 and 50% of the control amplitude. These effects of R indicate a basal phosphorylation resulting in a basal Ca permeability which can be augmented by β-adrenergic stimulation. When, in the control, the outward current was relatively large, it was depressed by R just contrary to C. In such cells the AP duration may be little affected for the decrease in calcium inward current is compensated by a decrease in potassium outward current.

The mechanism by which β-adrenergic stimulation brings about a larger Ca current was studied by measuring the activity of single Ca channels in a membrane patch [5]. Generally, the Ca current recorded from the whole cell can be increased by a larger amplitude of the current through the single channel (i) or by a larger number of channels in the patch (N) or a higher probability of the channel to be in the open state (p_o) or any combination of these three factors. The activity of a single channel in response to step depolarizations is burstlike, i.e. brief openings are separated by shorter or longer times in the closed state (Fig. 3Aa). Some traces, however, do not show activity at all (blanks), i.e. the channel is in an inactivated state. In the experiment of Fig. 3 the patch contained only one channel because no superposition of the activity of two channels is observed in the course of many depolarizations. Adrenaline did not increase the amplitude of the unitary currents (i) (Fig. 3Ba) nor did it produce superpositions of unitary currents, i.e. it did not increase the number of channels (N) in the patch. It did, however, greatly increase the probability of the channel to be in the open state (p_o) by both the increase of p_o in sweeps with channel ·openings and the decrease of the

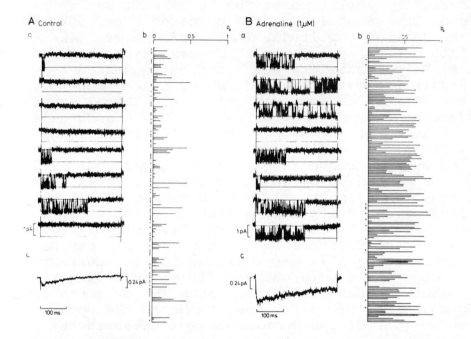

Fig. 3Aa and Ba: Ca channel activity in response to step depolarizations before and in presence of adrenaline. Horizontal lines obtained from amplitude histograms determine amplitude of single channel current. Ab, Bb open probability (integrated activity of each trace) on successive depolarizations. Dots mark blanks. c average currents of 200 traces (unpublished record from Cavalié, Pelzer and Trautwein).

proportion of blanks in the ensemble. The increase in p_O in sweeps was studied by computing distribution histograms of open and shut times. For the computations a threshold level was applied halfway between the baseline and the average open channel current. Shut-open transitions were detected as crossings of this threshold; sojourns in times were grouped in 0.13 ms bins and displayed as time histograms. Open or closed periods that lasted until the end of the depolarizing step pulse were disregarded. Open time distributions are monoexponential whereas the shut time distribution consists of the sum of 2 exponentials. The short shut times (>1ms) correspond to brief closures within bursts, the longer shut times (2-3 ms) separate bursts [6]. Adrenaline or cAMP injection alter these fast gating properties in several ways. The mean channel life time ($\geq$ 1ms) is prolonged by a factor of 1.5-2 and the frequency of openings is increased. The duration of the long closings between bursts is decreased by about one half without significant alteration of the short closures within bursts. Besides these drug channel interations on a ms-time scale β-adrenergic stimulation markedly decreases the proportion of empty sweeps where the channel is unavailable to open suggesting an inactivated state in the order of seconds. As a result of these changes the amplitude of the mean current obtained by averaging a large number of current traces like in Fig. 3Aa, Ba is increased (compare Fig. 3Bc with Ac). There is a strong correlation between the number of blanks and voltage dependent inactivation as well as the amplitude of the ensemble average current [7]. It seems then that β-adrenergic stimulation removes a chemical inactivation (dephosphorylation?), the removal beeing mainly responsible for the increase in average current. In addition channel gating is altered towards longer open (conducting) and shorter shut states.

REFERENCES

[1] Brum, G., Flockerzi, V., Hofmann, F., Oster-
    rieder, W., Trautwein, W. (1983). Injec-
    tion of catalytic subunit of cAMP-depen-
    dent protein kinase into isolated cardiac
    myocytes. Pflügers Arch. 398, 147-157

[2] Osterrieder, W., Brum, G., Hescheler, J.,
    Trautwein, W., Flockerzi, V., Hofmann, F.
    (1982). Injection of subunits of cyclic
    AMP-dependent protein kinase into cardiac
    myocytes modulates Ca^{2+} current. Nature
    298, 576-578

[3] Hofmann, F. (1980). Apparent constants for
    the interaction of regulatory and cataly-
    tic subunits of cAMP-dependent protein
    kinase I and II. J. Biol. Chem. 255,
    1559-1564

[4] Krebs, E.G., Beavo, J.A. (1979). Phosphory-
    lation-dephosphorylation of enzymes. Ann.
    Rev. Biochem. 48, 923-959

[5] Hamill, O.P., Marty, A., Neher, E., Sakmann,
    B., Sigworth, J. (1981). Improved patch-
    -clamp techniques for high-resolution cur-
    rent recording from cells and cell-free
    membrane patches. Pflügers Arch. 391,
    85-100

[6] Cavalié, A., Ochi, R., Pelzer, D., Traut-
    wein, W. (1983). Elementary currents
    through Ca^{2+} channels in guinea pig myo-
    cytes. Pflügers Arch. 398, 284-297

[7] Trautwein, W. and Pelzer, D. (1984). Vol-
    tage-dependent gating of single calcium
    channels in cardiac cell membranes and
    its modulation by drugs. In "Calcium and
    Cell Physiology" (Marmé, D., ed.) Springer
    Heidelberg, New York.

ADENYLATE CYCLASE AND GUANYLATE CYCLASE IN THE EXCITABLE CILIARY MEMBRANE FROM PARAMECIUM

SUSANNE KLUMPP, DORIS GIERLICH AND JOACHIM E. SCHULTZ

Pharmazeutisches Institut der Universität, Morgenstelle 8, 7400 Tübingen, FRG

Paramecium tetraurelia is a protozoon of about 150 x 30 μm. Its cellbody is covered by approximately 5,000 cilia of the 9+2 type which are necessary for motility. Paramecium has been nicknamed swimming neuron or swimming receptor since it is an electrically excitable cell. It responds to external stimuli with an alteration of its swimming speed and direction [1]. The behavior is governed by changes in membrane potential. Hyperpolarization results in forward speeding while depolarization causes a reversal of the ciliary power stroke, that is backward swimming. The depolarizing Ca-influx occurs via voltage operated calcium channels localized in the ciliary membrane [2]. Deciliation of Paramecium leads to loss of electrical excitability which is restored upon regrowth of the cilia [2]. Thus, the cilia can be considered an excitable organelle. The easily observed behavior and the accessibility of the cell to electrophysiological testing and genetic manipulation open a unique possibility to tie together biochemical, behavioral and electrophysiological events at a molecular level [3].

Very often, cyclic AMP and cyclic GMP are thought of as intracellular amplifier molecules. Therefore, we started to investigate whether adenylate cyclase (AC) and guanylate cyclase (GC) are present in the cilia of Paramecium and how they may be regulated and coupled to electrical and behavioral events.

MATERIALS AND METHODS

An extensive description of the methods to mass-culture Paramecium tetraurelia, wildtype 51s,

Proceedings of the 16th FEBS Congress
Part B, pp. 391–396
© 1985 VNU Science Press

without bacteria, to deciliate the cells and purify cilia has been presented and the reader is referred to the original literature [4]. Also, conditions for assays of AC and GC using [α-^{32}P] labelled trinucleotide phosphates have been detailed [5,6].

RESULTS AND DISCUSSION

A large capacity for biosynthesis of cAMP and cGMP was found in cilia from Paramecium. All enzyme activity was particulate. Separation of ciliary membranes from incompletely demembranated cilia and axonemes on a sucrose density gradient indicated that AC and GC were localized >90% in the excitable ciliary membrane (Table 1, [6]).

Table 1: Distribution of AC and GC in ciliary fragments from Paramecium.
Cilia were disintegrated with a French Press and the pellet of a high spin centrifugation was layered onto a sucrose gradient. IDC = incompletely demembranated cilia, [for details see 6].

Ciliary fragment	Total activity (pmol cNMP/min)	
	AC	GC
Membranes (5mg)	6670	6413
IDC (3.7mg)	388	438
Axonemes (1.6mg)	397	244

The ciliary membrane vesicles could be further separated on a Percoll density gradient. Surprisingly, a distinctive heterogeneity in AC and GC pattern of the ciliary membrane was observed [6]. While GC was found mainly in a fraction of high buoyant density, AC was observed in two fractions of membrane vesicles of different densities [6]. Electron microscopic inspection revealed that all vesicles were of a mean diameter of 300 nm, the heavier fraction having a multishell appearance [4]. Further biochemical differences other than AC and GC e.g. in distribution of protein kinases or phosphodiesterases, or in protein patterns on SDS/PAGE were not found.

Regulation of guanylate cyclase

In many tissues Ca-ions have been implicated in regulation of cGMP levels in unbroken cells. Yet, GCs which were sensitive to Ca-ions in a meaningful concentration range, were not identified. Often, nitroso compounds stimulate GC [7]. These were without potency on the GC from Paramecium. Since the voltage dependent calcium channels are localized in the ciliary membrane, we investigated an involvement of Ca. The Ca-chelator EGTA inhibited GC activity over a narrow concentration range. After removal of Ca-ions from all assay reagents, GC activity was about 20% of control. A dose response curve with Ca yielded an ED50 of only 8 μM, maximal activation was obtained at 50-100 μM (Fig. 1A, [5]). Higher concentrations were inhibitory. The activation of GC was remarkably specific for Ca. Sr was somewhat active, Ba not at all. Actually, the ED50 for Ca was not altered even in the presence of 1 mM Ba^{2+}. Many physiological effects of Ca-ions seem to be intracellularly mediated by the Ca-receptor protein calmodulin (CaM). Addition of CaM to GC assays had only a marginal effect, however, CaM antibodies raised against CaMs from pig brain, soybean, Tetrahymena and Paramecium strongly inhibited GC activity implicating the presence of endogenous CaM [8]. In an effort to replace Ca by La, it was found that La-ions inhibited GC irreversibly by dissociation of tightly bound CaM [8]. Enzyme activity in the washed membrane fraction could be restored by homologous and other CaMs, e.g. from pig brain, several plants or Tetrahymena [9].

The specificity for divalent alkaline earth metal ions to activate the reconstituted GC was changed compared to the native GC indicating that CaM could not completely fit into the original binding site at the catalytic entity [9]. Although it is most attractive to speculate that the Ca-influx into the cilia occurring during the Ca/K action potential is directly coupled to intraciliary cGMP production this idea must first be experimentally proved using pawn-mutants, which have a defect in the voltage gated Ca-current [3].

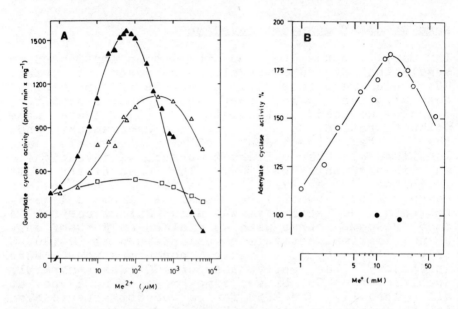

Fig. 1: Ionic regulation of GC (A) and AC (B) of the ciliary membrane from Paramecium.
(A): stimulation of GC by Ca (▲), Sr (△), and Ba (□)
(B): stimulation of AC by K (0—0). Na (●—●) was without stimulatory activity. (From references [5 and 10])

Adenylate cyclase in the cilia

The particulate AC activity in the cilia from Paramecium was a separate enzyme entity, not just a GC which happened to use ATP as substrate. This was evident from several observations [5,6,10]:
  a) AC and GC activity were differentially localized in the cilia
  b) AC was not affected by 100 μM lanthanum-ions which completely inhibited GC
  c) AC activity was not reduced by the presence of

EGTA in the assay while this turned off GC
d) antibodies against CaM had no effect on AC activity but inhibited GC (see above)
e) antibodies against GC from rat brain did not inhibit ciliary AC activity, yet, reduced GC activity by 50%
f) the temperature dependence and stability, pH-optimum and divalent cation requirement were different for AC and GC.

Most recently, we were able to solubilize AC and GC from the ciliary membrane in a two step procedure [10]. Treating the membrane preparation with 1% Brij 56, about 60% of the total protein was solubilized, yet, AC and GC activity remained in the pellet. Sonication with 0.5% Lubrol PX in the presence of mercaptoethanol and glycerol resulted in release of both enzymes into the supernatant. Subsequent chromatography on an Ultrogel AcA 22 column separated both enzyme activities, GC still retaining its bound CaM [10].
AC activity from the ciliary membrane of Paramecium was not influenced by several compounds which have powerful effects on ACs from many systems: GTP, GMPPNP, NaF, forskolin, cholera toxin, pertussis toxin [10]. It was found that cAMP concentrations in Paramecium in vivo are regulated by the Donnan ratio established specifically by potassium and calcium-ions [11]. Ca-ions >200 μM inhibited AC. K-ions had a rather unique stimulatory effect. Only 3 mM K^+ enhanced AC by 50%, the maximal effect was seen with 15 mM (Fig. 1B). Lithium and sodium-ions were without stimulatory effect (Fig. 1B, [10]).

Apart from the interesting question as to the detailed mechanism of regulation of AC and GC in the ciliary membrane the system lends itself to a molecular probe for the physiological function of cAMP and cGMP in regulation of ion fluxes and, consequently, of behavior of this unicellular organism.

REFERENCES

[1] Eckert, R., Brehm, P. (1979). Ionic mechanisms of excitation in Paramecium. Annu. Rev. Biophys.

Bioeng. 8,353-383.

[2] Dunlap, K. (1977). Localization of calcium channels in Paramecium caudatum. J. Physiol. (Lond.) 271,119-133.

[3] Kung, C., Chang, S.-Y., Satow, Y., van Houten, J. Hansma, H. (1975). Genetic disection of behavior in Paramecium.
Science (Wash.D.C.) 188,898-904.

[4] Thiele, J., Klumpp, S., Schultz, J.E., Bardele, C.F. (1982). Differential distribution of voltage-dependent calcium channels and guanylate cyclase in the excitable ciliary membrane from Paramecium tetraurelia. Eur.J. Cell Biol. 28,3-11.

[5] Klumpp, S., Schultz, J.E. (1982). Characterization of a Ca^{2+}-dependent guanylate cyclase in the excitable ciliary membrane from Paramecium. Eur. J. Biochem. 124,317-324.

[6] Schultz, J.E., Klumpp, S. (1983). Adenylate cyclase in cilia from Paramecium. FEBS Lett. 154,347-350.

[7] Murad, F., Arnold, W.P., Mittal, C.K., Braughler, J.M. (1979). Properties and regulation of guanylate cyclase and some proposed functions for cyclic GMP. Adv. Cycl. Nucl. Res. 11,175-204.

[8] Schultz. J.E., Klumpp, S. (1984). Calcium/Calmodulin-regulated guanylate cyclases in the ciliary membranes from Paramecium and Tetrahymena. Adv. in Cycl. Nucl. Prot. Phosph. Res. 17,275-283.

[9] Klumpp, S., Kleefeld, G., Schultz, J.E. (1983) Calcium/Calmodulin-regulated guanylate cyclase of the excitable ciliary membrane from Paramecium. J. Biol. Chem. 258,12455-12459.

[10] Klumpp, S., Gierlich, D., Schultz, J.E. (1984) Adenylate cyclase and guanylate cyclase in the excitable ciliary membrane from Paramecium: separation and regulation. FEBS Lett. 171,95-99.

[11] Schultz, J.E., Grünemund, R., von Hirschhausen, R., Schönefeld, U. (1984). Ionic regulation of cyclic AMP levels in Paramecium tetraurelia in vivo. FEBS Lett. 167,113-116.

Supported by the Deutsche Forschungsgemeinschaft (SFB 76).

CELL METABOLISM CONTROLS NEURON IONIC CHANNELS

E.A.Liberman, S.V.Minina
IPIT USSR Academy of Science, Moscow, USSR

In 1957 E.A.Liberman (1) discovered a complex code of nervous impulses sent by single neuron. Later a similar code was described by Hubel & Wiesel (2). They named the neurons sending such complicated codes "neuron detectors". According to this point of view, the neurons represented in (1) are color detectors. This implies that the cat's pattern in our brain is the consequence of excitation of a special neuron. But we see whole cat's pattern and at the same time hear its "meiow". We believe from this that it is necessary to develop a quite different description of the device responsible for our feeling. Now, we know that similar codes may arise from changes in intracellular metabolism of one neuron (Fig.1a,b). This finding was preceded by a theoretical

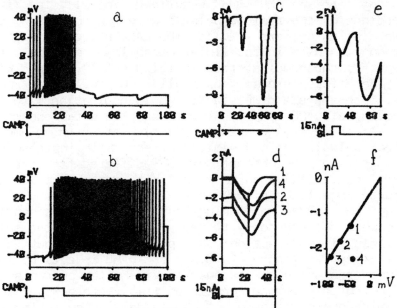

Fig.1 cAMP effect on potential & current in snail neuron

Proceedings of the 16th FEBS Congress
Part B, pp. 397–406

elaboration of the concept of a molecular computer (MC). This idea was stimulated by measurement of the membrane potential of mitochondria, submitochondrial particles and photophosphorylating particles (3,4).The mitochondrial membrane potential, measured by Liberman's method of penetrating ions (5), is changed during electron transfer from one protein to another (6) along the respiratory chain. The first idea was that the membrane was MC with an electron-carrier protein molecule as the element of memory and with DNA and RNA-dependent ATP-ase controlled by molecular words (7). The second idea (8) was that molecular stochastic language can work as MC. The proof of the universality of a stochastic language was shown in (9). These works predicted "splicing". The plenary lectures of K.Rajewsky and G.P.Georgiev provide excellent experimental proofs that MC really operates in living cells. Moreover, Georgiev's lecture shows that just the language described in (8-10) operates in the cell. We went in another direction to show that an intraneuronal MC takes part in brain function. The method used by us at present to investigate the effect of intraneuronal injection of cyclic AMP was described in (11). The first recordings of the rapid depolarizing effect of cAMP are shown in our papers (12,13). The cAMP effect is seen to be connected with intracellular metabolism and is prolonged by phosphodiesterase inhibitors ((13,14) and Fig. 1b). The effect is observed in all types of snail neurons. Ten years ago we started an investigation with the injection of cAMP by pressure. We saw the effect shown in Fig. 1; however, pressure injection of large volume of control solution gave a similar effect. With iontophoretic injection the effect of cAMP differed from that of other ions (12,14). Now we know that iontophoretic and pressure injections of cAMP give a similar effect. But to prevent the cAMP effect being masked a direct mechanical response it is necessary to use a more concentrated solution. Fig. 1 shows not only the potential (a,b) but also the current response (c,d,e) to cAMP injection. This response resembles the famous Hodgkin-Huxley currents in the potential-clamped condition (15).Note however that the existance of a maxim. is caused only by switching off the cAMP injection. This was shown clearly in the paper

(13), where the current restoring resting potential was measured. The shape of the current response to cAMP injected with a short pressure pulse (Fig. 1c,e) is caused by a complicate intracellular processes and cannot be used for such conclusion as in the Hodgkin-Huxley case. A more complex shape of current is induced by iontophoretic injection (Fig. 1d,e), so the dependence of the maximum of cAMP-induced current on different fixed potential levels did not allow any conclusion to be drawn about the underlying ionic mechanism, as was attempted in (16). Fig. 1d,f illustrates directly the mistake of drawing any such conclusion. Inspite of the values of current maximum (curves 1,2,3 in Fig.1d) corresponding to points on a straight line, curve 4 obtained 15 min after curve 1 has an altered shape and maximum value (compare with Fig.6,8,9,11 in (16)). Therefore, in order to determine what ions are involved in cAMP response it is necessary to measure the reversal potential of cAMP current (17-18). Such experiments lead us to the conclusion that cAMP effect is connected with an increase in Na-conductivity and decrease in K-conductivity (17,19). An important question is whether the mediator which hyperpolarize neurons acts through activation of adenylate cyclase resulting in an increase in cAMP production. The observed cAMP effect is caused by the cAMP concentration gradient and not by concentration alone. During intracellular injection this gradient is opposite to the gradient in the case in which adenylate cyclase at the plasma membrane is activated by mediators. To control this possibility we applied cAMP extracellularly by means of pressure,using a bathing solution in which all NaCl was replaced by NacAMP (80mM). The cAMP application evoked a transitory depolarization followed by hyperpolarization that lasted for the duration of the injection (Fig.2a). Intracellular cAMP injection caused the usual depolarization. Fig. 2b shows how spike duration changes during extracellular application of cAMP. A similar prolongation of spike duration can be observed during intracellular cAMP injection (Fig. 2c,d). The effect of intracellular injection of cAMP can be very strong (Fig. 2e,f), but it is reversible and reproducible (11). This change of membrane potential at the repetitive generation of nerve impulses and their

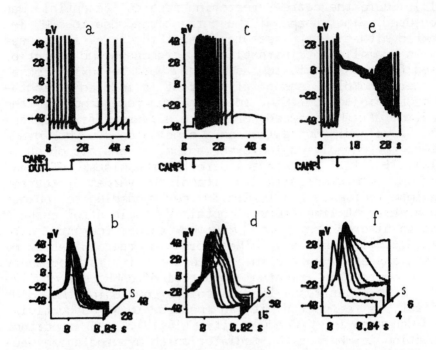

Fig.2 Effect of extra- and intracellular application of cAMP

shape changes may be described by Hodgkin-Huxley equations with a potential-independent increase in gNa and decrease in gK during cAMP injection. As stated above, the rapid response to cAMP is similar to the mechanical response of the neuron cell body (Fig. 3a). We believe that it is not artefact, but a real physiological effect. The neuron responds to inflation as mechanical receptor. Moreover, we suppose that the rapid response to cAMP injection is induced not by the usual biochemical process, involving activation of protein kinase and membrane protein phosphorylation, but direct interaction of cAMP with the cytoskeleton of the cell. Indeed, the delay of the rapid response to cAMP is so short that cAMP cannot be transported from electrode tip to neuron membrane by usual diffusional process (Fig.3d,e). When we investigated the delay of the effect of iontophoretic injection of cAMP (20,21), diffusional delay seems to be long enough

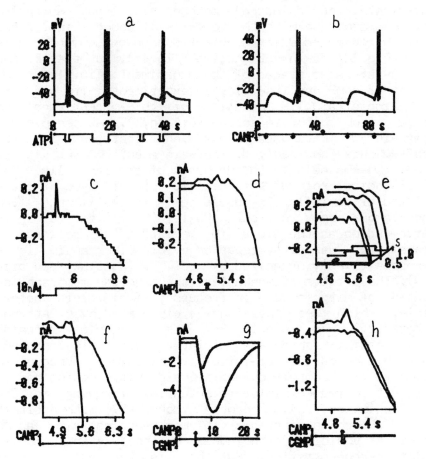

Fig.3 Mechanical response and delay of response to cAMP

(Fig.3c), but in experiments with injection of cAMP by means of a short pressure pulse applied by a micropipette in the middle of a large neuron delay is too short (Fig.3d,e). Therefore, we suggest that the rapid response of a neuron to cAMP is caused by a new type of biochemical and biophysical process. This process starts probably with direct interaction of cAMP with the cytoskeleton near the micropipette tip. It has been shown (22) that in neurons there is associated with microtubules a protein similar to the regulatory subunit of cAMP

401

dependent protein kinase. Binding of injected cAMP with this protein could induce a mechanical signal spreading to the membrane with the velocity of sound. Fig.3 shows that the observed delay does not depend on neuron diameter (Fig.3d) or injecting time (Fig.3e), but that it increases at later stages of the experiment (Fig.3f). The effect of cGMP and its delay in experiments with pressure injection of a 0.1 M solution of this drug does not differ from cAMP injection (Fig.3g,h). At the present symposium we have heard excellent lectures given by prof.H.Reuter and prof. W.Trautwain about the activity of single Ca-channels in the membrane of cardiac cells. The physiological role of this activity of this type of channel and of Ca-influx in muscle cells is well known from the famous work of sir A.Huxley (23). A role of Ca in nerve ending as the signal for mediating the release of transmitter was first reported by E.A.Liberman in Kiev's Symposia (1966), organized by prof. P.G.Kostyuk, see also (24). The effects of uncouplers shunting the membrane potential of mitochondria on frequency of miniature potentials, which were previously discovered by P.Fatt and B.Katz (25), was shown in (26). Nerve impulse reaching nerve ending increases a miniature potentials frequency only by means of Ca-influx activation. Uncouplers released Ca from mitochondria inside nerve ending and as a result increased miniature potentials frequency in Ca-free solution (26). Recently E.Neher (27) with a direct method showed an increase in membrane capacity as a result of vesicle fusion induced by increase in intracellular Ca-concentration. But what is the role of Ca-influx through the membrane channels demonstrated in the neuron body in reports of prof. P.G.Kostyuk and prof. H.D.Luxe? Both increasing and decreasing of Ca-concentration cause hyperpolarization. But in usual physiological conditions the high Ca-buffering capacity inside the cell body prevents such effects. Accordingly it is inferred that cyclic nucleotides but not calcium serves as the signal to switch on intracellular processes. Really if the interior of the neuron cell body works as a MC, Ca-ions could not play such role as in nerve endings and in muscle. The generatory potential producing code of nerve impulses is output of MC. Each

402

nerve impulse evokes Ca-influx. Therefore Ca-ion cannot serve as the input signal to MC. Calcium influx can serve for neuron MC as signal that nerve impulse was sent. But this influx cannot influence on generation of next impulses. Calcium activates phosphodiesterase and decrease cAMP level. A compensating process probably exist. The rapid electromechanical reaction described in this report seems to us to be very important for the MC. We think that the usual MC operating with molecular words (DNA and RNA)(8) is the system which constructs and controls the quantum molecular computer (QMC) (28). QMC operates with hypersound signals. The remarkable properties of QMC allows to understand the main miracle of quantum mechanics. Each phonon in this QMC searchs all molecular structure.As a result the neuron QMC can solve physical problems on real three-dimensional holographic system of the cell's cytoskeleton. The QMC of the living cell is the simplest mathematical system.The usual computer with macroscopic elements is a physical device because all of its operations can be predicted. The QMC operations can not be predicted by external measurements. According to our hypothesis the QMC of living cell is the system with inner point of view and free will. The both this properties arise from quantum structure and existence of molecular language. Molecular language allows to put a question about inner point of view of QMC. It is like our conscience. According to the hypothesis (29) our soul (conscience) is not chemical, rather physical device - quantum regulator (QR). A brain sends information in this device by modulated hypersound waves. QR of our conscience is the place with cat's pattern and with its "meiow" and with our seeing and hearing personality. Just for the description of QR it is necessary to unite (consolidate) all physical fields and mathematics. Such unification is necessary since there are the contradictions between physics and mathematics.The physics postulates that the past determines the future of system-state and its behaviour, but mathematics prepose the full control. A biological systems can really changes the future. But it is necessary take into account the physical limit of control. First of all there are the losts of energy and time for calculation (30,31). Quantum properties of QMC

of living cell and QR of our conscience give not only the
minimal prize of action (30), but also unity and personality of living system. Only quantum computers can
serve as real mathematical devices and as controlling
system. Of course we can have dialogue so with quantum,
as with usual computers. But there is no inner point of
view in usual computer. Really, all responses of macroscopic computer can be predicted, principally, by means of
usual physical measurements without a change the state of
its macroscopic elements. The hypothesis about QMC and QR
will be check experimentally. Usual way is investigation
of complex spectrum of this system. The second way is
psychological test: you can ask a cell by molecular words
and read the molecular answer about its future behavior.
But we shall investigate role of cAMP and intracellular
mechanical movement in intraneuronal information processing.

1. Liberman, E.A. (1957). On the character of information
   entering the brain of a frog over one nerve fibre from
   two receptors of the retina. Biofizika 2, 427-430.
2. Hubel, D.H., Wiesel, T. N. (1959). Receptive fields of
   single neurones in the cat's striate cortex.J.Physiol.
   (L.) 148, 574-591.
3. Liberman, E. A., Tsofina, L. M. (1969). Active transport of penetrating anion by fragments of mitochondria
   and photophosphorylating bacteria. Biofizika 14, 1017-
   1022.
4. Liberman, E. A., Topaly, V. P., Tsofina, L. M., Jasai-
   tis, A. A., Skulachev, V.P. (1969). Mechanism of coupling of oxidative phosphorylation and the membrane potential of mitochondria. Nature 222, 1076-1078.
5. Liberman, E. A., Topaly, V.P. (1968). Selective transport of ions through bimolecular phospholipid membranes. Biochim. Biophys. Acta 163, 125-136.
6. Ernster, L., Lee, C. P. (1964). Biological oxidoreduc-
   tions. Annual Rev. Biochem. 33, 729-740.
7. Liberman, E. A. (1969). Hypothesis about the role of
   cell membranes in controlling system of cell. Biofizika membran, Kaunas Med. Institut, pp. 147-154.
8. Liberman, E. A. (1972). Cell as a molecular computer

(MCC). Biofizika 17, 932-943.
9. Waintswaig, M. N., Liberman, E. A. (1973). Formal description of the cell molecular computer. Biofizika 18, 939-942.
10. Liberman, E.A. (1972). Ionic and electronic transport through membranes and possible role of these processes in the operating of cell molecular computer. Proc. of IY International Biophysical Congress, Nauka, Moscow, pp. 360-394.
11. Liberman, E. A., Minina, S. V., Shklovsky-Kordi, N.E., Conrad, M. (1982). Change of mechanical parameters as a possible means for information processing by the neuron. Biofizika 27, 863-870.
12. Liberman, E.A., Minina, S. V., Golubtsov, K.V. (1975). The study of metabolic synapse. I. Effect of intracellular microinjection of $3',5'$-AMP. Biofizika 20, 451-456.
13. Liberman, E. A., Minina, S. V., Golubtsov,K.V. (1977). II.Comparison of cyclic $3',5'$-AMP and cyclic $3',5'$-GMP effects. Biofizika 22, 75-81.
14. Liberman, E.A., Minina, S. V., Shklovsky, N.E. (1978). Neuron membrane depolarization by cyclic $3',5'$-adenosine monophosphate and its possible role in neuron molecular cell computer action. Biofizika 23, 305-311.
15. Hodgkin, A. L., Huxley, A. F. (1952). Current carried by sodium and potassium ions through the membrane of the giant axon of Loligo. J. Physiol. (L.) 116, 449-472.
16. Kononenko, N. I., Kostyuk, P. G., Shcherbatko, A. D. (1983). The effect of intracellular cAMP injection on stationary membrane conductance and voltage- and time-dependent ionic currents in identified Snail neurons. Brain Res. 268, 321-338.
17. Liberman, E. A., Minina, S. V., Shklovsky-Kordi, N. E. (1981). Cyclic nucleotides control the permeability of neuron membrane inside the cell. III Sovjet-Sweden Symposium "Phys. Chem. Biol." Theses of reports. Tbilisi, pp. 200-201.
18. Liberman, E. A., Minina, S. V., Shklovsky-Kordi, N. E. (1982). Effect of intracellular cyclic nucleotide injection on ionic current under the voltage-clamp conditions. Biofizika 27, 542-545.

19. Liberman, E. A., Minina, S. V., Shklovsky-Kordi, N.E., Conrad, M. (1982). Microinjection of cyclic nucleotides provides evidence for a diffusional mechanism of intraneuronal control. BioSystems 15, 127-132.
20. Liberman, E. A. (1979). Analog-digital molecular cell computer. BioSystems 11, 111-124.
21. Liberman, E. A., Minina, S. V., Shklovsky-Kordi, N. E. (1980). The study of diffusional modelling system of neuronal molecular computer. Biofizika 25, 445-461.
22. Miller, P., Walter, U., Theurkauf, W. E., Vallee,R.B., De Camilli, P. (1982). Frozen tissue sections as an experimental system to reveal specific binding sites for the regulatory subunit of type II cAMP-dependent protein kinase in neurons. Proc. Natl. Acad. Sci.USA. 79, 5562-5566.
23. Hyxley A. F., Taylor R.E. (1958). Local activation of striated muscle fibres. J. Physiol. (L.) 144, 426-441.
24. Blioch, Zh. L., Glagoleva, I. M., Liberman, E. A., Nenashev, V. A. (1968). The study of the mechanism of quantal transmitter release at a chemical synapse. J. Physiol. (L.) 199, 11-35.
25. Glagoleva, I. M., Liberman, E. A., Khashaev, Z. Kh. (1970). The effect of uncouplers of oxidative phosphorylation on the release of acetylcholine from nerve endings. Biofizika 15, 76-83.
26. Fatt, P., Katz, B. (1952). Spontaneous subthreshold activity at motor nerve endings. J. Physiol. (L.) 117, 109-128.
27. Neher, E., Marty, A., Fenwyk, E. (1983). Influence of inner Ca concentration on the jumps of the capacity. Progrress in Brain Res. 58, 39-44.
28. Liberman, E. A. (1983). Quantum molecular regulator. Biofizika 28, 183-186.
29. Liberman, E.A. (1979). Biological physics and the physics of the real world. BioSystems 11, 323-327.
30. Liberman, E. A. (1974). IY. Price of action is a value characterized the "difficulty" of the problem solution for the computer. Biofizika 19, 148-150.
31. Liberman, E. A. (1978). Biological physics and physics of real world. Biofizika 23, 1118-1121.

ACTIVATION OF SINGLE NEURONAL CALCIUM CHANNELS

H.D. LUX and A.M. BROWN[*]
Max-Planck-Institut für Psychiatrie, Am Klopferspitz 18A,
8033 Planegg, R.F.G.
[*]University of Texas Medical Branch, Galveston, TX 77550

SUMMARY

Activation of Ca channels has been described as a Hodgkin-Huxley process in which the time constants have ratios of two or greater (1,2,3) or as a three-state linear sequential process with two very different time constants (4). This was examined by measuring the turn-on and turn-off of macroscopic Ca currents and the discharge of single Ca channels in Helix neurons. The results show that neither a literal Hodgkin-Huxley mechanism nor a three-state model applies. A minimum model of activation requires at least four states.

This type of Ca channel is also present in vertebrate neurons. Some of these (dorsal root ganglionic cells (DRG) but not sympathetic neurons) exhibit in addition the activity of another type of Ca channel which shows a longer mean open time and larger conductance. This channel is activated at low depolarization, but only from a sufficiently negative membrane potential. It completely inactivates in a strongly voltage-dependent manner.

METHODS

The experiments on Helix were done using isolated nerve cell bodies of Helix. A combined voltage clamp was used (5) in which potential was measured with a microelectrode and current was delivered by a suction pipette. The latter also allowed dialysis of the cell's interior. Single Ca-channel currents were measured with the patch-clamp method in the cell- attached configuration. In these experiments the neurons were voltage-clamped using a conventional two microelectrode clamp and the patch was

Proceedings of the 16th FEBS Congress
Part B, pp. 407–414
© 1985 VNU Science Press

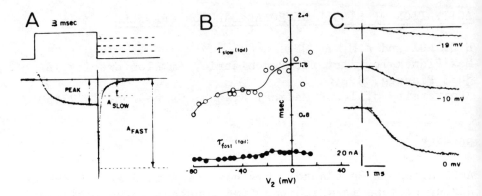

Figure 1. A, example of the Ca current obtained from
stepping to +30 mV and returning to a holding potential
of -50 mV. The tail current is fit with a sum of two
exponentials with τ's of 0.15 and 1.2 ms. The peak current during the step is indicated as well as the amplitudes associated with the fast and slow exponentials. B,
time constants of similar fits to tail currents obtained
at various return potentials following strong activation.
C, turn-on of Ca current obtained at the potentials shown.
Currents are corrected for asymmetry currents obtained
after substitution of Co for Ca. Superimposed are fits to
the data with an m^2 model (Data from 8).

held at the bath potential, for details see (6). K currents were suppressed by Cs substitution, TEA and 4-AP.
Na currents were suppressed by Tris substitution and/or
TTX. Linear components of leakage and capacitance were
removed by subtraction of hyperpolarizing pulses. Extracellular Ca concentration was 10 or 40 mM. The DRG experiments on single channels utilized isolated (outside
out) membrane patches as described previously (7).

RESULTS AND DISCUSSION

The capacitive current transient in the combined clamp
experiments (5) in Helix was 95% complete within ~50 μs
and R_s was found to be ~ 5 KΩ. The membrane was thus
clamped within 2 mV during times when tail currents were

408

measured (8). The tail currents following a voltage-clamp step to +30 mV for 5 ms had two time constants in a ratio of ~8 at a return potential of -50 mV (Fig. 1A). At this potential channel activity is zero in the steady-state (6). This result excludes a literal Hodgkin-Huxley model, which predicts only a single exponential in the tail currents at potentials where activation is zero. The slow component was clearly voltage-dependent whereas the fast component was only slightly voltage-dependent (Fig. 1B). These two tail 's could not account for the delay in the turn-on at similar potentials (Fig. 1C) as would be required by a sequential three-state model. Turn-on was well-described by an m^2 model, however, see also (1). It thus may be composed of a weighted sum of exponential functions with τ_m and $\tau_m/2$ which decreases with increased depolarization (see Fig. 1C). But $\tau_m/2$ (0.4 to 1.1 ms) is always found to be considerably larger than τ_f of the fast tail (Fig. 1A) and both τ_m and $\tau_m/2$ display a voltage-dependence that is inverse to that of the tail τ's. Taken together, these results indicate that at least three τ's are necessary to describe the data: a result that requires a minimum of four states.

Fig. 2A shows single Ca-channel currents following a depolarizing step in potential. Only single level openings were observed from this patch at various potentials. The binomial theorem predicted a significant number of multiple openings if more than one channel were present. We thus concluded that the openings came from one channel. The openings were repetitive and the briefer intervals gave rise to bursts. The amplitudes had a normal distribution around a single current value. The open times were distributed as a single exponential function and the mean values were relatively independent of potential between -20 and zero mV (6,9). Bursts and intervals between bursts (including single openings) are characterized by at least two closed states. In order to account for the apparent probability density function (PDF) of the two closed times, a sequential three state model may be assumed (4). However, the analysis of the waiting times or the latencies until the first opening following the voltage step reveals discrepancies with a three-state model of activation (see Fig. 2B,C).

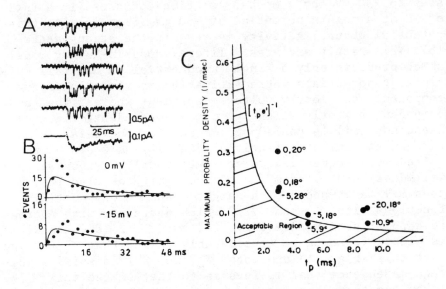

Figure 2. A, example of some Ca single channel records
following a step from −50 to −5 mV. The averaged current
at the bottom came from summing 68 records. B, two waiting time distributions for records such as those in A.
Data points are the number of points in a 2 ms bin. The
smooth curve is a theoretical curve computed with parameters from a three-state model which were obtained from a
stationary analysis of the single-channel data. Note that
the model predicts a "faster" waiting time distribution
than is measured; this is interpreted as evidence that a
higher-order model involving more closed states is required to describe turn-on from rest. C, The smooth curve
for $\rho_1 = \rho_2$ is the maximum allowable value of the peak
of the waiting time probability density plotted as a
function of the time to peak (t_p) as obtained for a three-
state model. Measured values must lie in the "acceptable
region" in order for the data to be consistent with a
three-state model (see 9). Data obtained under various
conditions are plotted with the potential and temperature
indicated. Note that all but one of the data points lie
outside this region, indicating an inconsistency with the
model.

410

The waiting time PDF was evaluated to relate maxima with times to peak (t_p) and eigenvalues ($\beta_{1,2}$). In Fig. 2B two waiting-time distributions are plotted and the smooth curve is predicted from estimates of the parameters from a stationary analysis of the data using open- and close-time histograms. Note that many of the measured waiting times are "slower" than the predicted values, indicating that a higher order model involving more closed states may be required to describe turn-on from rest. Best fitting but otherwise arbitrary three-state PDFs for waiting times showed eigenvalues that tended to be identical. These values strongly disagreed with those calculated from rate constants derived from the open- and close-time histograms. The peak of the data was also not fit well. This is displayed by the results shown in Fig. 2C in which all but one of the measured maximum values of the waiting time distribution fall in the unacceptable region for a three-state model indicating that the measured responses are not realizable with this model (9). An error in data display lends support to the argument. In Fig. 2, maximum values were taken from histogrammed data with finite bin widths (2 ms), and these would tend to be smaller than a true peak value. Single-channel data indicate a single open state from observations of the amplitude distributions as well as from the single exponential open time distribution. We conclude that for a sequential model at least four states are required to describe activation of Ca channels.

The opening frequency declined at longer times as shown in Fig. 2A and this was proof that single Ca channels can inactivate. Moreover, they must reopen from the inactivated state. Inactivation is not necessarily a consequence of channel opening (10). It can thus also prolong the waiting times. The effect on times to peak and β's are found to be quite small, however, since inactivation of this type of channel occurs at rates which are much lower than those of activation.

Two components of an inward-going Ca current were observed in cultured DRG cells of chick and rat (11) but not in Helix. Both currents in DRG cells persisted in the presence of 30 μM TTX or when external Na was replaced by choline. They were fully blocked by millimolar additions of Cd^{2+} and Ni^{2+} to the bath. In 5 to 10 mM external Ca, a current of small amplitude, turned on already during steps changes to -60 mV membrane potential, leveled off at -30 mV to a value of 0.2 nA. A second, larger current component, which resembled the previously described Ca current appeared at more positive voltages (-20 to -10 mV). The current component activated at the more negative membrane potentials showed the stronger dependence on external Ca. Time- and voltage-dependent activation is also complex as manifested by the current's sigmoidal rise (11), which became faster with increased depolarization. Its tail currents were generally slower than those associated with the more common Ca current. From -60 mV holding potential, the maximum obtainable amplitude of the low depolarization-activated current was only one tenth of that achieved from a holding potential of -90 mV. Voltage-dependent inactivation of this current component was fast compared with that of the other component. The properties of this low voltage-activated and fully inactivating Ca current suggest it is the same as the inward current that has been postulated in several central neurons to produce depolarizing potential waves and burst-firing only when membrane hyperpolarization precedes (12).

Recently a distinct Ca channel was found (7) with time- and voltage-dependent properties closely corresponding to the activation-inactivation behavior of this Ca conductance (Fig. 3). The mean lifetime of this channel is 4 to 6 times longer and its conductance considerably larger than those of the common Ca channel. Openings also occur in the form of bursts but activation necessitates strongly negative holding potentials. Activation as well as inactivation of this channel is greatly speeded with increased depolarization. Inactivation results in eventually complete closures. This channel coexists in isolated membrane patches with the previously described Ca channel which is less sensitive to changes in holding potential and shows a much slower inactivation time course.

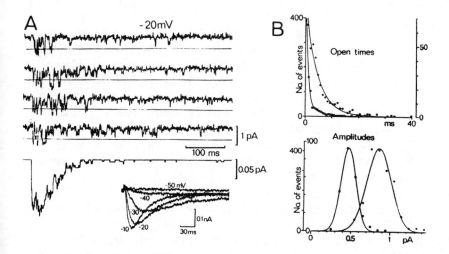

Figure 3. A, Ca channel currents in an outside-out patch
from a rat DRG cell, recorded during steps to -20 mV from
a holding of -90 mV. Events were averaged (last trace)
over 27 trials. Large- and small-amplitude events appear
in the recordings, with the larger unitary currents occurring predominantly in the initial periods. The detection level (lines) for the large-amplitude events was by
2 x s.d. set beyond the mean amplitude of the smaller
unitary currents. Inset in A, whole-cell Ca currents
recorded from a rat DRG cell at the potentials indicated.
Holding potential, -90 mV. Note the voltage-dependent
time courses of activation and inactivation. B, Amplitude
and open time histograms of the two unitary Ca currents
at -40 mV. The amplitude distributions were fitted by
Gaussian curves. The left-hand side distribution (left
scale) has a maximum of 0.45 pA. It contains some large-
amplitude events that escaped inactivation and thus contribute to the overlapping of the two distributions. The
large-amplitude distribution (right scale) has a maximum
of 0.86 pA. Exponential functions were fitted to the open
time histograms, with resulting time constants of 0.72
and 4.67 ms for the small and large unit, respectively.
The considerable differences between these values streng-
then the conclusion that tow different populations of Ca
channels were separated (7).

REFERENCES

1. Kostyuk, P.G. and O.A. Krishtal. (1977). Effects of and calcium calcium-chelating agents on the inward and outward currents in the membrane of mollusc neurones. J. Physiol. (Lond.) 270, 569-580.
2. Hencek, M. and J. Zachar. (1977). Calcium currents and conductance in the muscle membrane of the crayfish. J. Physiol. (Lond.) 268, 51-71.
3. Llinas, R., I.Z. Steinberg and K. Walton. (1981). Presynaptic calcium currents in squid giant synapse. Biophys. J. 33, 289-322.
4. Fenwick, E.M., A. Marty and E. Neher. (1982). Presynaptic calcium channels in bovine chromaffin cells. J. Physiol. (Lond.) 331, 559-636.
5. Brown, A.M., K. Morimoto, Y. Tsuda and D. Wilson. (1981). Calcium current-dependent and voltage-dependent inactivation of calcium channels in Helix aspersa. J. Physiol. (Lond.) 320, 193-218.
6. Lux, H.D. and A.M. Brown. (1984). Patch and whole cell calcium currents recorded simultaneously in snail neurons. J. Gen. Physiol. 83, 727-750.
7. Carbone, E. and H.D. Lux. (1984). A low voltage-activated, fully inactivating Ca channel in vertebrate sensory neurones. Nature 310, 501-503.
8. Brown, A.M., Y. Tsuda and D.L. Wilson, D.L. (1983). A description of activation and conduction in calcium channels based on tail and turn-on current measurements. J. Physiol. (Lond.) 344, 549-583.
9. Brown, A.M., H.D. Lux and D.L. Wilson. (1984). Activation and inactivation of single calcium channels in snail neurons. J. Gen. Physiol. 83, 751-769.
10. Lux, H.D. and A.M. Brown. (1984). Single channel studies on inactivation of calcium currents. Science 225, 432-434.
11. Carbone, E. and H.D. Lux. (1984). A low voltage-activated calcium conductance in embryonic chick sensory neurons. Biophys. J. 46, 413-418.
12. Llinas, R., and Y. Yarom. (1981). Properties and distribution of ionic conductances generating electroresponsiveness of mammalian inferior olivary neurons in vitro. J. Physiol. (Lond.) 315, 569-584.

Symposium XIV

STRUCTURE AND FUNCTION OF PEPTIDES AND PROTEINS

STRUCTURAL AND FUNCTIONAL ORGANIZATION
OF PEPTIDE AND PROTEIN LIGANDS

GUNAR CHIPENS
Institute of Organic Synthesis, Latvian SSR
Academy of Sciences, Riga, USSR

The selectivity of ligand-receptor interaction relies on
the complementarity of stereoelectronic structures of active regions of the ligand and the receptor system. Since
the forces of intermolecular interaction are subject to
rapid fading with increasing distance between the molecules (i.e. the energy of interaction is inversely proportional to the distance with high exponent) the first prerequisite for complex formation is the strict complementarity of the geometric profiles of the active sites involved in interaction. Peptide molecules in aqueous solution represent a mixture of different conformers existing
in equilibrium. For the contact between the ligand and
receptor molecule to be effective, i.e. leading to complex
formation, fixation, if only short-term, on the active
site structure of the ligand complementary to the receptor
"pocket" is required.
According to our working model, the formation and fixation
of biologically active space structures of ligands is
often brought about upon transition of the molecule from
aqueous environment to the less polar medium existing in
the receptor biophase or on direct interaction between
the ligand and receptor molecules when the contacting
surfaces undergo dehydration. The charged and polar groups
of peptides and proteins are hydrated in water. Water dipoles act as protective groups that screen the electro-
magnetic fields of the ions. During dehydration, the
"protective" groups are removed and the exposed ions and
dipoles become involved in bonding. The energies of such
bonds, e.g. resulting from the interaction of the Arg
side-chain and COOH groups,

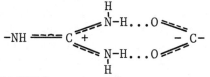

Proceedings of the 16th FEBS Congress
Part B, pp. 417–422
© 1985 VNU Science Press

are comparable with the energy of covalent bonds, such as disulphide. Hydrogen bonds become also considerably strengthened in apolar medium. The formation of salt, hydrogen and other intramolecular bonds leads to the quasicyclization of active sites in the molecule, viz. to the formation of "biologically active" space structures complementary to the active site of the receptor:

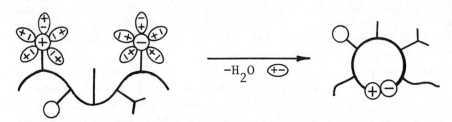

The sites for quasicyclization in peptide and protein molecules often involve the so-called common fragments discovered by us by using the systems and matrix analysis [1,2]. The nucleus of the common fragments consists of a basic amino acid (Arg or Lys) or its functional equivalents – aminodicarboxylic acid amides in juxtaposition to one or several proline or valine residues. In the structure of pituitary hormones and kinins the common fragments are always located next to the minimal specifically active fragment. This is suggestive of a certain structural organization of the molecules which has important functional implications, since removal of the common fragment decreases the specific activity of peptides, on an average, by 3-4-fold [1,2]. The first data suggesting possible involvement of the common fragments in the formation and fixation of space structures of peptides were obtained by means of semiempirical conformation calculations for bradykinin. The most stable conformation was found to have quasicyclic structure [3]. Another site for quasicyclization in peptides and proteins is generally represented by the carboxyl or amide groups of the C-terminal amino acids or Asp, Glu residues and their amides. New evidence in favour of possible participation of common fragments in the formation of space structures of peptides and proteins was obtained following the demonstration of cysteine-containing common fragments [4] in which the functions of basic amino acids are fulfilled by cysteine. The structures of common fragments and their cysteine-containing analogues of two types are shown below:

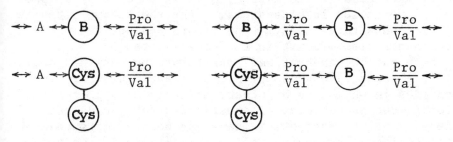

(A is aminodicarboxylic acid or glycine; B is Arg, Lys, Asn or Gln; ⟷ indicates the direction of peptide chain acylation). Both the disulphide and ionic bond confer to the ligand molecule its unique steric configuration essential for ligand-receptor interaction. This leads to assume the equifunctionality of disulphide bonds in cyclic peptides and salt bridges or hydrogen bonds in quasicyclic ones:

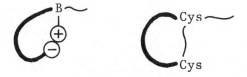

This assertion gains support from the study of evolution of protein structures, e.g. microbial proteinases where nonvalent, salt, hydrogen and other bonds of Arg...Asp, Glu...Lys type become gradually replaced by disulphide bridges [4]. Disulphide bond breakage (synthesis of acyclic analogues by substituting Cys for Ala or Cys(Me)) results in a dramatic loss of biological activity by oxytocin, vasopressin, somatostatin, etc. Changes in biological activity are comparable with the effects of removal of common fragments from linear quasicyclic peptides and are mainly due to peptide space structure disruption (abrupt reduction in the specific weight of the corresponding conformer). Parameter analysis for the commonest disulphide cycles and potential quasicycles in peptide and protein structures demonstrates that cyclic and quasicyclic structures containing 6–8 amino acid residues are prevalent in both cases. This size of the "active" ligand loop apparently reflects some universal principles of peptide/protein interaction in biosystems, since the active sites in peptide substrates, enzyme inhibitors and antigenic determinants also lie within the same limits [4].

To bear out the theoretical considerations outlined above it is expedient to synthesize cyclic analogues for linear peptides in which the hypothetical ionic or hydrogen bond, closing the quasicycle, is substituted for a covalent, peptide one. At present, we have synthesized more than 60 cycloanalogues belonging to 11 biologically active groups of peptides. They include pituitary hormones (ACTH, MSH), neuropeptides (substance P, neurotensin), immunopeptides (tuftsin and other Ig fragments), toxins (wasp venom kinin, bradykinin-potentiating peptides), tissue hormones (angiotensin, bradykinin, kallidin), etc. Biologically active cycloanalogues have been obtained in all cases corroborating the universality or quasicyclization principle [5]. Some examples of cyclopeptide structures – analogues of linear peptides or their fragments are given below:

$$\overline{\text{KPPGFGPGR}^{\rfloor}} \ (1), \quad \overline{\text{KKKLRGKPPGFGPFR}^{\rfloor}} \ (\text{II})$$

$$\overline{\text{TKPRG}^{\rfloor}} \ (\text{III}), \ \overline{\text{TKPR}^{\rfloor}} \ (\text{IV}), \ \overline{\text{KHFRWG}^{\rfloor}} \ (\text{V}),$$

$$\overline{\text{KHFRWGG}^{\rfloor}} \ (\text{VI}), \ \overline{\text{KRPPGFSPFR}^{\rfloor}} \ (\text{VII}),$$

$$\overline{^{\lfloor}\text{KPPGFGPFR}^{\rfloor}} \ (\text{VIII}), \ \overline{\text{KPRRPYIF}^{\rfloor}} \ (\text{IX}),$$

$$\overline{\text{KNKPRRPYIL}^{\rfloor}} \ (\text{X}), \ \overline{\text{EHFGWGKPVG}} \ (\text{XI})$$

The most conspicuous features of cyclopeptides distinguishing them from their linear precursors are as follows: (1) Alterations in the biological spectrum of peptides and greater selectivity of action. E.g., cyclobradykinin (1) retaining the high depressor activity of the natural hormone has no effect on the extravasal smooth muscle. (2) Many, but not all, cyclopeptides have distinctly prolonged duration of action in vivo. Compound I, a cycloanalogue of wasp venom kinin II and other cyclokinins affect blood pressure for several hours, whereas their linear precursors are effective during tens of seconds. (3) Changes in peptide cycle size are accompanied by altera-

tions in the spectrum and character of action. Compound
III, unlike its cycloanalogue IV, acts as tuftsin antagonist. ACTH cycloanalogue V exhibits pronounced melanotropic activity, but is completely devoid of steroidogenic
properties, while cycloanalogue VI displays both types of
activity. In some cases, considerable variation in the
cycle size is possible without affecting the biological
activity (e.g. macrocyclobradykinin [5]). (4). A significant factor for the manifestation of biological activity
of cyclopeptides is the presence of a basic amino acid in
the common fragment. Among the cycloanalogues of bradykinin and kallidin, the myotropic activity is present only
in compounds containing the common fragment with a basic
amino acid, e.g. cyclokallidin VII and α-cyclobradykinin
VIII. (5) If a linear peptide has several potential sites
for quasicyclization (neurotensin, substance P, tachyki-
nins, etc.), the corresponding cyclopeptides show a differential spectrum of biological activity. E.g., a neurotensin fragment cycloanalogue IX affects the central nervous system, but exerts no effect on blood pressure or
extravasal smooth muscle. Conversely, the other fragment
cycloanalogue X studied was characterized by high depres-
sant activity, but was only slightly myotropic, etc. (6)
On some cases, cyclopeptides possess extremely high biological activity. E.g., the melanotropic activity of the
cyclic analogue of MSH fragment XI is by three orders of
magnitude higher than that of the linear precursor.
Rational synthesis of cycloanalogues for linear peptides
based on the application of systems, matrix and conformation analysis of peptide/protein structures [2,4] and
the results of bioassays obtained for cycloanalogues cor-
roborate the expediency of the present approach to the
study of the mechanism of action of natural bioregulators.
The ultimate goal of these investigations is to develop
new biochemical reagents and drugs.

REFERENCES

1. Chipens, G., Auna, Z.P., Kluša, V.E. (1973). Some concepts of the molecular mechanism of action of peptide hormone at receptor level. In: Peptides 1972,

H. Hanson, H. Jakubke (eds), North-Holland, Amsterdam, pp. 437-449.
2. Chipens, G., Kriķis, A., Polevaja, L.K. (1979). Physico-chemical principles of information transfer at
molecular level. In: Biophysical and Biochemical
Information Transfer if Recognition. J.G. Vassi-
leva-Popova, E.V. Jensen (eds). Plenum Press, New
York, pp. 23-47.
3. Ivanov, V.T., Filatova, M.P., Reissman, Z., Reutova, T.O., Efremov, E.S., Pashkov, V.S., Galaktio-
nov, S.G., Grigorian, G.L., Ovchinnikov, Yu.A.
(1975). In: Peptides: Chemistry, Structure, Biology. R. Walter, J. Meienhofer (eds). Ann Arbor
Science, Ann Arbor, Michigan, pp. 151-157.
4. Chipens, G., Polevaja, L., Veretennikova, N., Kriķis, A. (198+). Structure and Function of Low Molecular Peptides. Zinātne, Riga, pp. 1-323 (in Russian).
5. Ovchinnikov, Yu., Chipens, G., Ivanov, V. (1983).
Peptides 1982. K.Blaha, P. Malon (eds). Walter de
Gruyter. Berlin, pp. 1-18.

SCORPION TOXINS : A STRUCTURE-ACTIVITY RELATIONSHIPS STUDY RELATED BOTH TO NEUROTOXIC AND ANTIGENIC PROPERTIES OF THESE TOXINS

DARBON, H., SAMPIERI, F., EL AYEB, M. and ROCHAT, H.

INSERM U 172 and CNRS UA 553
Laboratoire de Biochimie Faculté de Médecine Nord
Boulevard P. Dramard 13326 MARSEILLE CEDEX 15

Toxic activities of scorpion venoms are due to small basic proteins which are extensively purified in view to define their structures and, in this way, to reach a better molecular understanding of their interactions with their pharmacological receptors related to the voltage sensitive sodium channels. According to the test animal used during purification, toxins have been called mammal toxins (mouse), insect toxins (fly larva) or crustacean toxins (isopod). They form a family of proteins made of one single chain of 60 to 70 amino acid residues cross-linked by four disulfide bridges (1). Based on sequence homologies, several structural groups are defined (table 1), a classification strictly confirmed on the level of the antigenic properties of these proteins : an antiserum prepared against one toxin is able to react with every toxin belonging to the same group when no cross-reactivity is observed with toxins of other groups (2). According to different pharmacological effects and specific binding to two separate sites on rat brain synaptosomes, scorpion toxins may also be divided in two types named α- and β-toxins (3-4).
So, it was really tempting to study the structure activity relationships both at the pharmacological and the immunological levels in order to define the regions of the toxins involved in these two activities.

1. Structure-toxicity relationship.
Taking the tridimensional structure of CsE V3 (5) as a structural model for all toxins was really helpfull.

Proceedings of the 16th FEBS Congress
Part B, pp. 423–429
© 1985 VNU Science Press

Schematically, scorpion toxins show two faces : one containing the α–helix and the β–turn, the other a conserved hydrophobic surface made of three regions in which conserved streches of amino acids are found, i.e. regions 2–7, 51–54 and 58–61[1], clustered together and forming a large continuous patch (6).

```
                 1    10      20       30       40      50       60      70

        AaH I    KRDGYIVYPN-NCVYHCVP--P---CDGLCKKN-GGSSGS-CSFLVPSGLACWC-KDLP-DNVPIKDT--SRKCT-
I       AaH I'                  I                                                            R
        AaH I''  V    NSK                            AK     G I     V-A           P  Y HS
        AaH III

        AaH II   VKDGYIVDDV-NCTYFCGR---NAYCNEECTKL-KGESG-YCQWASPYGNACYCYK-LP-DHVRTKGP---GRCH-
        BoT III            R                                            V                N
II      Lqq V    L       K    F       D  K K G                W       R SI EK          N
        Amm V    L    I  L    F       DD K K G                W       R SI EK          N
        Be M10   R    A  K D A        D   K G GA  K WY GQ     W       W PI QKV S K N

III     BoT I    GRDAYIAQPE-NCVYECAQ---NSYCNDLCTKN-GATSG-YCQWLGKYGNACWC-KDLP-DNVPIRIP---GKCHF
        BoT II             K                      K        RW   Y I-   K     E

IV      Lqq IV   GVRDAYIADDK-NCVYTCGS---NSYCNTECTKN-GAESG-YCQWLGKYGNACWCIK-LP-DKVPIRIP---GKC-R

        Css II   -KEGYLVSKSTGCKYECLKLGDNDYCLRECKQQYGKSSGGYCYAF-----ACWC-THLY-EQAVVWPLPNKT-CN-
V       CsE I    - D  E-    KT Y  E F N   WKHIGG Y   G    G Y EG P DSTQT       - T
        Ts VII     MDHE    LS F-IRPSG  G   GIKK - -  -AW P   Y Y-G P NWVK  DR-ATNK --

VI      CsE v3   -KEGYLVKKSDGCKYGCLKLGENEGCDTECKAKNQGGSYGYCYAF-----ACWC-EGLP-ESTPTYPLPNK-SC--

        AaH IT   KKNGYAVDSS-GKAPECLL---SNYCNNQCTKV-HYADKGYCCLL-----SCYCFGLNDDKKVLEISDTRKSYCDTTIIN
```

Table 1: Amino acid sequences of toxins from scorpions.
AaH: Androctonus australis Hector; Amm: Androctonus mauritanicus mauritanicus; Be: Buthus epeus; BoT: Buthus occitanus Tunetanus; Lqq: Leiurus quinquestriatus quinquestriatus; Css: Centruroides suffusus suffusus; CsE: Centruroides sculpturatus Ewing; Ts: Tityus serrulatus.

When the position of the four disulfide bridges is unchanged in all mammal toxins, it was found that, due to the shift of the half–cystine in position 13 to position 43, one upon the four disulfides of the insect toxin (i.e. 43–74) is in a different position : the corresponding bridge being 13–74 in mammal toxins. This may produce a conformational difference probably involved in the specificity to insects of this toxin (7). The methylation or carboxymethylation of a reduced toxin completely destroys its toxicity, which means that the native conformation is needed for the activity of the toxin. A partially reduced AaH II preparation was methylated in the way to open statistically 0.4 disulfide bridge. This modification leads to a loss of 38 % of toxicity suggesting that the

1. *Amino acid residues are numbered in Table 1 according to positions in the aligned sequences.*

424

opening of one disulfide bridge induces a complete loss of activity (8). More recently it was shown that, in AaH IT, the bridge 43-74 was more easily reduced than the others (7). This bridge is the only one which is not buried in the molecule, is probably involved in the specificity of this toxin to insect and is homologous to bridge 13-74 in mammal toxins.

When comparing the sequences of α-toxins (groups I to IV) and β-toxins (groups V and VI), it is obvious that homologies are greater between toxins of two α-groups or two β-groups than between toxins of the α-type and toxins of the β-type. It is noteworthy that stretch 20 to 23 is specific to β-toxins and stretch 46 to 50 to α-toxins. It is tempting to attribute, at least partially, the difference in the pharmacological effects of α - and β-toxins to these specific sequences. To determine more precisely which part of the toxins is involved in the pharmacological and antigenic activities, punctual modifications were performed. Basic residues are good targets for such a study because of their relative high reactivity towards chemicals and their exposure to the solvent. Lysine residues were modified using succinimidyl-ester activated reagents and arginine residues using 1-2 cyclohexanedione. Each modification was followed systematically by some purification steps and identification of the modified residue(s). 1) $\underline{\alpha\text{-toxins}}$: the modification of the lysine residue in position 66, the unique lysine in the C-terminal region of AaH II, leads to a non-active derivative whatever the size of the reagent used : biotin, azido-nitrophenyl-amino acetate (8) or acetate. These modifications lead to the loss of one positive charge. Thus this toxin needs such a charge in this position to be active. Steric constraint seems unrelevant since acetylation of the toxin gives the same absence of activity and as circular dichroism analysis of the biotin derivative shows no major conformational perturbation (9). Lqq V shows a 78 % of sequence homology with AaH II : lysine 66 is present but a lysine replace the proline 68. The $\varepsilon\text{-NH}_2$ of this lysine skim the α-helix face, opposed to the conserved-hydrophobic face. When modifying either residue 66 or 68, 90 % and 50 % of the activity is lost. It means that both residues are involved in the toxicity of the toxin, position 68 at a lower degree than position 66. An other α-toxin, i.e. AaH III, has been modified on its unique arginine residue in position 2, close to lysine 66 on the hydrophobic surface, leading to a complete loss of activity. So, this basic residue is directly involved in the toxin-receptor interaction. Position 2 is highly conserved. It is occupied either by a lysine or an arginine. Although we were unable to obtain Lqq V derivatives monomodified on lysine 2, dimodified derivatives on residues 2 and 66 or 2 and 68 are completely inactive (9). 2) β-toxins : two lysines have been modified on Css II, lysines 14 and 71 (10). Modification of lysine 14 leads to a toxin 10 % still active when modification of lysine 71 gives a non active derivative. Position 14 is located in the conserved-hydrophobic surface when position 71 may be placed at the upper junction of this surface with the α-helix surface, near the exposed disulfide bridge 13-74. Arginine 28, located in the middle of the α-helix, has been modified without modification of the activity : thus this position is probably not involved in the β-toxin-receptor interaction. Modification of the unique arginine residue 70 of AaH IT leads to a non-active derivative. Taking into account the structural modification due to the presence of the specific 43-74 disulfide bridge, arginine 70 may well be present near the hydrophobic surface.

2. Structure-antigenicity relationship

This study has been possible thanks to the availability of several antigenically polymorphic α-toxins with known amino acid sequences and of chemically modified derivatives of AaH II. The approach followed to obtain information about toxin antigenic sites involved several steps. Firstly, four Fab anti-toxin fragments were demonstrated to bind simultaneously on the surface of a given toxin, suggesting the presence of at least four major antigenic sites or domains (11). Secondly, competition of ^{125}I-AaH II and Bot III for an anti-AaH II serum in one hand and partial saturation of Bot III surface with three Fab anti-AaH II fragments in another hand have allowed to attempt the localization of an antigenic region around the disulfide bridge 13-74 and to point out the role of valine 10 and histidine 75 of AaH II (11). Thirdly, a predictive method established by Hopp and Woods (12) was applied to 13 α-toxins. The highest hydrophilic peaks predicted are associated exclusively with four regions, which is in full agreement with the proposed number of major antigenic sites (13). Finally, the antigenic sites are dependent on conformation since reduction and carboxy-methylation of the four disulfide bridges abolish the antigenicity of AaH II. However, a significant antigenicity (20 %) is conserved when cysteine residues are methylated. This result is interpreted by the existence of native-like conformation in the reduced and S-methylated toxin. The acetylation of the amino groups of AaH II reduces the antigenicity to 25 %. The observed residual antigenicity could possibly be attributed to the antigenic site(s) without immunodominant lysine residue. Selective biotinylation of lysine 66 and carboxymethylation of histidines 62 and 75 suggest that these residues, although important, are not dominant for the antigenicity (13). The N- terminal pentapeptide sequence seems to be excluded from the antigenicity of scorpion toxins since it was demonstrated a similar antigenicity between native Buthus occitanus mardochei toxin III and the same protein shortened from the N- terminal pentapeptide (14).

From the above data, it is possible to draw a picture localizing structures responsible for both toxic and antigenic activities. It appears that residues mainly involved in the toxic activity are located at or near the "conserved-hydrophobic surface" which may be, by this way, at least part of the interaction site between toxins and their receptor, the voltage-dependent sodium channel. Furthermore, the structure responsible for the antigenic activities are located on the highly variable and exposed regions of the toxins, regions which do not overlap the "conserved-hydrophobic region". Nevertheless, this last region may be either an immunosilent or an hyporesponsive antigenic one. Why this exposed region, conserved through evolution, is not a major antigenic site is a question under investigation.

1. ROCHAT, H., BERNARD, P. and COURAUD, F. (1979) Scorpion toxins : chemistry and mode of action. Adv. Cytopharmacol. 3, 325-334.
2. DELORI, P., VAN RIETSCHOTEN, J. and ROCHAT, H. (1981) Scorpion venoms and neurotoxins : an immunological study. Toxicon 19, 393-407.
3. JOVER, E., COURAUD, F. and ROCHAT, H. (1980) Two types of scorpion neurotoxins characterized by their binding to two separate receptor sites on rat brain synaptosomes. Biochem. Biophys. Res. Comm. 95, 1607-1614.
4. COURAUD, F., JOVER, E., DUBOIS, J.M. and ROCHAT, H. (1982). Two types of scorpion toxin receptor sites, one related to the activation, the other to the inactivation of the action potential sodium channel. Toxicon 20, 9-16.
5. FONTECILLA-CAMPS, J., ALMASSY, R.J., SUDDATH, F.Z., WATT, D.D. and BUGG, C.E. (1980). Three-dimensional structure of a protein from scorpion venom. A new structural class of neurotoxins. Proc. Natl. Acad. Sci. USA 77, 6496-6500.
6. FONTECILLA-CAMPS, J., ALMASSY, R.J., EALICK, S.E., SUDDATH, F.L., WATT, D.D., FELDMANN, R.J. and BUGG, C.E. (1981). Architecture of scorpion neurotoxins : a class of membrane binding proteins. TIBS 6, 291-296.
7. DARBON, H., ZLOTKIN, E., KOPEYAN, C., VAN RIETSCHOTEN, J. and ROCHAT, H. (1982). Covalent structure of the insect toxin of the north african scorpion Androctonus australis Hector. Int. J. Peptide Protein Res. 20, 320-330.
8. HABERSETZER-ROCHAT, C. and SAMPIERI, F. (1976). Structure-function relationships of scorpion neurotoxins. Biochemistry 15, 2254-2261.
9. DARBON, H., JOVER, E., COURAUD, F. and ROCHAT, H. (1983). Alpha-scorpion neurotoxin derivatives suitable as potential markers of sodium channels : preparation and characterization. Int. J. Peptide Protein Res. 22, 179-186.
10. DARBON, H. and ANGELIDES, K.J. (1984). Structural mapping of the voltage-dependent sodium channel : distance between the tetrodotoxin and Centruroides

suffusus suffusus II β-scorpion toxin receptors. J. Biol. Chem. 259, 6074-6084.

11. EL AYEB, M., MARTIN, M.F., DELORI, P., BECHIS, G. and ROCHAT, H. (1983). Immunochemistry of scorpion α-neurotoxins. Determination of the antigenic site number and isolation of a highly enriched antibody specific to a single antigenic site of toxin II of Androctonus australis Hector. Mol. Immunol. 20, 697-708.

12. HOPP, T.P. and WOODS, K.R. (1981). Prediction of protein antigenic determinants from amino acid sequences. Proc. Natl. Acad. Sci. USA, 78, 3824-3828.

13. EL AYEB, M., BAHRAOUI, E.M., GRANIER, C., DELORI, P., VAN RIETSCHOTEN, J. and ROCHAT, H. (1984). Immunochemistry of scorpion α-toxins : purification and characterization of two functionnally independent IgG populations raised against toxin II of Androctonus australis Hector. Mol. Immunol. 21, 223-232.

14. VARGAS-ABARCA, O. (1982). Contribution à l'étude du venin du scorpion Buthus occitanus mardochei. Thèse de 3ème cycle, Université d'Aix-Marseille II.

GENES FOR PROTON TRANSLOCATING ATPases

JOHN E. WALKER, VICTOR L.J., TYBULEWICZ, GUNNAR FALK, NICHOLAS J. GAY and ANNIE HAMPE[1]
Medical Research Council Laboratory of Molecular Biology, Hills Road, Cambridge CB2 2QH, England

ABSTRACT

Genes for subunits of eukaryotic H^+-ATPases are distributed between plastid and nuclear DNA. Mitochondrial enzymes are mostly nuclear encoded. The gene for one subunit, the proteolipid, is mitochondrially coded in yeast, but is a nuclear gene product in other fungi and mammals. Chloroplast ATPase genes show a constant pattern of distribution between chloroplast and nuclear DNA. Genes for prokaryotic ATPases cluster in operons. Those for the eight subunits of the E. coli enzyme are organised in the unc operon, in which the genes for F_0 and F_1 are in the order $a:c:b:\delta:\alpha:\gamma:\beta:\epsilon$. This operon contains two subclusters corresponding to F_0 and F_1 genes. In the photosynthetic bacteria Rhodopseudomonas blastica and Rhodospirillum rubrum F_0 genes are not associated with F_1 genes. In both organisms F_1 genes form an operon in which the gene order is the same as that in the E. coli F_1 subcluster. In R. blastica an additional unidentified gene is interposed between γ and β. The clustering reflects the evolution of the genes by duplication and divergence.

INTRODUCTION

Proton translocating ATPase catalyses phosphorylation of ADP to form ATP in a reaction that is driven by a membrane proton potential gradient. In bacteria and mitochondria the gradient is generated by electron

[1] Present address : Centre Hayem, Hopital St-Louis, Paris, France

Proceedings of the 16th FEBS Congress
Part B, pp. 431–442

transfer resulting from respiration and in chloroplasts and in photosynthetic bacteria by photosynthetic electron transfer (1-3). The structures of the enzymes from these diverse sources are similar in many respects (4-6). They are composed of two major structural domains, a globular assembly F_1 which is bound to the second domain, and an intrinsic membrane assembly F_o. F_1 contains catalytic sites where ADP, ATP and P_i bind; F_o has a transmembranous proton channel through which the proton potential membrane gradient is coupled to ATP synthesis in F_1. Under a variety of conditions intact F_1 can be released from the membrane sector: it is an ATP hydrolase. Gel electrophoresis of F_1, F_o and F_1F_o isolated from bacteria, chloroplasts and mitochondria has demonstrated that similarities are to be found in composition and size of subunits from these various sources. The E. coli complex appears to be simplest. Here F_1 is a complex of five subunits, α, β, γ, δ and ϵ, assembled with stoicheiometries of 3:3:1:1:1 respectively (7). Equivalent subunits are present in similar relative amounts in mitochondria and probably also in chloroplasts although this remains controversial (5). E. coli F_o has three-subunits a, b and c for which stoicheiometries of 1a:2b:10-12c-: have been advanced (8). In many cases equivalence of subunits in bacteria, mitochondria and chloroplasts has now been established by sequence analysis. The mammalian mitochondrial enzyme is more complex than the bacterial one, having at least four more polypeptides associated with it. These include mitochondrial 6 (which is not equivalent to bacterial 6), an inhibitor protein (9) and factor 6 (10). In yeast mitochondria a proteolipid component of H^+-ATPase, aap1, has been described that may be related to the A6L gene product of bovine mitochondria (11,12). These proteins may have

Synonyms: (a) H^+-ATPase, proton translocating ATPase complex, F_1F_o ATPase or ATP synthase; (b) subunit c, proteolipid, DCCD binding protein, ATPase-9 (yeast), subunit III (chloroplasts); (c) subunit a, ATPase-6 (yeast), subunit I (chloroplasts). Abbreviation : aap1 = ATPase associated protein.

similar secondary structures (12) and sequence homologies between the two proteins can also be detected.

GENES FOR EUKARYOTIC H$^+$-ATPase

They are divided between nuclear and plastid DNAs (Table 1). In the mitochondrial enzymes of mammals, insects and fungi the genes for the a subunit, a component of F$_o$, is in mt-DNA. Upstream of this gene in yeast and Aspergillus is a gene encoding a hydrophobic protein of 48 amino acids (aapl) (11,12). The A6L gene, possibly related to it, occupies a similar position in juxtaposition to the a subunit gene in mammalian and Drosophila mitochondria (13-16). With the exception of the yeast ATPase-9 gene (encoding the DCCD binding protein), also found in mt-DNA (17) all other genes for H$^+$-ATPase subunits appear to be in nuclear DNA. In yeast and fungi some of them have been demonstrated to be translated on soluble ribosomes as longer precursors (18-20).

GENES FOR PROKARYOTIC ATPase

The eight genes for the E. coli complex form the unc operon and are co-transcribed from a single promoter (21). Additionally this operon contains a ninth gene, uncI, which appears not to encode a component of the enzyme complex (21-23) ; it can be deleted without apparent effect on the enzyme (24) and its function remains obscure.

A second interesting feature of the unc operon (discussed below) is that the genes are arranged in an order related to the structure of the enzyme complex in so far as F$_o$ genes and F$_1$ genes cluster.

Clustering of genes for proteins that assemble with each other has been observed previously in coliphages, for instance, in bacteriophage lambda (25). Here the order of action of the gene products is very similar (but not identical) to the order of the genes within

TABLE 1. Location of genes for eukaryotic H^+-ATPase

| | Genes in | | |
Species	Plastid	Nucleus	References

A. Mitochondria

Man	a, A6L	See footnote 1	13
Cow	a, A6L	"	14
Mouse	a, A6L	"	15
Drosophila	a, A6L	"	16
Neurospora	a	c	28,42
Yeast	a,c,aapl	β, [the rest]	29,17,12,11, 30
Aspergillus	a,aapl		31,12
Wheat	[α,c]		32

B. Chloroplasts

Spinach	βε[I] III		33,5,34
Tobacco	α		35,36
Barley	βε		37
Wheat	αβε[I] III		22,23,24, 38–40
Maize	βε		41

Footnotes: 1. mt-DNA sequence is known, as are protein sequences of many H^+-ATPase subunits, so absence from mt-DNA is taken to imply presence in nuclear DNA. Sequence are known for all subunits explicitly mentioned except for those in parentheses.

these clusters (26). This led to the suggestion that gene order may be related to the assembly pathway (25) although other explanations of clustering also have been advanced (27).

In order to find out if clustering and gene order of ATPase genes is maintained in other prokaryotes and to try and see if the uncI gene is present in other organisms we have investigated two members of the Rhodospirillaceae, or photosynthetic non-sulphur bacteria, Rhodopseudomonas blastica and Rhodospirillum rubrum.

RHODOPSEUDOMONAS BLASTICA ATP OPERON

A region of the genome of R. blastica containing genes for H^+-ATPase was cloned by employing a 983 bp EcoRI-PvuII fragment from the uncD gene (β-ATPase) of E. coli as a hybridisation probe (43). The probe extended from amino acid 17 to amino acid 344 of the β subunit. This encompasses a region that is highly conserved in sequence in the E. coli and bovine enzymes (44).

By screening 250 individual recombinants of a library of R. blastica in bacteriophage λ two positive clones were found. In one of these the DNA sequence of a region of 12,268bp was determined. Genes encoding subunits of H^+-ATPase were identified by comparison with E. coli protein sequences using the computer program DIAGON. Highly significant homologies were detected between each of the five E. coli F_1 proteins and the individual protein sequences predicted from the genes delineated in the R. blastica DNA. It was also noted that as in other species (45) that the sequences of R. blastica α and β are related to each other, but this homology is much weaker than that found between any pairs of α (or β) sequences.

A second search with the protein sequences of E. coli F subunits and the uncI protein sequence failed to reveal homologous sequences amongst the R. blastica genes. Moreover, inspection of the predicted R. blastica protein sequences showed that none of them had either the overall hydrophobicity associated with the a, c and uncI proteins in E. coli (21,46) or the characteristically bipartite sequence, hydrophobic in

435

the N-terminal region, highly charged in the remainder, that has been found in the E. coli b protein (22, 47). Hence, genes for F_o subunits and uncI are not associated with genes for F_1 subunits in R. blastica. The F_1 genes were found to cluster except for an 825 bp gap between α and β. This appears to encode a globular protein of unknown function.

In a further attempt to locate the uncI (and possibly F_o genes), a nick-translated fragment from gene 1 of the E. coli atp operon was used as a probe on a Southern blot of a genomic digest of R. blastica. No hybridisation was observed. This implies either poor conservation of nucleotide sequence between the UncI of E. coli and R. blastica, or that R. blastica does not have an analogue uncI. The five F_1 genes and the intervening unknown gene constitute a single transcriptional unit that has been named the R. blastica atp operon (48).

RHODOSPIRILLUM RUBRUM H^+-ATPase GENES

A region of the genome of R. rubrum was found to hybridise to DNA probes prepared from parts of the α and β genes of R. blastica. A lambda recombinant hybridising to both probes was isolated by plaque hybridisation. A region of 8.8 kb of the DNA of this phage has been sequenced and found to contain five genes encoding proteins homologous to the five E. coli F_1 subunits (G. Falk, A. Hampe and J.E. Walker, unpublished work). These genes are arranged as shown in Fig. 1. As yet there is no direct evidence that these genes form an operon, although this seems likely.

EVOLUTIONARY CONSIDERATIONS

Our present knowledge of the organisation of H^+-Atpase genes is summarised in Fig. 1. A number of striking features are evident. Firstly, the order of genes within the R. blastica atp operon is the same as that found for the corresponding genes in the E. coli unc operon, with the exception that an extra gene has

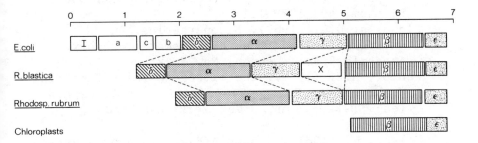

Figure 1. Organisation of H^+-ATPase genes in prokaryotes and chloroplasts. The scale is in kilobases.

apparently been interposed between γ and β in the photosynthetic bacterium. In R. rubrum the same order of F_1 genes as in E. coli is also maintained and β and ε are associated in chloroplasts (33,41). However, the lack of association of F_o genes with F_1 genes in the two photosynthetic bacteria implies that the maintenance of the genes for the whole complex in a single operon is not an obligatory arrangement. This is reminiscent of the trp operon, specifying enzymes in the tryptophan pathway. In E. coli and other enteric bacteria all the genes are co-transcribed, whereas in other organisms they may be split up into two or three subclusters (49). It is more likely that the specific order of genes in the F_1 clusters reflect the evolution of F_1 genes which in at least the cases of α and β appear to have evolved from a common ancestor by gene duplication and divergence. Further experiments in progress should demonstrate whether the F_o genes in photosynthetic bacteria form a second cluster or whether they are further split up into smaller transcriptional units.

REFERENCES

1. Hinkle, P.C. and McCarty, R.E. (1978). How cells make ATP. Scientific American 238, 104-123.
2. Fillingame, R.H. (1980). The proton translocating

pumps of oxidative phosphorylation. Ann. Rev. Biochem. 49, 1079-1113.

3. Nicholls, D.G. (1982). Bioenergetics. An introduction to the chemiosmotic theory. Academic Press, London, New York.

4. Senior, A.E. (1979). The mitochondrial ATPase. In: Membranes in Energy Transduction, R.A. Capaldi (ed). Dekker, Inc., New York and London, pp. 233-276.

5. Nelson, N. (1981). Proton ATPase of chloroplasts. Curr. Topics Bioenerg. 11, 1-34.

6. Racker, R. (1981). Subunit functions of ATP driven pumps. In: Mitochondria and Microcosmes, C.P. Lee, G. Schatz and G. Dallner (eds). Addison-Wesley, Reading, Mass., USA, pp. 337-356.

7. Fillingame, R.H. (1981). Biochemistry and genetics of bacterial H^+-translocating ATPases. Curr. Topics Bioenerg. 11, 35-105.

8. Foster,D.L. and Fillingame, R.H. (1982). Stoicheiometry of subunits in H^+-ATPase complex of Escherichia coli. J. Biol. Chem. 257, 2009-2015.

9. Pullman, M.E. and Monroy, G.C. (1963). A naturally occurring inhibitor of mitochondrial adenosine triphosphatase. J. Biol. Chem. 238, 3762-3769.

10. Kanner, B.I., Serrano, R., Kandrach, M.A. and Racker, E. (1976). Preparation and characterisation of homogeneous coupling factor 6 from bovine heart mitochondria. Biochem. Biophys. Res. Commun. 69, 1050-1056.

11. Macreadie, I.G., Novitski, C.E., Maxwell, R.J., John, U., Ooi, B.G., McMullen, G.L., Lukins, H.B., Linnane, A.W. and Nagley, P. (1983). Biogenesis of mitochondria. The mitochondrial (aap1) coding for mitochondrial ATPase subunit 8 in Saccharomyces cerevisiae. Nucl. Acids Res. 11, 4435-4451.

12. Velours, J., Esparza, M., Hoppe, J., Sebald, W. and Guerin, B. (1984). Amino acid sequence of a new mitochondrially synthesized proteolipid of

the ATP-synthase of <u>Saccharomyces cerevisiae</u>. EMBO J. 3, 207-212.

13. Anderson, S., Bankier, A.T., Barrell, B.G., de Bruijn, M.H.L., Coulson, A.R., Drouin, J., Eperon, I.C., Nierlich, D.P., Roe, B.A., Sanger, F., Schreier, P.H., Smith, A.J.H., Staden, R. and Young, I.G. (1981). Sequence and organisation of the human mitochondrial genome. Nature 290, 457-465.

14. Anderson, S., de Bruijn, M.H.L., Coulson, A.R., Eperon, I.C., Sanger, F. and Young, I.G. (1982). Complete sequence of bovine mitochondrial DNA. Conserved features of the mammalian mitochondrial genome. J. Mol. Biol. 156, 683-717.

15. Bibb, M.J., van Etten, R.A., Wright, C.T., Salberg, M.W. and Clayton, D.A. (1981). Sequence and gene oganisation of mouse mitochondrial DNA. Cell 26, 167-180.

16. de Bruijn, M.H.L. (1983). <u>Drosophila melanogaster</u> mitochondrial DNA, a novel organisation and genetic code. Nature 304, 234-241.

17. Macino, G. and Tzagoloff, A. (1979). Assembly of the mitochondrial membrane. The DNA sequence of a mitochondrial ATPase gene in <u>Saccharomyces cerivisiae</u>. J. Biol. Chem. 254, 4617-4623.

18. Nelson, N., Nelson, H. and Schatz, G. (1980). Biosynthesis and assembly of the proton-translocating adenosine triphosphatase complex from chloroplasts. Proc. Natl. Acad. Sci. USA 77, 1361-1364.

19. Lewin, A.S., Gregor, I., Mason, T.L., Nelson, N. and Schatz, G. (1980). Cytoplasmically made subunits of yeast mitochondrial F_1-ATPase and cytochrome c oxidase are synthesised as individual precursors not as polypeptides. Proc. Natl. Acad. Sci. USA 77, 3998-4002.

20. Maccecchini, M.L., Rudin, Y., Blobel, G. and Schatz, G. (1980). Import of proteins into mitochondria : precursor forms of the extra mitochondrially made F_1-ATPase subunits in yeast. Proc. Natl. Acad. Sci. USA 76, 343-347.

21. Walker, J.E., Saraste, M.. and Gay, N.J. (1984). The unc operon : nucleotide sequence, regulation and structure of ATP synthase. Biochem. Biophys. Acta Bioenerg. Rev. 768,164-200.

22. Gay, N.J. and Walker, J.E. (1981). The unc operon: nucleotide sequence of the promoter and genes for the membrane proteins and the δ subunit of Escherichia coli ATP synthase. Nucl. Acids. Res. 9, 3919-3926.

23. Brusilow, W.S.A., Porter, A.C.G. and Simoni, R.D. (1983). Cloning and expression of uncIm the first gene of the unc operon. J. Bact. 155, 1265-1270.

24. Gay, N.J. (1984). Construction and characterisation of an E. coli strain with a mutation of the uncI gene. J. Bact. 158, 820-825.

25. Katsura, I. (1983). In: Lambda II, R.W. Hendrix, J.W. Roberts and F.W. Stahl (eds). Cold Spring Harbor (1980).

26. Casjens, S. and Hendrix, R. (1974). Comments on the arrangement of the morphogenetic genes of bacteriophage lambda. J. Mol. Biol. 90, 20-23.

27. Stahl, F.W. and Murray, N.E. (1966). The evolution of genes clusters and genetic circularity in micro-organisms. Genetics 53, 569-576.

28. Sebald, W. (1977). Biogenesis of mitochondrial ATPase. Biochim. Biophys. Acta 463, 1-27.

29. Macino, G. and Tzagoloff, A. (1980). Assembly of the mitochondrial membrane system: sequence analysis of a yeast mitochondrial ATPase gene containing the oli-2 and oli-4 loci. Cell 20, 507-517.

30. Salzgruber-Muller, J., Kunapuli, S.P. and Douglas, M.G. (1983). Nuclear genes coding the yeast mitochondrial adenosine triphosphatase complex. Isolation of ATP2 coding for the F_1-ATPase β subunit. J. Biol. Chem. 258, 11465-11479.

31. Grisi, E., Brown, T.A., Waring, R.B., Scazzocchio, C. and Davies, R.W. (1982). Nucleotide sequence of a region of the mitochondrial genome of

    <u>Aspergillus nidulans</u> including the gene for the
    ATPase subunit 6. Nucl. Acids Res. 10,3531-3539.
32. Hack, E. and Leaver, C.J. (1983). The α subunit of
    the maize F_1-ATPase is synthesised in the
    mitochondrion. EMBO J. 2, 1783-1789.
33. Zurawski, G., Bottomley, W. and Whitfeld, P.R.
    (1982). Structures of the genes for the β and ε
    subunits of spinach chloroplast ATPase indicate
    a dicistronic mRNA and an overlapping
    translation stop/start signal. Proc. Natl. Acad.
    Sci. USA 79, 6260-6264.
34. Alt, J., Winter, P., Sebald, W., Moser, J.G.,
    Schedel, R., Westhoff, P. and Herrmann, R.G.
    (1983). Localisation and nucleotide sequence of
    the gene for the ATP synthase proteolipid
    spinach plastid chromosome. Curr. Genet. 7,
    129-138.
35. Deno, H., Shinozaki, K. and Sugiura, M. (1983).
    Nucleotide sequence of tobacco chloroplast gene
    for the α subunit of proton translocating
    ATPase. Nucl. Acids Res. 11, 2185-2191.
36. Shinozaki, K. and Sugiura, M. (1982). Sequence of
    the intercistronic region between the ribulose
    1,5 bisphosphate carboxylase/oxygenase large
    subunit and the coupling factor β subunit gene.
    Nucl. Acids Res. 10, 4923-4934.
37. Zurawski, G. and Clegg, M.T. (1984). The barley
    chloroplast DNA <u>atp</u> BE, <u>trn</u> M2 and <u>trn</u> V1 loci.
    Nucl. Acids Res. 12, 2549-2559.
38. Howe, C.J. Personal communication.
39. Bird, C. Personal communication.
40. Howe, C.J., Auffret, A.D., Doherty, A., Bowman,
    C.M., Dyer, T.A. and Gray, J.C. (1982). Location
    and nucleotide sequence of the gene for the
    proton translocating subunit of wheat
    chloroplast ATP synthase. Proc. Natl. Acad. Sci.
    USA 79, 6903-6907.
41. Krebbers, E.T., Larrinua, I.M., McIntosh, L. and
    Bogorad, L. (1982). The maize chloroplast genes
    for the β and ε subunits of the photosynthetic
    coupling factor CF_1 are fused. Nucl. Acids Res.
    10, 4485-5002.

42. Viebrok, A., Perz, A. and Sebald, W. (1982). The imported preprotein of the proteolipid subunit of the mitochondrial ATP synthase from Neurospora crassa. Molecular cloning and sequencing of the mRNA. EMBO J. 1, 565-571.

43. Saraste, M., Gay, N.J., Eberle, A., Runswick, M.J. and Walker, J.E. (1981). The atp operon: nucleotide sequence of the γ, β, and ε subunits of Escherichia coli ATP-synthase. Nucl. Acids Res. 9, 5287-5296.

44. Runswick, M.J. and Walker, J.E. (1983). The amino acid sequence of the β subunit of ATP-synthase from bovine heart mitochondria. J. Biol. Chem. 258, 3081-3089.

45. Walker, J.E., Saraste, M., Runswick, M.J. and Gay, N,J, (1982). Distantly related sequences in the α and β subunits of ATP synthase, myosin, kinases and other ATP-requiring enzymes and a common nucleotide binding fold. EMBO J. 1, 945-951.

46. Sebald, W. and Hoppe, J. (1981). On the structure and genetics of the proteolipid subunit of the ATP synthase complex. Curr. Topics Bioenerg. 12, 1-64.

47. Walker, J.E., Saraste, M. and Gay, N.J. (1982). E. coli F_1-ATPase interacts with a membrane protein component of a proton channel. Nature 298, 867-869.

48. Tybulewicz,V.L.J., Falk, G. and Walker, J.E. (1984). The Rhodopseudomonas blastica atp operon: nucleotide sequence and transcription. J. Mol. Biol. in press.

49. Crawford, I.P. (1975). Gene arrangements in the evolution of the tryptophan synthetic pathway. Bact. Rev. 39, 87-102.

A CONTRIBUTION TO THE CHEMICAL PROTEIN SYNTHESIS AS

EXEMPLIFIED BY HUMAN PROINSULIN

VINOD KUMAR NAITHANI, HANS GREGOR GATTNER AND HELMUT ZAHN
Deutsches Wollforschungsinstitut an der TH Aachen
Veltmanplatz 8, 51 Aachen

INTRODUCTION

Human proinsulin is a tridisulfide protein comprising of 86 residues (1,2) (Fig. 1). Due to the scarcity of native human proinsulin its primary structure was inferred from the sequence of human insulin and C-peptide. Our group (3) and also Yanaihara and his coworkers (4) have attempted the total synthesis of proinsulin. Despite the enormous progress made in synthetic methodology and in purification, the chemical synthesis of such a protein of 9000 dalton is still a big challenge. Recently human proinsulin has been produced in bacteria by recombinant DNA technology (5), thus making it available for biomedical investigations.

The following paper discusses the results of the total syntheses and semisynthesis of human proinsulin.

RESULTS

Total synthesis

Yanaihara et al. (4) reported two syntheses of human proinsulin in 1977 and 1980. In the second improved synthesis the minimally protected 1-86 was assembled from sixteen segments bearing 3-8 residues by the azide procedure. After quantitative removal of the protecting groups, proinsulin hexa S-sulfonate was reduced and oxidized. Ion exchange chromatography gave a major proinsulin fraction contaminated with impurities.

In contrast to Yanaihara's approach, we applied nearly maximum protection (for review see 3). From the four main segments 1-23, 24-45, 46-70 and 71-86) two big-segments 1-45 and 46-86 were prepared (Fig. 2). The final coupling

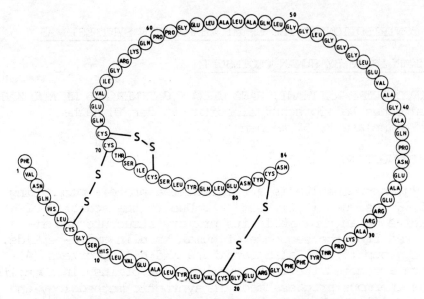

Fig. 1 Primary structure of human proinsulin (1,2).

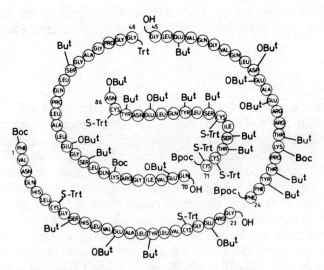

Fig. 2 Four main protected segments of human proinsulin.

444

of the two segments using DCC/HOBt proceeded poorly. The
quantitative deblocking and purification, according to our
previously established procedure with semisynthetic hexa
S-trityl bovine proinsulin (6), yielded only traces of
human proinsulin hexa S-sulfonate contaminated with impurities. As a result, the folding experiment to obtain
human proinsulin could not be conducted.

Semisynthesis

Earlier our laboratory reported the semisynthesis of a
proinsulin analogue with a shortened connecting peptide
(7). The semisynthesis was made possible by the application of mixed anhydride procedure (8) which enabled
rapid and specific N-acylations of minimally protected
native chains with protected single amino acids as well as
large segments. This procedure also proved efficient to
attach protonated arginine. Also, the minimally protected
B-chain was activated and condensed by this procedure
(7,8). However, in the semisynthesis of human proinsulin
the B-chain derivative was coupled by the azide procedure.

Mixed anhydride acylations were performed in aqueous-
organic solution (80% dimethylformamide-water) at pH 7-7.2
(apparent pH as measured with glass electrode). In general, a 5 fold excess of mixed anhydride was allowed to
react with amine components (minimally protected native
A-chain and its elongated derivatives) for 1 min. The
reaction was stopped with hydroxylamine. Excess carboxyl
component was separated by counter current distribution
or by Sephadex G-25 chromatography after treatment with
trifluoroacetic acid. Final purification was accomplished
by ion exchange chromatography.

The purity of intermediate products was checked by end
group determination, thin layer electrophoresis at pH 2.2
and 4.8 as well as by amino acid analysis.

Porcine insulin A-chain and des Ala^{30}-B-chain were
utilized as the starting material as these are identical
to the N-terminal (residues 1-29) and the C-terminal
(66-86) regions of human proinsulin. The thiol functions
were protected as cyclic disulfides [A(SS)$_2$ or des Ala^{30}-
B(SS)]. The two amino groups (Phe-1 and ε-Lys-29) of the

B-chain were blocked with the Msc-groups (Fig. 3).

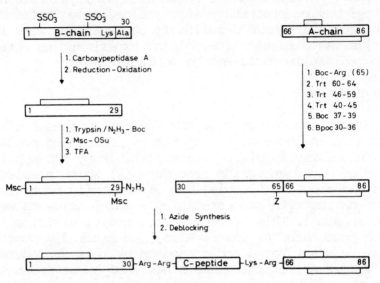

Fig. 3 Semisynthetisis of human proinsulin cyclic
tri-disulfide 1-86(SS)$_3$.

Preparation of segment 30-86(SS)$_2$. Amongst the various
procedures investigated to attach Arginine (65) the mixed
anhydride method gave the highest yield (70%). The elongated Arg-A(SS)$_2$ (65-86) was purified by chromatography
on SP-Sephadex.

The remaining synthetic peptides Trt-Gly-Ser(Bu^t)-Leu-
Gln-Lys(Z) (60-64), Trt-Gly-Gly-Pro-Gly-Ala-Gly-Ser(Bu^t)-
Leu-Gln-Pro-Leu-Ala-Leu-Glu(OBu^t) (46-59), Trt-Gly-Gln-
Val-Glu(OBu^t)-Leu-Gly (40-45), Boc-Leu-Gln-Val (37-39) and
Bpoc-Thr(Bu^t)-Arg-Arg-Glu(OBu^t)-Ala-Glu(OBu^t)-Asp(OBu^t)
(30-36) were also attached by the mixed anhydride procedure. The minimally protected intermediates 60-86, 46-86,
40-86 and 37-86 were purified by DEAE-cellulose chromatography and the segment 30-86 was purified by SP-Sephadex
chromatography.

Preparation of Msc$_2$-1-29(SS)-N$_2$H$_3$. The preparation of this
derivative was straightforward and was obtained as shown

in Fig. 3.

Preparation of 1-86(SS)$_3$. The final elongation of the segment 30-86 with a 10 fold excess Msc$_2$-1-29(SS) was achieved by the azide method. The protecting groups were then removed by treatment with NaOH and methansulfonic acid-m-cresol mixture. The purification of the deblocked mixture by Sequadex G-50f and SP-Sephadex chromatography yielded human proinsulin as tri-disulfide. This product was characterized by amino acid analysis, electrophoresis before and after performic acid oxidation. The folding experiment to obtain proinsulin with correct disulfide bonds has so far not been performed.

CONCLUSION

The total synthesis of well characterized homogeneous proinsulin is not yet complete. We believe that the tactics of near maximal protection and coupling of the two large segments is not suitable for the synthesis of human proinsulin. Instead, we recommend Yanaihara's strategy of assembling the molecule by coupling minimally protected small peptides. A similar approach, which was applied by Fujii and Yajima (9), led to the synthesis of a larger protein ribonuclease A. Semisynthesis using insulin chains enabled the preparation of open chain human proinsulin and an analogue with shortened connecting peptide. This approach seems feasible for semisynthesis of proinsulin analogues.

ACKNOWLEDGEMENT

This work was financially supported by the ministerium für Wissenschaft und Forschung des Landes NRW and Deutsche Forschungsgemeinschaft.

REFERENCES

1. Oyer, P.E., Cho, S., Peterson, J.D. and Steiner, D.F. (1971). Studies of human proinsulin: Isolation and amino acid sequence of human pancreatic C-peptide.

J. Biol. Chem. <u>246</u>, 1375-1386.

2. Ko, A.S.C., Smyth, D.G., Markussen, J. and Sundby, F. (1971). The amino acid sequence of the C-peptide of human proinsulin. Europ. J. Biochem. <u>20</u>, 190-199.

3. Naithani, V.K. and Zahn, H. (1984). Synthesis of pro-insulin. In: Peptide and Protein Reviews, Vol. 3, Hearn, M.T.W. (ed), Marcel Dekker, Inc., New York and Basel, pp. 81-146.

4. Yanaihara, N., Sakagamin, M., Sakura, N., Hashimoto, T. and Yanaihara, C. (1977). On total synthesis of human proinsulin. In: Peptide Chemistry, Shiba, T. (ed), Protein Research Foundation, Osaka, Japan, pp. 195-200; Yanaihara, N., Sakagami, M. and Yanaihara, C. (1980). Alternative approach for human proinsulin synthesis. In: Insulin, Brandenburg, D. and Wollmer, A. (eds), Walter de Gruyter, Berlin-New York, pp. 81-89.

5. Frank, B.H., Pette, J.M., Zimmermann, R.E. and Burck, P.J. (1981). The production of human proinsulin and its transformation to human insulin and C-peptide. In: Peptides: Synthesis-Structure-Function, Rich, D.H. and Gross, E. (eds), Pierce Chemical Co., Rock-ford-Illinois, pp. 729-738.

6. Büllesbach, E.E., Danho, W., Helbig, H.-J. and Zahn, H. (1980). Human proinsulin VIII: Studies on the S-tritylation of reduced insulin A- and B-chains and their detritylation. Hoppe-Seyler's Z. Physiol. Chem. 361, 865-873.

7. Büllesbach, E.E. (1982). Semisynthesis of a shortened open-chain proinsulin. Tetrahedron Letters <u>23</u>, 1877-1880.

8. Naithani, V.K., Gattner, H.-G., Büllesbach, E.E., Föhles, J. and Zahn, H. (1979). Mixed anhydrides as reagents in semisynthesis. In: Peptides: Structure and biological function, Gross, E. and Meienhofer, J. (eds), Pierce Chemical Co., Rockford, Illinois, pp. 571-576.

9. Fujii, N. and Yajima, H. (1981). Total synthesis of bovine pancreatic ribonuclease A, Part 6, Synthesis of RNase A with full enzymatic activity, J. Chem. Soc. Perkin I, 831,841.

STRUKCTURE - CONFORMATION - ACTIVITY RELATIONSHIP OF THE BRADYKININ POTENTIATING PEPTIDE BPP$_{9\alpha}$

S. REISSMANN, M. P. FILATOVA, N. A. KRIT,
T. A. ALEKSANDROVA, E. BIRCKNER, M. FRIED-
RICH, I. FRIC, I. PAEGELOW, W.-E. SIEMS,
G. HEDER and H. AROLD

Friedrich-Schiller-University Jena, GDR,
Institute of Biological and Medicinal
Chemistry, AMN, USSR and
Institute of Organic Chemistry and Bioche-
mistry, CSAV, CSSR

INTRODUCTION

The bradykinin potentiating nonapeptide BPP$_{9\alpha}$ at first isolated from the venom of the snake Bothrops jararaca, potentiates the action of bradykinin and is a very potent inhibitor of the enzyme peptidyl dipeptide hydrolase. This enzyme is known as angiotensin converting enzyme. Because of its important role in the blood pressure regulation the development of highly effectiv inhibitors is of great interest for diagnosis and treatment of some kinds of the hypertension. Our goal in this field is to obtain a better understanding of the chemical and physical bases for the biological action of the bradykinin potentiating peptides.

SYNTHESIS

As a prerequisite for these studies we have synthesized analogues with amino acid exchanges in all positions - except position 9 - some partial sequences and labelled compounds.

Proceedings of the 16th FEBS Congress
Part B, pp. 449–455
© 1985 VNU Science Press

The syntheses of the nonapeptide analogues
were carried out by a conventional method
via fragment condensation. By this route
of synthesis the side chain of arginin was
blocked by protonation. The condensation
steps were accomplished by activated esters
(1, 2).

Figure 1: Synthesis of $BPP_{9\alpha}$ and analogues

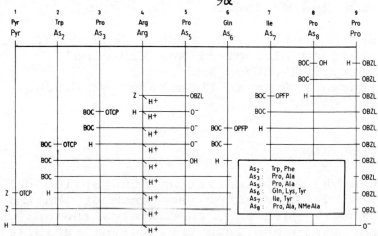

STRUCTURE – ACTIVITY – RELATIONSHIP

Studies of the structure activity relationship indicate the importance of the N-terminal sequence in addition to the C-terminus
(compounds 2 and 3). This fact was supported
by the enhanced biological activity of some
acylated nonapeptide analogs. In some cases
(analogues 2,4,7,11) exist great differences
between the bradykinin potentiating activity
and the inhibition of the isolated and purified enzyme on the other hand. Especially
partial sequences show differences between
these two kinds of activities, in some cases
in 1 or 2 orders of magnitude. Furthermore,
it seems that the inhibition of enzyme is
more sensitive to changes in the sequence
and other modifications on the molecule.

These results indicate different structural requirements for potentiating and inhibiting action and have us encouraged to further biochemical investigations about the different action mechanism.

Table 1 : Biological activity of BPP$_{9\alpha}$ and some analogues (2)

| No | Compound | | Potentiation of the brandykinin action on guinea pig ileum (perc.) | Inhibition of the peptidyl dipeptid hydrolase IC$_{50}$ (M) |
	Sequence	Abbrevation		
1	Pyr – Trp – Pro – Arg – Pro – Gln – Ile – Pro – Pro	BPP$_{9\alpha}$	100	3×10^{-9}
2	Pro – Trp – Pro – Arg – Pro – Gln – Ile – Pro – Pro	[1 – Pro] – BPP$_{9\alpha}$	115	5×10^{-9}
3	Glu – Trp – Pro – Arg – Pro – Gln – Ile – Pro – Pro	[1 – Glu] – BPP$_{9\alpha}$	20	n.d.
4	Pyr – Phe – Pro – Arg – Pro – Gln – Ile – Pro – Pro	[2 – Phe] – BPP$_{9\alpha}$	80	4×10^{-8}
5	Pyr – Trp – Pro – Phe – Pro – Gln – Ile – Pro – Pro	[4 – Phe] – BPP$_{9\alpha}$	25	4×10^{-7}
6	Pyr – Trp – Pro – Tyr – Pro – Gln – Ile – Pro – Pro	[4 – Tyr] – BPP$_{9\alpha}$	70	5×10^{-8}
7	Pyr – Trp – Pro – Leu – Pro – Gln – Ile – Pro – Pro	[4 – Leu] – BPP$_{9\alpha}$	80	10^{-7}
8	Pyr – Trp – Pro – Lys – Pro – Gln – Ile – Pro – Pro	[4 – Lys] – BPP$_{9\alpha}$	65	2×10^{-8}
9	Pyr – Trp – Pro – Arg – Pro – Lys – Ile – Pro – Pro	[6 – Lys] – BPP$_{9\alpha}$	60	$2,5 \times 10^{-8}$
10	Pyr – Trp – Pro – Arg – Pro – Tyr – Ile – Pro – Pro	[6 – Tyr] – BPP$_{9\alpha}$	110	10^{-8}
11	Pyr – Trp – Pro – Lys – Pro – Lys – Ile – Pro – Pro	[4,6-DiLys] – BPP$_{9\alpha}$	80	2×10^{-6}
12	Pro – Trp – Pro – Arg – Pro – Lys – Ile – Pro – Pro	[1-Pro,6-Lys]-BPP$_{9\alpha}$	50	7×10^{-8}
13	Pyr – Trp – Pro – Arg – Pro – Gln – Tyr – Pro – Pro	[7- Tyr] – BPP$_{9\alpha}$	75	10^{-8}

The replacement of proline residues by alanine in the positions 3, 5 or 8 enhances the flexibility of the peptide backbone.

Table 2 : Biological activities of analogues with substitutions of the proline residues (2)

| No | Compound | | Potentiation of the bradykinin action on guinea pig ileum (perc.) | Inhibition of the peptidyl dipeptid hydrolase IC$_{50}$(M) |
	Sequence	Abbrevation		
1	Pyr – Trp – Ala – Arg – Pro – Gln – Ile – Pro – Pro	[3 – Ala] – BPP$_{9\alpha}$	65	5×10^{-8}
2	Pyr – Trp – Pro – Arg – Ala – Gln – Ile – Pro – Pro	[5 – Ala] – BPP$_{9\alpha}$	35	6×10^{-8}
3	Pyr – Trp – Pro – Arg – Pro – Gln – Ile – Ala – Pro	[8 – Ala] – BPP$_{9\alpha}$	45	$5,5 \times 10^{-7}$
4	Pyr – Trp – Ala – Arg – Ala – Gln – Ile – Ala – Pro	[3,5,8 – Ala] – BPP$_{9\alpha}$	0,3	—
5	Pyr – Trp – Pro – Arg – Pro – Gln – Ile – NMeAla – Pro	[8-NMeAla]– BPP$_{9\alpha}$	10	6×10^{-7}

The biological activity of the compounds 1, 2 and 3 is only slightly reduced. But the simultaneous replacement of all 3 proline residues in compound 4 leads practically to a complete loss of activity. It seems that to some degree folding and stabilization of the molecule by proline residues is necessary for the biological activity.

CONFORMATIONAL STUDIES

Conformational shape

Circular dichroism studies. The influence of the amino acid exchanges on the general conformational shape of the molecule was estimated by CD spectra (2). These spectra show chiroptical effects at 200 nm, at 220-240 nm and in the region of aromatic bands. Position and intensity of the strong negative band at 200 nm are only weakly influenced by the polarity of the solvents and by pH-values in the range from 2 to 9. However drastic changes are to be seen in the region of tryptophane transitions, indicating that different types of indolyl orientation seems to be prefered in water and in ethanol. All the estimated analogues with modifications in the side chains give CD curves similar to the original sequence in water as well as in ethanol (Fig. 2). From this finding we might conclude, at first that the pyroglumatic acid in position 1 is not essential for the characteristic conformational shape and secondly that the guanido group in position 4 makes only a weak contribution in stabilizing the conformation. Contrary to the slight influence of modifications in the side chains some analogues with alterations in the backbone of the peptide show drastic changes in the CD spectra. Whereas the analog with alanine in the place of proline in position 5 show the characteristic CD curve, the analogues with alanine in position 8 or 3 give changes in position

and intensity (Fig. 2). The changed conformational shape results from the enhanced
flexibility of the backbone including
alterations in the population of cis-trans
isomers on proline peptide bonds. Except the
des-pyroglutamic acid octapeptide the other
shortened sequences show a changed conformational shape, too.

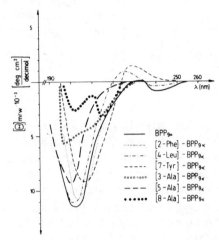

Figure 2:
CD-spectra of
BPP$_{9\alpha}$ and some
analogues in
C_2H5OH

In addition to these informations about the
general shape of the peptide it would be
highly desirable to evaluate intramolecular
distances. For this purpose we have used two
methods: electron spin resonance and fluorescence measurements.

Electron spin resonance studies. The use of
the ESR technique requires the introduction
of two spin labels into the peptide molecule
(3). For this reason the iminoxyl radical has
been covalently bound to functional groups in
specially synthesized analogues. In a good
aggreement with the estimated values from
the fluorescence measurements, the distance
between the positions 1 and 6 is significantly shorter than between 1 and 4.

Figure 3: Intramolecular distances in spin-labelled analogues of BPP$_{9\alpha}$

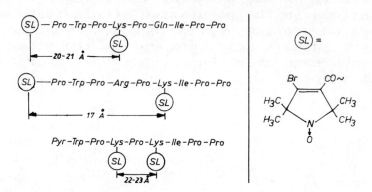

Fluorescence studies. In analogues with tyrosine in the positions 4, 6 or 7 intramolecular distances were estimated from the energy transfer between tyrosine and tryptophane (4). These values are determined in water at room temperature. The most stricking finding is the short distance between tryptophane in position 2 and tyrosine in position 6.

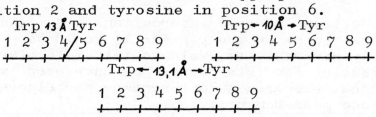

The estimated intramolecular distances give no indication for an approximation between the side chains of tryptophane and arginine. On the other hand the shortened distances between the positions 2 and 6 or 1 and 6 appear to provide evidence for an interaction between these side groups.

Flexibility of the side chains

These assumptions were supported by estimations of the mobility of the side chains in different positions. For this reason we have studied the correlation times in spin labelled analogues (5) and the influence of amino acid exchanges on the polarization of the tryptophane fluorescence. The estimated correlation times in mono spin-labelled analogues show an immobilization of the iminoxyl radical in all positions (1, 4 and 6). From fluorescence polarization studies on the original nonapeptide sequence, analogues with different modifications and some partial sequences we may draw the conclusion, that there are only slight interactions between the side chains in position 4 and 2.

REFERENCES

(1) Filatova, M.P., Krit, N.A., Kovaltschuk, O.V., Komarova, O.M. and Reissmann, S. (1980). Sintes deviatischlenovo peptidnovo ingibitora peptidyldipeptidasi. Bioorg. Khim. $\underline{6}$, 1605 - 1614
(2) Reissmann, S. et. al., in preparation
(3) Filatova, M.P., Reissmann, S., Reutova, T.O., Ivanov, V.T., Grigoryan, G.L., Shapiro, A.M. and Rosanzev, E.G.(1977) Konformazionnije sostojanija bradikinina i jevo analogov v rastworach. Spektri EPR-spin-metschenich analogov. Bioorg. Khim. $\underline{3}$, 1181 - 1189
(4) Schiller, P.W. (1980). Determination of the average end-to-end distance of two angiotensin II analogs by resonance energy transfer. Int.J.Peptide Protein Res. $\underline{15}$, 259 - 266
(5) Kuznetsov, A.N., Wassermann, A.M., Volklow, A.U. and Korst, N.N. (1971) Determination of Rotational Correlation Time of Nitric Oxyde Radicals in Viscous-Medium. Chem. Phys. Lett. $\underline{12}$ 103 - 109

ACTIVITY PROFILES OF CONFORMATIONALLY RESTRICTED OPIOID PEPTIDE ANALOGS

PETER W. SCHILLER, JOHN DIMAIO AND THI M.-D. NGUYEN
Laboratory of Chemical Biology and Peptide Research
Clinical Research Institute of Montreal
110 Pine Avenue West, Montreal, Que., Canada H2W 1R7

INTRODUCTION

Since the discovery of the enkephalins (H-Tyr-Gly-Gly-Phe-Met(or Leu)-OH) in 1975 an unprecedented effort has been made to determine the conformation(s) of these opioid peptides in various environments (for a review see ref. [1]). The outcome of these studies indicates that the natural enkephalins are flexible molecules capable of adopting several different conformations. This molecular flexibility permits adaptation to different receptor topographies and, therefore, explains the lack of specificity of the enkephalins toward the various types of opioid receptors (μ, δ, $\varkappa$, etc.). The receptor selectivity of linear peptides can be enhanced through incorporation of local conformational constraints at specific peptide bonds or side-chains or through more drastic restriction of the overall conformation by synthesis of cyclic analogs [2]. In the present paper we describe three families of cyclic enkephalin analogs which were designed on the basis of structure-activity relationships and conformational considerations. The activity profiles of the analogs were determined in bioassays based on inhibition of electrically evoked contractions of the guinea pig ileum (GPI) and the mouse vas deferens (MVD), which are representative for μ- and δ-opioid receptor interactions, respectively.

RESULTS AND DISCUSSION

A first type of cyclic enkephalin analog was obtained

Proceedings of the 16th FEBS Congress
Part B, pp. 457–462
© 1985 VNU Science Press

through substitution of a D-α, ω-diamino acid residue in position 2 of enkephalin and cyclization of the ω-amino group to the C-terminal carboxyl group [3] (Table I, compounds I-IV). Since these analogs showed high potency in the GPI-assay and low activity on the MVD, they are μ-receptor selective, as indicated by their high MVD/GPI IC50-ratios (Table I). Lengthening of the side-chain in position 2 resulted in a gradual increase in μ-receptor selectivity. The open-chain analog IVa is distinguished from cyclic analog IV merely by the opening of a single carbon-nitrogen bond. Since compound IVa is non-selective, it can be concluded that the μ-receptor selectivity of IV is exclusively due to the conformational constraint introduced through ring closure and that μ- and δ-receptors have indeed different conformational requirements. Analogs I and II contain rather rigid 13- and 14-membered ring structures precluding the formation of various β-bend structures which have been proposed as bioactive conformations of enkephalin. A conformational comparison of analogs III and IV by NMR spectroscopy revealed a difference in intramolecular hydrogen bonding between the two compounds, indicating that more than one conformation of the peptide backbone is tolerated for activity at the μ-receptor, and supporting the concept that the correct spatial disposition of the side-chains rather than the backbone conformation is crucial for the interaction with the receptor [4]). Whereas cyclic analog IV was found to be 5 times more potent than its linear correlate IVa in the GPI-assay, an exactly reversed potency relationship between the two compounds was observed in the [3H]naloxone binding assay which is also representative for μ-receptor interactions. This discrepancy between bio- and binding assay suggests that the conformational restriction introduced in IV through ring closure has a divergent effect on receptor affinity and the ability to activate the receptor ("efficacy"). Since compound IV has the same configurational requirements at residues 1,2,4 and 5 as [Leu5]enkephalin and shows a similar potency increase upon substitution of p-nitrophenylalanine in position 4, it can be assumed

Table I. Potencies of Opioid Peptide Analogs in the GPI- and MVD-assay

Compound		GPI IC50 [nM]	MVD IC50 [nM]	MVD/GPI IC50-ratio
I	H-Tyr-c[-N$^\beta$-D-A$_2$pr-Gly-Phe-Leu-]	23.4	73.1	3.12
II	H-Tyr-c[-N$^\gamma$-D-A$_2$bu-Gly-Phe-Leu-]	14.1	81.4	5.77
III	H-Tyr-c[-N$^\delta$-D-Orn-Gly-Phe-Leu-]	48.0	475	9.90
IV	H-Tyr-c[-N$^\epsilon$-D-Lys-Gly-Phe-Leu-]	4.80	141	29.4
IVa	H-Tyr-D-Nle-Gly-Phe-Leu-NH$_2$	24.6	25.2	1.02
V	H-Tyr-D-Glu-Gly-Phe-Lys-NH$_2$	42.7	699	16.4
VI	H-Tyr-D-Lys-Gly-Phe-Glu-NH$_2$	1.13	0.648	0.573
VII	H-Tyr-D-Glu-Phe-Lys-NH$_2$	7.99	101	12.6
VIII	H-Tyr-D-Lys-Phe-Glu-NH$_2$	2.93	5.21	1.78
IX	H-Tyr-D-Cys-Gly-Phe-Cys-NH$_2$	1.51	0.760	0.503
X	H-Tyr-D-Cys-Gly-Phe-D-Cys-NH$_2$	0.780	0.298	0.382
XI	H-Tyr-D-Cys-Gly-Phe-Cys-OH	3.06	0.190	0.0621
XII	H-Tyr-D-Cys-Gly-Phe-D-Cys-OH	1.48	0.122	0.0824
XIII	[Leu^5]enkephalin	246	11.4	0.0463

that the mode of binding to the receptor is the same for the cyclic and the linear analog. However, in a few cases analogous substitutions in analogs IV and IVa had a different effect on potency, indicating a possible difference in the binding process between the cyclic and the linear analog (cf. ref. [5]). Finally, cyclic analog IV was found to be highly stable against enzymatic degradation and at a dose of 20 nanomoles (i.c.v.) it produced long lasting analgesia and catatonia in rats.

A family of side-chain to side-chain cyclized opioid peptide analogs has recently been obtained [6] through substitution of an α, ω-diamino acid and a glutamic or aspartic acid residue in appropriate positions followed by amide bond formation between the side-chain amino and carboxyl groups (Table I, compounds V-VIII). H-Tyr-D-Glu-Gly-Phe-Lys-NH$_2$ (V) shows about the same potency and μ-receptor selectivity in the two bioassays as cyclic analog III. Transposition of the Gly and Lys residue results in a highly potent cyclic analog (VI) which, however, is non-selective, as indicated by its MVD/GPI-IC50-ratio of 1.78. Analogs V and VI both contain relatively large 18-membered ring structures. The differences in potency and receptor selectivity shown by these two compounds is likely to be due to the different position and direction of the side-chain connecting amide bond which may produce dissimilar intramolecular hydrogen bonding and thereby different ring conformations. The des-Gly^3 analog of compound V, H-Tyr-D-Glu-Phe-Lys-NH$_2$ (VII) is about 6 times more potent than its parent compound (V) on both preparations and, therefore, shows similar preference for μ-receptors over δ-receptors. In comparison to cyclic analog VI, its des-Gly^3 analog (VIII) shows similar high potency and lack of selectivity. Since cyclic analogs VII and VIII contain a phenylalanine residue in the 3-position, they show structural resemblance with morphiceptin and dermorphin.

A different type of side-chain to side-chain cyclized enkephalin analog was prepared by substitution of a D-Cys residue in position 2 and a D- or L-Cys residue in positon 5 of the peptide sequence followed by oxidative disulfide bond formation [7] (Table I, compounds IX to XII). The cyclic enkephalinamide analogs IX and X were found to be extremely potent in both the GPI- and MVD-assay and, therefore, showed no significant receptor selectivity. A receptor binding mode of these cyclic analogs similar to that of the natural enkephalins was again suggested by the results of structure-activity studies which indicated that the cystine bridge-containing analogs have the same configurational requirements at the individual residues as linear enkephalins [5]. In contrast to the non-selective cystine bridged enkephalinamide analogs (IX and X) the corresponding analogs with a free C-terminal carboxyl group (XI and XII) show moderate δ-receptor selectivity. The same difference in receptor selectivity is observed between linear enkephalins and enkephalinamides. Thus, the cyclic analogs XI and XII show preference for δ-receptors over μ-receptors comparable to that of [Leu^5]enkephalin but are about two orders of magnitude more potent on both preparations. Substitution of the half-cystine residues in compound XI and XII by half-penicillamine residues results in analogs showing high preference for δ-receptors [8], most likely as a consequence of the enhanced rigidity of their 14-membered ring structures. Taken together, these results demonstrate that various types and degrees of conformational restriction can have a pronounced effect on receptor affinity and selectivity, "efficacy", structure-activity patterns and stability of opioid peptides. In conclusion, the introduction of conformational constraints has emerged as a promising new tool in peptide analog design, as it is also illustrated by the interesting properties shown by cyclic analogs of several other biologically active peptides prepared by Prof. Chipens and his colleagues (see chapter by G.I. Chipens, this volume).

(Work supported by the Medical Research Council of Canada (grant MT-5655) and the Quebec Heart Foundation).

REFERENCES

[1] Schiller, P.W. (1984). Conformational analysis of enkephalins and conformation-activity relationships. In: The Peptides, Vol. 6, S. Udenfriend and J. Meienhofer (eds). Academic Press, New York, pp. 219- 268.

[2] Hruby, V.J. (1983). Conformational restrictions of biologically active peptides via amino acid side chain groups. Life Sci. 31, 189-199.

[3] DiMaio, J., Nguyen, T.M.-D., Lemieux, C. and Schiller, P.W. (1982). Synthesis and pharmacological characterization in vitro of cylic enkephalin analogs: effect of conformational constraints on opiate receptor selectivity. J. Med. Chem. 25, 1432-1438.

[4] Kessler, H., Hölzemann, G. and Zechel, C. (1984). Conformational analysis of cyclic enkephalin analogs of the type Tyr-cyclo(-N$^{\omega}$-Xxx-Gly-Phe-Leu-); Xxx = L-Orn, D-Orn, L-Lys, D-Lys. Int. J. Peptide Protein Res., in press.

[5] Schiller, P.W. and DiMaio, J. (1983). Aspects of conformational restriction in biologically active peptides. In: Peptides: Structure and Function, V.J. Hruby and D.H. Rich (eds). Pierce Chemical Company, Rockford, Ill., pp. 269-278.

[6] Schiller, P.W., Nguyen, T.M.-D. and Miller, J. (1984). Synthesis of side-chain to side chain cyclized peptide analogs on solid supports. Int. J. Peptide Protein Res., in press.

[7] Schiller, P.W., Eggimann, B., DiMaio, J., Lemieux, C. and Nguyen, T.M.-D. (1981). Cyclic enkephalin analogs containing a cystine bridge. Biochem. Biophys. Res. Commun. 101, 337-343.

[8] Mosberg, H.I., Hurst, R., Hruby, V.J., Gee, K., Yamamura, H.I., Galligan, J.J. and Burks, T.F. (1983). Bis-penicillamine enkephalins possess highly improved specificity toward opioid receptors. Proc. Natl. Acad. Sci. USA 80, 5871-5874.

462

NMR OF GRAMICIDIN A DOUBLE HELICES

Vladimir Bystrov and Alexandr ARSENIEV
M.M.Shemyakin Institute of Bioorganic Chemistry,
USSR Academy of Sciences, Ul. Vavilova, 32,
Moscow V-334, USSR

Gramicidin A (GA) is a linear polypeptide antibiotic consisting of 15 alternating L and D amino acid residues:

HCO-L-Val^1-Gly-L-Ala-D-Leu-L-Ala-D-Val-L-Val-
-D-Val-L-Trp-D-Leu^{10}-L-Trp-D-Leu-L-Trp-D-Leu-
-L-Trp^{15}-NHCH$_2$CH$_2$OH.

This compound has attracted much attention due to its ability to form monovalent cation selective pores, or channels in biological and artificial planar bilayer membranes (for reviews see [1,2]).

The problem of spatial structure of the channel is dramatically complicated because of diversity of energetically allowed conformations of GA [1,3-5]. Although the dimeric structure is well established [6], still many forms have to be considered, including single-stranded and double-stranded helical conformations with different relative orientation of N- and C-terminals, different handeness, and different number of residues per turn.

In some organic solvents GA forms an equilibrated set of several conformers with so slow rates of interconversion that they could be isolated separately [3]. For instance, after crystalization from ethanol of purified by countercurrent distribution GA and subsequent dissolving in dioxane-d$_8$, the proton NMR spectrum of the 0.01 M solution was found to correspond to a single conformer [7,8], named species 3 after Veatch et al [3]. By using two-dimensio-

Proceedings of the 16th FEBS Congress
Part B, pp. 463–471
© 1985 VNU Science Press

nal (2D) high-field 500 MHz proton NMR spectroscopy all signals were resolved and assigned to specific positions in the chemical structure of GA [8]. The three sets of NMR data were taken into consideration: a) vicinal spin-spin couplings for $H-NC^{\alpha}-H$ protons [9], which have L-D alternating relatively high values (Table), that witness of extended backbone structure, b) halftimes of deuterium exchange, which are very long

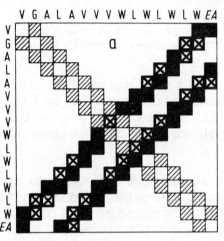

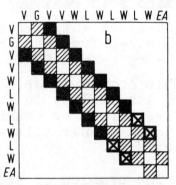

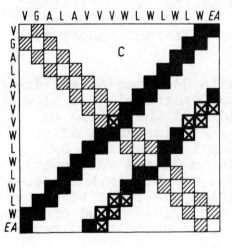

Fig.1. Diagrams of NOE connectivity between backbone protons of a) GA species 3 in dioxane, b) des-Ala^3-D--Leu^4-Ala^5-D-Val^6-GA in dioxane and c) 1:1 Gs$^+$GA complex in $CD_3OH/CDCl_3$ solution. The filled and crossed squares correspond to respectively identified and impeded NOESY spectrum cross-peaks for interchain connectivities, the hatched squares - to interchain connectivities.

464

TABLE. Observed vicinal proton H-NC -H coupling constants (^3J, Hz) and the deuterium exchange half-times ($t_{1/2}$, hours) of the backbone NH groups for species 3 of gramicidin A (GA-3) in dioxane-d_8, des-L-Ala^3,D-Leu^4,L-Ala^5,D-Val^6-gramicidin A (des$^{3-6}$-GA) in dioxane-d_8, and the Cs$^+$-gramicidin A complex 1:1 (Cs$^+$-GA) in the CD$_3$OH/CDCl$_3$ (1:1) solution, 30°C. EA- ethanolamine group.

Residue	GA - 3		des$^{3-6}$-GA		Cs$^+$-GA	
	^3J	$t_{1/2}$	^3J	$t_{1/2}$	^3J	$t_{1/2}$
L-Val-1	9.2	1.5	10.3	2.5	9.0	<0.2
Gly-2		1.5		15		0.2
L-Ala-3	7.8	8	-	-	8.4	0.6
D-Leu-4	8.0	8	-	-	8.8	23
L-Ala-5	6.6	6	-	-	6.0	0.2
D-Val-6	9.2	27	-	-	7.2	64
L-Val-7	7.5	46	9.6	>100	9.4	>100
D-Val-8	9.2	33	8.8	>100	8.4	>100
L-Trp-9	7.0	35	8.8	>100	8.4	>100
D-Leu-10	9.3	83	5.9	>100	7.6	>100
L-Trp-11	7.4	49	9.9	>100	9.2	>100
D-Leu-12	9.0	59	6.6	>100	6.4	>100
L-Trp-13	7.0	11	8.8	>100	9.6	>100
D-Leu-14	9.2	28	7.4	>100	8.8	
L-Trp-15	7.2	26	8.1	>100	9.6	>100
EA		46		10		7.7

for the majority of the NH backbone groups (Table), that correspond to their participation

465

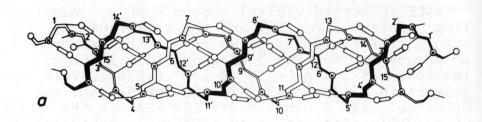

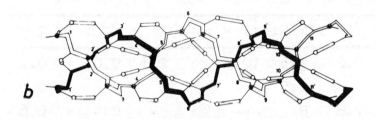

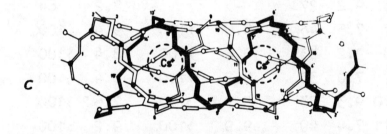

Fig.2. Conformations of gramicidin A double helices: a) left-handed antiparallel $\uparrow\downarrow \pi\pi_{LD}^{5.6}$ b) right-handed parallel $\uparrow\uparrow \pi\pi_{LD}^{5.6}$ and c) right-handed antiparallel $\uparrow\downarrow \pi\pi_{LD}^{7.2}$ with assumed positions of two Cs+ cations.

in hydrogen bonding and c) the interproton nuclear Overhausser effect (NOE)connectivities (Fig.1a), which demonstrate the dimeric double helical structure of the GA species 3.

By computer treatment of these results with
distance geometry algorithm [10], modified to
include vicinal couplings and hydrogen bonding
information, the spatial structure of the GA
species 3 was unequivocally evaluated [7,8] as
a left-handed antiparallel double helix
with 5.6 residues per turn (Fig.2a). This is a
rigid structure with 26 interstrand NH...O=C
hydrogen bonds and hydrophobic external surface,
forming a cylinder of 36 Å lenght that is long
enough to penetrate through bilayer membrane and
with 3 Å diameter of internal axial cavity that
could accomodate such alkali metal cations as
Li^+, Na^+ and K^+. Thus, in principle, this structure meets the general requirements of the
transmembrane channel. The conformation looks
reasonably fixed as soon as the peptide backbone
chain is concerned, but the side chains are subjected to considerable degree of flexibility.

Other conformational forms of GA were not so
easy to isolate in enough for NMR quantity and
thus to imitate the GA species 4 [3] conformation
we made use of synthetic shortened derivative -
des-L-Ala^3,D-Leu^4,L-Ala^5,D-Val^6-gramicidin A
[11]. Freshly dissolved in dioxane-d$_8$, this compound contains a mixture of slow interconverted
conformational forms, but after 12 hours at 30°C
the sample reaches an equilibrium for one predominant (> 90%) conformer. This form, according
to the IR and CD spectra [11], has a stable conformation, similar to structure of the GA species 3. Every signal in the NMR spectrum was
assigned by COSY, NOESY, RELSY, as well as in
complicated cases by double-quantum 2D-NMR and
NOERELSY techniques. Details will be published
in Bioorganicheskaya Khimia (USSR) . Although
the obtained vicinal H-NC$^\alpha$-H coupling constants
and the NH deuterium exchange half-times (Table)
are similar to those for the GA species 3, the
NOE-connectivity map (Fig.1b) has completely

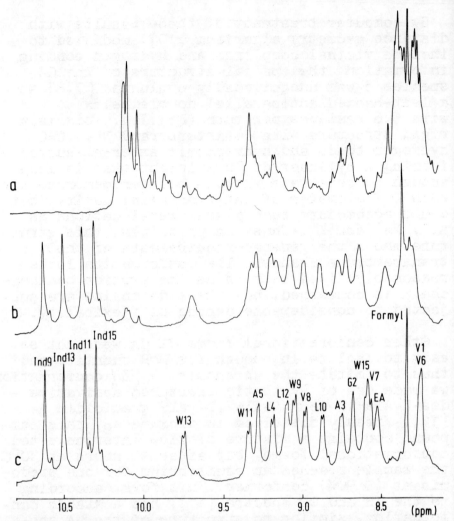

Fig.3. Low field region of the 500 MHz proton
NMR spectra of a 0.03 M solution of gramicidin A
in CD₃OH/CDCl₃ (1:1), 30°C at different
[Cs⁺]/[GA] molar ratio: a) 0.0, b) 0.6 and
c) 1.1. The backbone NH resonance assignments
are indicated by one letter code for amino acid
residues and the number in the primary structure
of gramicidin A. EA - amide proton of ethanolamine moiety, Ind - indole NH protons of tryptophan residues.

different appearance, which leads to conclusion, that the solution structure of the shortened GA analog is a right-handed parallel double helix $\uparrow\uparrow \pi\pi_{LD}^{5.6}$ with 5.6 residues per turn (Fig.2b). The dimensions of this helix, when adjusted to the full length of the GA amino acid sequence, are the same as for the GA species 3 structure discussed above. Thus it also could be considered as candidate for transmembrane channel.

Finally we were lucky to imitate the metal-GA complex in membrane-like environment by titration in the mixture of methanol and chloroform. With addition of caesium salt (CsCNS) the intensity and chemical shift of signals, arising from the complexed form are growing (Fig.3) in confirmity with a two-site binding reaction, in which the first metal binding step is a slow process, while the second step is fast in NMR time scale. Association and dissociation rates of the second cation binding is faster than for the first cation presumably due to electrostatic repulsion between cations. By combined consideration of the obtained NMR data (Table and Fig.1c) the structure of Cs^+-GA complex was evaluated as right-handed antiparallel double helix $\uparrow\downarrow \pi\pi_{LD}^{7.2}$ with 7.2 residues per turn, which is shown in Fig.2c with the most plausible positions of Cs^+ cations as infered from titration dependencies of the NH proton chemical shifts. This cylindrical structure with 27 Å lenght and 4 Å diameter of the internal axial cavity is well suited to accomodate the caesium cations, which are 3.3 Å in diameter and demonstrate greater than other alkali metal cations permeability via GA channels in bilayer phospholipid membranes [12].

The presented NMR study of GA conformations in organic solvents reveals stability of double helical structures (Fig.2), which have to be taken into account in further consideration of mechanism of GA induced membrane ion conductance and biological action of GA as endogenous inhibitor of RNA polymerase of the producing microorganism [13].

REFERENCES

1. Ovchinnikov, Yu.A. and Ivanov, V.T. (1982). Helical structures of gramicidin A and their role in ion channeling. In: Conformation in Biology, R.Srinivasan and R.H.Sarma (eds). Academic Press, New York, pp. 155-174.
2. Andersen, O.S. (1984). Gramicidin channels. Ann. Rev. Physiol. 46, 531-548.
3. Veatch, W.R., Fossel, E.T. and Blout, R. (1974). The conformation of gramicidin A. Biochemistry 13, 5249-5256.
4. Chandrasekaran, R. and Prasad, B.V.V. (1978). The conformation of Polypeptides containing alternating L and D amino acids. CRC Crit. Rev. Biochem. 5, 125-161.
5. Urry, D.W., Trapane, T.L. and Prasad, K.U. (1983). Is the gramicidin A transmembrane channel single-stranded or double-stranded helix? A simple unequivocal determination. Science 221, 1064-1067.
6. Veatch, W.R. and Stryer, L. (1977). The dimeric nature of the gramicidin A transmembrane channel: conductance and fluorescence energy transfer studies of hybrid channels. J.Mol.Biol. 113, 89-102.
7. Arseniev, A.S., Bystrov, V.F., Ivanov, V.T. and Ovchinnikov, Yu.A. (1984). NMR solution conformation of gramicidin A double helix. FEBS Lett. 165, 51-56.
8. Arseniev, A.S., Barsukov, I.L., Sychev, S.V., Bystrov, V.F., Ivanov, V.T. and Ovchinnikov, Yu.A. (1984). Double helical conformation of gramicidin A. Biol.Membr. (USSR) 1, 5-17.

9. Bystrov, V.F. (1976). Spin-spin coupling
   and conformational states of peptide systems. Progr. NMR Spectr. 10, 41-81.
10. Braun, W., Bosh, C., Brown, L.R., Go, N.
   and Wüthrich, K. (1981) Combined use of
   proton-proton Overhauser enhancements and
   a distance geometry algorithm for determination of polypeptide conformations.
   Biochim. Biophys. Acta 667, 377-396.
11. Sychev, S.V., Nevskaya, N.A., Jordanov, St.,
   Shepel, E.N., Miroshnikov, A.I. and Ivanov, V.T. (1980). The solution conformations of gramicidin A and its analogs.
   Bioorg. Chem. 9, 121-151.
12. Eisenman, G. and Sandblom, J.P. (1984). Mo-
   deling the gramicidin channel. Interpretation of experimental data using rate
   theory. Biophys. J. 45-90.
13. Sarkar, N., Langley, D. and Paulus, H.
   (1977). Biological function of gramicidin:
   selective inhibition of RNA polymerase.
   Proc. Natl. Acad. Sci. USA 74, 1478-1482.

MEMBRANE ORGANIZATION AND FUNCTION

USE OF LIPID-SPECIFIC PROBES IN MEMBRANE RESEARCH. AN ALTERNATIVE WAY OF BIOLOGICAL SIGNAL AMPLIFICATION

L.D. BERGELSON
Shemyakin Institute of Bioorganic Chemistry,
Academy of Sciences of the USSR, Moscow

In some systems hormones or hormone-like substances may generate large biological effects at extremely low effector concentrations. Traditionally the supersensitivity is explained by high positive cooperativity or by induction of an enzyme cascade which amplifies the primary response of the target to low levels of stimuli. Actually, however, the observed effector concentrations are so small that they may have represented one effector molecule per thousands of cells. Naturally, the question arises:what molecular mechanism can explain the capability of a single effector molecule to "excite" a large number of target cells?

We are attempting to address this question by studying effector induced fluorescence changes using new types of fluorescent probes synthesized in our laboratory [1-3]. These probes are modified natural lipids carrying an anthrylvinyl or perylenoyl group at the end of one of the aliphatic chains. Because such probes retain the head group structure and general molecular shape of their natural prototypes we call them lipid-specific probe (LSP).

In comparison with the widely used nonlipid probes such as diphenylhexatriene, ANS or pyrene, the LSP proved to have important advantages [4,5]. They truly reflect the phase behavior of their host lipids and in complex systems, where lateral phase separation is possible, co-localize with their natural prototypes. Lateral phase separations can be caused by many factors including proteins which frequently induce formation of a boundary phase.

Proceedings of the 16th FEBS Congress
Part B, pp. 475–481
© 1985 VNU Science Press

In such systems the LPS easily enter the boundary region. The boundary lipids since they are flexible molecules, must follow the shape changes of the protein. Therefore LSP, in principle, could be used to detect subtle conformational changes of membrane embedded proteins, such as changes occuring when a ligand binds to a site of the protein.

These considerations led us to develop a new binding assay based on measurement of fluorescence changes of the lipid-specific probes caused by conformational changes of the receptor protein. The assay stands from the assumption that the change of the fluorescence anisotropy of an LSP induced by ligand-receptor binding is proportional to the number of occupied binding sites. If this is true, the plot of the change of the fluorescence anisotropy against the reversed value of the free ligand concentration should have a linear regression and should intersect the axis of ordinates in the region of 1.0. This proved, indeed, to be the case for the binding of the B chain of the plant toxin ricin to Burkitt's lymphoma cells (Fig. 1). The binding constant and the number of ricin receptors found by the fluorescence method were in reasonable agreement with those derived from direct binding analysis. However, in comparison with

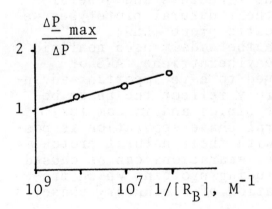

Fig. 1. Dependence of the fluorescence polarization (P) of Burkitt's lymphoma cells labeled with fluorescent sphingomyelin on the concentration of the B chain of ricin.

binding analysis, the fluorescence analysis is
more sensitive: even the effect of one ricin B
molecule per cell could easily by registered.
   We further used the fluorescence assay method
to study the binding of prostaglandins (PGs)
[6]. In the course of these studies we made an
observation which at the first glance was not
easy to explain. In order to make my story easier
to tell, I here shall present results obtained
with a simple model, the high density serum lipoproteins (HDL).
   The structure of HDL has been extensively studied
by many investigators, and a fairly consisted
model has emerged. According to that model, the
HDL globule has an apolar core of triglycerides
and cholesterol esters. The core is covered by
polar monolayer consisting of phospholipids,
proteins and free cholesterol. Strangely enough,
up to now nobody attempted to study the interaction of PGs with HDL despite the fact that both

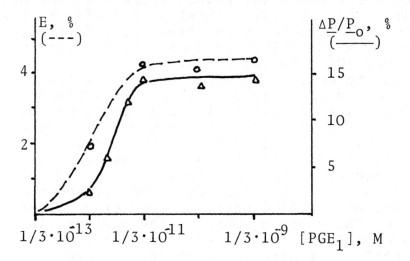

Fig. 2. Changes of the fluorescence polarization
($\underline{P}$) and tryptophan-to-probe energy transfer
parameter ($\underline{E}$) upon addition of prostaglandin E_1
to fluorescent labeled HDL.

are involved in the development of atherosclerosis.

When small amounts of PGE$_1$ were added to HDL labeled with fluorescent sphingomyelin, the fluorescence parameters gradually changed demonstrating that some type of rearrangement of the surface lipids had taken place (Fig. 2). The effect appeared to be highly specific: PGE$_2$ which differs from PGE$_1$ only by an additional double bond had no influence on the fluorescence parameters and did not interfere with PGE$_1$. Appearantly the effect was due to specific interaction of PGE$_1$ with one of the apoproteins because the PG had no effect on liposomes prepared from HDL lipids.

The rearrangement caused by PGE$_1$ appeared to be reversible. When the PG was removed by dialysis or addition of excess albumin, the fluorescence parameters returned to the initial values and then could be raised again by adding a new portion of the PG. However, that cycle could be repeated only a limited number of times and after a few hours the responsiveness of the HDL towards PGE$_1$ was lost. Finally, the effect proved to be saturable. Saturation occured already at 10^{-10} M PG. This corresponds to 1 molecule PGE$_1$ per $10^2 - 10^3$ globules.

Thus the action of PGE$_1$ on HDL resembles the interaction of a ligand with a high affinity binding site because it is specific, saturable and (seemingly) reversible. However, in contrast to classical ligand-receptor interactions, one PG molecule appearantly induces changes in a large number of HDL paticles.

A possible explanation could be derived from another of our findings: the very slow relaxation of the rearrangement of the surface lipids caused by the effector. After removal of the PG, both the fluorescence anisotropy and the tryptophan-to-probe energy transfer assume their initial values, however, they relax at different rates: the energy transfer decreases much faster than the fluorescence anisotropy (Fig. 3). This is understandable because the energy transfer reflects the interaction between only two molecules, the protein and the probe, whereas changes in the fluorescence anisotropy result from the cooperative rearrangement of many lipid molecules occupying a large area. In this sense we can say that the memory of membrane lipids is longer than that of the proteins.

A simple calculation shows that during the relaxation of the fluorescence parameters, a single PG molecule will collide several hundred times with each HDL globule, provided that the PG-receptor interation is weak. In a reversible system characterized by (1) short life-time of the effector-target complex, (2) high diffusion rates of the effector in the medium and (3) slow relaxation of the changes induced by the effector, a type of "excited" state of the target could be maintained despite the lack of detectable effector binding. In this way even a macro-

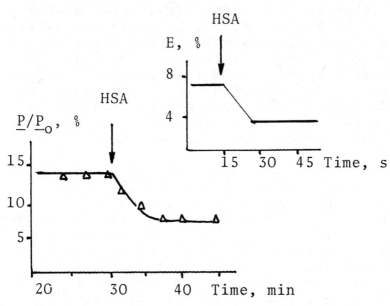

Fig. 3. Relaxation of P and E values after removal of PGE_1 from the sample of Fig. 2.

scopic multicomponent system could be responsive
to a single effector molecule. Such mechanism,
of course, would require energy which must be
provided by a secondary coupled process. In the
case of HDL which are metastable structures, a
likely energy source is the exothermic aggregation of lipoprotein particles. We found, indeed,
that the spontaneous aggregation of HDL is much
enhanced by traces of PGE_1. With cells or sucel-
lular particles the energy could be gained from
metabolic reactions.

The principles outlined here could form the
basis for a new theory of signal amplification.
However, whether they apply to cells has yet to
be shown. Other mechanisms for transmitting a
signal from a single molecule to a large number
of cells, such as inthermolecular enzyme cas-
cades (e.g. [7]) should also be considered.

REFERENCES

1. Molotkovsky, J.G., Dmitriev, P.I., Nikuli-
   na, L.F. and Bergelson, L.D. (1979). Synthesis of new fluorescent labeled phosphatidyl-
   cholines. Bioorgan. Khim. 5, 588-594.
2. Molotkovsky, J.G., Dmitriev, P.I., Molotkov-
   skaya, I.M., Bergelson, L.D. and Manevich,
   Y.M. (1981). Synthesis of new fluorescent
   phospholipids and a study of their behaviour
   in model membranes. Bioorgan. Khim. 7, 586-
   600.
3. Molotkovsky, J.G. and Bergelson, L.D. (1982).
   Perylenoyl-labeled lipid-specific fluorescent
   probes. Bioorgan. Khim. 8, 1256-1262.
4. Molotkovsky, J.G., Manevich, Y.M., Gerasimo-
   va, E.N., Polessky, V.A. and Bergelson, L.D.
   (1982). Differential study of phosphatidylcholine and sphingomyelin in human high-
   density lipoproteins with lipid-specific
   fluorescent probes. Eur. J. Biochem. 122,
   573-579.

5. Molotkovsky, J.G., Manevich, Y.M., Babak, V.I and Bergelson, L.D. (1984). Anthryl and perylenoyl labeled lipids as membrane probes. Biol. Membranes (USSR) 1, 33-43.
6. Molotkovsky, J.G., Manevich, Y.M., Bezuglov, V.V., Kulikov, V.I., Muzia, G.I., Prokazova, N.V. and Bergelson, L.D. (1984). Influence prostaglandin E_1 on the structure of high density lipoproteins. Abstracts of 16-th FEBS Meeting (Moscow, June 25-30, 1984), III-134.
7. Pankova, T.G., Idonina, T.A., Deribas, V.I., and Salganic, R.I. (1983). Biochemical cascade mediating the estradiol action. Exp. Clin. Endocrinol. 82, 131-139.

STUDIES ON THE STRUCTURE AND FUNCTION OF THE MITOCHONDRIAL ATPase COMPLEX

Sequence homology of the oligomycin sensitivity conferring protein (OSCP) and factor F_6 with other subunits of H^+-ATPases

V.A. Grinkevich[*], N.A. Aldanova[*], P.V. Kostetsky[*], N.N. Modyanov[*], Yu.A. Ovchinnikov[*], T. Hundal["], L. Ernster["]

[*]Shemyakin Institute of Bioorganic Chemistry, USSR Academy of Sciences, Moscow, USSR; ["]Department of Biochemistry, Arrhenius Laboratory, University of Stockholm, Stockholm, Sweden.

"Oligomycin sensitivity conferring protein" (OSCP) (1) and coupling factor 6 (F_6) (2) are components of the mitochondrial H^+-ATPase, participating in the interaction between the catalytic (F_1) and the proton-translocating (F_0) moieties of the enzyme.

Determination of the complete amino acid sequence of OSCP (3) confirms the notion that this protein is a counterpart of the δ-subunit of E.coli F_1 (4,5). As reported elsewhere (6,7,8) there is also a functional similarity between OSCP and the δ-subunit of E. coli F_1, both requiring an intact α-subunit in order to be bound to F_1.

The N-terminal region of OSCP is more hydrophobic (75% hydrophobicity) than the corresponding segment of the δ-subunit (60%):

OSCP/7-26/ PPVQIYGIEGRYATALYSAA

δ /1-18/ MSEFITVARPYAKAAFDFA

and may serve to anchor OSCP in the membrane (9). This may explain why OSCP remains bound to the membrane sec-

Proceedings of the 16th FEBS Congress
Part B, pp. 483–488
© 1985 VNU Science Press

tor while the δ-subunit in E.coli accompanies F$_1$ when the latter is removed from the membrane.

Comparative analysis of the OSCP sequence with itself reveals a striking pattern of a homologous repeat (9):

```
  1- 52  FAKLVRPPVQIYGIEGRYATALYSAASKQNKLEQVEKELLRVGQILK*EPKMA
105-155  FSTMMSVHRGEVPCTVTTASALNEATLTELK**TVLKSFLKKGQVLKLEVKID


 53-104  ASLLNPYVKRSVKVKSLSDMTAKEKFSPLTSNLINLLAENGRLTNTPAVISA
156-190  PSIMGGMIVRIGE*KYV*DMSAKTKIQKLSRAMRQIL
```

Comparison of the amino acid sequences of OSCP and the b-subunit of E.coli F$_0$F$_1$-ATPase (10-12) also shows a homology between the repeating portion of OSCP and the central part of the b-subunit (9):

```
OSCP / 1- 48/  FAKLVRPPVQIYGIEGRYATALYSAASKQNKLEQVEKELLRVGQILKE
  b  /21- 67/  CMKYVWPPL*MAAIEKRQKEIADGLASAERAHKDLDLAKASATDQLKK


OSCP /49- 94/  PK*MAASLLNPYVKRSVKVKSLSDMTAK*EKFSPLTSNLINLLAENGR
  b  /68-115/  AKAEAQVIIEQANKRRSQILDEAKAEAEQERTKIVAQAQAEIEAERKR
```

Thus mitochondrial OSCP appears to contain structural elements of both the δ- and the b-subunits of E.coli F$_0$F$_1$-ATPase.

A considerable sequence homology was unexpectedly found between the repeating parts of OSCP/1-89/ and the ADP/ATP carrier/15-105/ (13,14).

The amino acid sequence of beef heart F$_6$ has recently been completed (15); it differs from that obtained by Fang et al. (16) in position 62: threonine vs phenylalanine. The polypeptide chain of F$_6$ as determined by Grinkevich et al. (15) consists of 76 residues and contains an internal repeat:

```
 1-35   NKELD*PVQKLFVDKIR*EYRTKRQ*TSGGPVDAGPEY
36-76   QQDLDRELFKLKQMYGKADMNTFPNFTFEDPKFEVVEKPQS
```

The internal homology is not as pronounced as in the case of OSCP; however, both proteins appear to have evolved by a process of gene duplication. In addition, OSCP and F_6 have homologous structural elements, mostly manifested when comparing the following regions:

```
OSCP  / 1-40/   FAKLVRPPVQIYGIEGRYATALYSAASKQNKLEQVEKELL
F6   /39-76/   LDRELFKLKQMYG*KADMNT*FPNFTFEDPKFEVVEKPQS
```

The N-terminal part of F_6 is homologous with the C-terminal region of the E.coli subunit c (15), including the DCCD-binding site (Asp-61):

```
F6 / 1-39/   NKELDPVQKLFVDKIREYRTKRQTSGGPVDAGPEYQQDL
c  /33-70/   GKFLEGAARQP*DLIPLLRTQFFIVMGLVDAIPMIAVGL
```

A certain homology is also found between F_6 and other H^+-ATPase subunits such as the mitochondrial ATPase inhibitor (18), the E.coli ε-subunit (19) and its mito-chondrial counterpart δ (4), as well as the amino acid sequence that can be deduced from URF A6L of mitochondrial DNA (20).

Further investigations will have to establish whether these structural homologies are of functional significance.

Acknowledgements.

This work has been supported by the Swedish Natural-Science Research Council. V.A. Grinkevich and N.N. Modyanov have been exchange fellows of the Royal Swedish Academy of Sciences and the USSR Academy of Sciences.

References.

1. MacLennan, D.H. and Tzagoloff, A. (1968). Studies on mitochondrial adenosine triphosphatase system. IV. Purification and characterization of the oligomycin sensitivity conferring protein. Biochemistry, 7, 1603-1610.
2. Fessenden-Raden, J.M. (1972). Purification and properties of a new coupling factor required for oxidative phosphorylation in silicotungstate-treated submitochondrial particles. J. Biol. Chem., 247, 2351-2357.
3. Ovchinnikov, Yu.A., Modyanov, N.N., Grinkevich, V.A., Aldanova, N.A., Trubetskaya, O.E., Nazimov, I.V., Hundal,T., Ernster, L. (1984). Amino acid sequence of the oligomycin sensitivity-conferring protein (OSCP) of beef heart mitochondria and its homology with the δ-subunit of the F_1-ATPase of Escherichia coli. FEBS Lett. 166, 19-22.
4. Walker, J.E., Runswick, M.J., Saraste, M. (1982). Subunit equivalence in Escherichia coli and bovine heart mitochondrial F_1F_0 ATPases. FEBS Lett. 146, 393-396.
5. Grinkevich, V.A., Modyanov, N.N., Ovchinnikov, Yu.A., Hundal, T., Ernster, L.(1982). Studies of the structure and function of the oligomycin sensitivity conferring protein (OSCP) from beef heart mitochondria. EBEC Reports 2, 83-84.
6. Hundal, T., Norling, B., Ernster, L. (1983). Lack of ability of trypsin-treated mitochondrial F_1-ATPase to bind the oligomycin-sensitivity conferring protein (OSCP). FEBS Lett. 162, 5-10.

486

7. Norling, B., Hundal, T., Sandri, G., Glaser, E., Ernster, L. (1984). Resolution and reconstitution of the mitochondrial F_1F_0-ATPase. In: H^+-ATPase (ATP-synthase): Structure, Function, Biogenesis. S. Papa, K. Altendorf, L. Ernster and L. Packer (eds). ICSU Press and Adriatica Editrice, Bari, pp. 295-312.
8. Hundal, T., Norling, B., Ernster, L. (1984). The oligomycin sensitivity conferring protein (OSCP) of beef heart mitochondria. Studies of its binding to F_1 and its function. J. Bioenerg. Biomembr. 16, 535-550.
9. Grinkevich, V.A., Aldanova, N.A., Kostetsky, P.V., Trubetskaya, O.E., Modyanov, N.N., Hundal, T., Ernster, L. (1984). Structural characteristics of the oligomycin sensitivity conferring protein (OSCP). In: H^+-ATPase (ATP-synthase): Structure, Function, Biogenesis. S. Papa, K. Altendorf, L. Ernster and L. Packer (eds). ICSU Press and Adriatica Editrice, Bari, pp. 153-160.
10. Gay, N.J., Walker, J.E. (1981). The atp operon: nucleotide sequence of the promoter and the genes for the membrane proteins, and the δ-subunit of Escherichia coli ATP-synthase. Nucleic Acids Res. 9, 3919-3926.
11. Kanazawa, H., Mabuchi, K., Kayano, T., Noumi, T., Sekiya, T. and Futai, M. (1981). Nucleotide sequence of the genes for F_0 components of the proton-translocating ATPase from Escherichia coli: Prediction of the primary structure of F_0 subunits. Biochem. Biophys. Res. Commun. 103, 613-620.
12. Nielsen, J., Hansen, F.G., Hoppe, J., Friedl, P., von Meyenburg, K.(1981). The nucleotide sequence of the atp genes coding for the F_0 subunits a, b, c and the F_1 subunit δ of the membrane bound ATP synthase of Escherichia coli. Mol. Gen. Genet. 184, 33-39.
13. Aquila, H., Misra, D., Eulitz, M., Klingenberg, M. (1982). Complete amino acid sequence of the ADP/ATP carrier from beef heart mitochondria. Hoppe-Seyler's Z. Physiol. Chem. 363, 345-349.

14. Saraste, M., Walker, J.E. (1982). Internal sequence repeats and the path of polypeptide in mitochondrial ADP/ATP translocase. FEBS Lett. 144, 250-254.

15. Grinkevich, V.A., Modyanov, N.N., Ovchinnikov, Yu.A, Hundal, T., Ernster, L. (1984). Sequence homology of the oligomycin sensitivity conferring protein (OSCP) and factor F_6 with other subunits of H^+-ATPase. EBEC Reports 3, pp. 307-308.

16. Fang, J., Jacobs, J.W., Kanner, B.I., Racker, E. and Bradshaw, R.A. (1984). Amino acid sequence of bovine heart coupling factor 6 (F_6). Proc. Natl. Acad. Sci. USA (in press).

17. Sebald, W., Hoppe, J. (1981). On the structure and genetics of the proteolipid subunit of the ATP synthase complex. Curr. Top. Bioenerg. 12, 1-64.

18. Frangione, B., Rosenwasser, E., Penefsky, H.S., Pullman, M.E. (1981). Amino acid sequence of the protein inhibitor of mitochondrial adenosine triphosphatase. Proc. Natl. Acad. Sci. USA 78, 7403-7407.

19. Saraste, M., Gay, N.J., Eberle, A., Runswick, M.J., Walker, J.E. (1981). The atp operon nucleotide sequence of the genes for the γ-, β- and ε-subunits of Escherichia coli ATP synthase. Nucleic Acids Res. 9, 5287-5296

20. Anderson, S., de Bruijn, M.H.L., Coulson, A.R., Eperon, I.C., Sanger, F., Young, I.G. (1982). Complete sequence of bovine mitochondrial DNA (conserved features of the mammalian mitochondrial genome). J. Mol. Biol. 156, 683-717.

TUMOR SPECIFIC INHIBITION OF DNA SYNTHESIS AND CELL PROLIFERATION BY A FACTOR FROM BOVINE PLACENTA

K. Letnansky, Institute for Applied And Experimental Oncology, University of Vienna, Vienna, Austria

It has been previously reported that components are found in placental tissue which inhibit DNA synthesis and cell division of fibroblasts, lymphocytes, and epidermis (1). Other authors described an inhibition of the growth rate of some rodent tumors, including the Walker carcinoma, the Brown-Pearce carcinoma, and the Ehrlich ascites carcinoma, growing on rats, rabbits, and mice, respectively (2, 3).

Although these components had been partially purified, attempts for their characterization had been undertaken only to a limited degree and there are some indications that the inhibitory action described in the earlier papers is due to the action of different compounds.

It was the aim of our investigations therefore, to separate these factors one from another and to find out if there possibly exists some specificity of certain components directed against tumor cells. Actually it could be demonstrated that there are more than one inhibitor in the preparations, which are bound specifically to receptors of the cell surface.

The first step in the separation procedure was the mechanical separation of the maternal from the fetal part of the placenta. Bovine placenta, which was used in our experiments, is one of the few materials where this procedure may be easily performed. According to the observations of Geipel (4) this step appeared to be very important to us, since this author described significant differences in the action of

Proceedings of the 16th FEBS Congress
Part B, pp. 489–499
© 1985 VNU Science Press

these two placental components on the uptake of
inorganic phosphate by explants of different
organs and by tissue culture cells. Similar results had been obtained by Jacherts et al. (5)
who investigated protein synthesis by a cell-
free HeLa system.
In our experiments, the further separation by
Sephadex chromatography of biologically active
components in the extracts of the fetal and the
maternal parts, respectively, demonstrated the
existence of several stimulators of protein
synthesis. Only the extracts obtained from the
decidua, the maternal part of the placenta,
additionally showed an inhibitory action in two
different regions of the chromatogram. This result prompted us to concentrate primarily on
these components in the following experiments.
Fig.1 demonstrates the separation of an extract
obtained from the maternal part of bovine placenta on a Sephadex G-100 column. The lower
curve of this diagram represents the absorption
of the eluted material. The upper curves were
obtained by testing the action of individual
fractions on thymidine incorporation of rat
bone marrow or ascites tumor cells. In this experiment cells of the Ehrlich ascites tumor of
the mouse had been used; essentially the same
results are obtained with rat tumors, including
the Yoshida ascites tumor.
It is particularly striking that there are two
regions within this profile, where an almost
90% inhibition of thymidine incorporation is
observed: In the low molecular weight region
between fractions 45 and 57 inhibitory action
is demonstrated with normal cells and tumor
cells as well. However, in the high molecular
weight region from fraction 10 to fraction 17
two inhibitors with differing specificity may
be partially resolved one from another: While
fraction 15 shows maximum inhibition of bone
marrow DNA synthesis, fractions 10 and 11 are
most effective in the tumor system, due to the

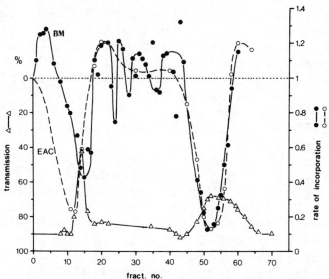

Fig.1: Fractionation of bovine maternal placenta on a Sephadex G-100 column by elution with TKM buffer (10 mM Tris-HCl, pH 7.4, 10 mM KCl, 1.5 mM MgCl$_2$). Lower curve: transmission of the eluting material at 260 nm, upper curves: influence of individual fractions on the incorporation of ^{3}H-thymidine into the DNA of Ehrlich ascites carcinoma cells (EAC) or bone marrow (BM)

presence of the tumor specific decidua inhibitory factor (DIF).
Further purification of this factor was performed by ion exchange chromatography on Dowex 50W and gel electrophoresis on 15% polyacrylamide gels in presence of urea or SDS. This resulted in the removal of most of the contaminating components from the inhibitor.
The activity of DIF is not influenced by treatment with nucleases. However, preincubation with proteolytic enzymes, including trypsin and papain, results in a significant loss of its inhibitory capacity, indicating the protein nature of the factor.

491

A comparison with other tumors proved the effectiveness of the inhibitor not only for
transplantation tumors but also for human tumors, grown in tissue culture. This is demonstrated in Fig.2 for a bronchogenic carcinoma
(E14) and for an osteosarcoma (2T). On the contrary, fibroblasts show no significant depres-
sion of DNA synthesis by the inhibitor, as do
bone marrow cells.
Prolonged incubation of tumor cells with DIF
obviously results in a severe damage of the
cells, as can be seen in Fig.3. In this experiment Ehrlich ascites tumor cells had been
incubated for 2 h at 37^3C in presence and in
the absence of the inhibitor. After the inocu-
lation of this material into mice, only those
cells which had been incubated without inhibitor produce rapidly growing tumors leading to
an early death of the animals. Significantly
slower growing tumors result from the damaged

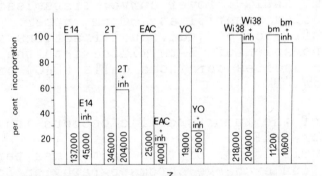

Fig.2:   Inhibition of ^{3}H-thymidine incorporation into the DNA of tumor and normal cells.
Figures within the columns represent absolute
values (counts per minute); thymidine uptake
in the absence of the inhibitor was set 100%.
E14 and 2T, established cell lines of human
bronchogenic carcinoma and osteosarcoma, respectively; EAC, Ehrlich ascites carcinoma;
Yo, Yoshida ascites sarcoma; Wi38, fibroblasts;
bm, rat bone marrow; inh, presence of inhibitor

cells, as shown by the greatly retarded death
rate.
The extent of the inhibition is proportional
to the amount of DIF added to the test system
until a constant final value is reached (Fig.
4). This might be an indication for the involvement of receptor-ligand reactions on the
cell surface and a subsequent internalization

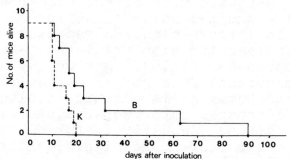

Fig.3: Survival of mice, inoculated with Ehrlich ascites tumor cells, which had been incubated in the presence (B) or absence (K) of
DIF for 2 h at 37°C.

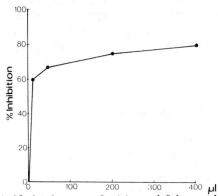

Fig.4: Inhibition of thymidine incorporation
as a function of the amount of DIF added to the
test system (10 - 400 µl of fraction 11 after
Sephadex-separation according to Fig.1). Investigations were made with Ehrlich carcinoma
cells.

493

of the complex. Two further experimental results are in favour with this explanation:
1) substances known for enhancing cell permeability, including lysolecithin, do not
   influence the action of the inhibitor
2) mild digestion of cells with proteolytic
   enzymes, which obviously remove receptor
   proteins from the surface, significantly
   reduces the action of the inhibitor.
In order to obtain more direct evidence in
elucidating the mechanism of action we prepared an inhibitor which was radioactively
labeled by reaction with tritiated N-succin-
imidylpropionate (fig.5). Then we isolated
surface membranes from normal cells (rat bone
marrow) and tumor cells (Yoshida ascites tumor) and incubated both preparations with the
labeled compound. Actually it turned out that
the tumor membranes bound significantly more
radioactivity than the membranes prepared from
normal cells, namely 5,600 dpm/μg of membrane
protein compared to 3,500.
A better insight into the binding characteristics of both models was achieved by performing
binding studies with varying amounts of tritiated inhibitor (20 - 500 μl) added to constant amounts of tumor or normal cell surface

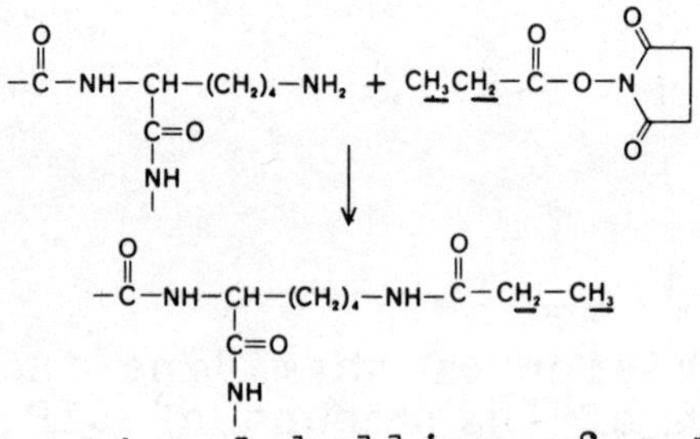

Fig.5: Radioactive labelling of a peptide by
reaction with N-succinimidyl(2,3-^{3}H)propionate
(tritium atoms are underlined) for 13 h at 4°C
in 0.1 M borate buffer, pH 8.5

494

membranes (50 µg). The results of these experiments had been evaluated according to Scatchard (6) as shown in Fig.6. There it is clearly demonstrated that membranes from liver cells do not bind the inhibitor as efficiently as do tumor membranes. Although there is no significant difference in the affinities of the membranes from both tissues, the biphasic binding characteristics of the tumor membranes indicate not only higher binding capacities but also the existence of additional receptor classes. Taken together, this results in the stimulated formation of receptor-ligand complexes observed on tumor cells, which is a prerequisite for an enhanced internalization of the inhibitor.

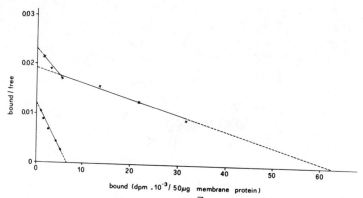

Fig.6: Scatchard plot of ^{3}H-propionylated DIF binding to membranes of liver (•) and Yoshida tumor cells (x). Labeled inhibitor was added in amounts ranging from 20 to 500 µl to 50 µg of plasma membranes from liver or tumor cells, suspended in 50 µl of phosphate buffered saline, pH 7.4. After adjusting the end volume to 550 µl the mixtures were incubated for 60 min at 30°C and centrifuged for 2 h at 100,000 xg. The pellet was rinsed with ice-cold saline, solubilized in Soluene and counted for radioactivity.

The completely different binding processes
taking place with liver and tumor membranes,
respectively, are demonstrated also in Fig.7.
After the separation of membrane components of
both tissues on 15% polyacrylamide urea gels,
gels were sliced into disks of 1 mm thickness,
which were incubated with the tritiated inhibitor. The receptor-inhibitor complexes having
formed during this procedure were precipitated
and counted for radioactivity. While the components of the liver membranes show only limited binding of DIF, the tumor preparation
clearly demonstrates significantly stimulated
complex formation and the existence of additional receptor sites.
All these experiments strongly support the idea
that a higher concentration of DIF in tumor

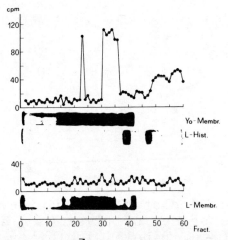

Fig.7: Binding of ^{3}H-labeled DIF to components
of surface membranes from Yoshida tumor cells
(Yo-Membr.) and liver cells (L-Membr.) separated on 10% polyacrylamide urea gels. Gels were
stained with amido black or sliced into disks
which were counted for radioactivity. One gel
with liver histones (L-Hist.), run under the
same conditions, served as a standard. Direction of the run was from left to right

cells compared to that one found in normal cells is a basic requirement for the different magnitude of the inhibitory action. Moreover, they offer an explanation concerning the mechanisms by which this may be achieved. They give no explanation, however, which reactions within the cells ultimately result in the observed inhibition of DNA synthesis. This question is completely open to discussion, although recent experiments from Pardee's laboratory (7, 8, 9) are tempting to speculate. According to these authors the inhibition of DNA synthesis caused by cycloheximide, which primarily inhibits protein synthesis, is due to the exhaustion of the cells with respect to a labile protein with a molecular weight of about 53,000 dalton. Since this protein is involved in the formation of the DNA polymerase multi-enzyme complex, the unsufficient supply of the cell caused by an inhibition of a continuously occurring resynthesis must necessarily result in a disturbed DNA production. Interestingly enough, two nuclear proteins with molecular weights in this range are diminished significantly also in our experiments after the incubation of Yoshida tumor cells with the inhibitory factor (Fig.8). This could be interpreted in a similar way, leading to the assumption that the primary point of attack might be some step during the process of protein synthesis. Although earlier experiments from our laboratory actually demonstrated an inhibition of protein synthesis, additional information must be awaited before the action of this inhibitor will be fully understood.

ACKNOWLEDGEMENT

I wish to thank Professor K. Theurer, Vitorgan, Stuttgart, for providing placental preparations prepared by special, mild procedures of tissue disintegration (DBP 10 33 37 4)

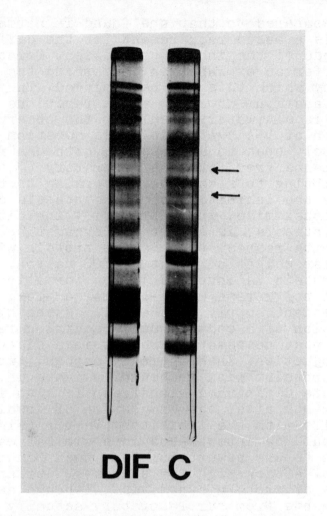

Fig.8: Separation of nuclear proteins of Yoshida cells which had been incubated for 1 h
at 37°C in the presence (DIF) and in the absence (C) of DIF on 15% polyacrylamide gels.
Gels are stained with amido black. Arrows indicate peptides disappearing during incubation in the presence of DIF.

References

1. Baden, H.P. (1973). J. Natl. Canc. Inst. 50, 43-48
2. Rauch, S., Zender, R., and Köstlin, A. (1956). Helv. med. acta 23/A, 75-109
3. Profitlich, H., Resch, E., and Wulf, W. (1955). Z. Krebsforsch. 60, 390-398
4. Geipel, A. (1965). Z. Gynäkol. 87, 1433-1436
5. Jacherts, D., Jacherts, B., and May, G. (1963). Mediz. Klin. 58, 752-754
6. Scatchard, G. (1949). Ann. N. Y. Acad. Sci. 51, 660-672
7. Pardee, A. B., Dubrow, R., Hamlin, J.L., and Kletzien, F. (1978). Ann. Rev. Biochem. 47, 715-750
8. Medrano, E.E., and Pardee, A.B. (1980). Proc. Natl. Acad. Sci. USA 77, 4123-4126
9. Campisi, J., Medrano, E.E., Morreo, G., and Pardee, A.B. (1982). Proc. Natl. Acad. Sci. USA 79, 436-440

THE MOLECULAR STRUCTURE OF THE MUSCARINIC ACETYLCHOLINE RECEPTOR

H. REPKE
Institute of Drug Research, Academy of Sciences
of GDR, 1136 Berlin, Alfred Kowalke Strasse 4

1. INTRODUCTION

The present research on muscarinic receptors
is mainly focused on two problems, the molecular
structure and the subtyp heterogeneity. The
current knowledge might be roughly summarized
as follows:
a) The muscarinic receptor is considered to be
a 80 000 D protein (1) which might consist of
two covalently linked identical subunits. In
certain tissues a 160 000 D dimer has been detected which is supposed to explain a subtyp
heterogeneity of agonist binding properties (2).
b) Two subtypes of muscarinic receptors can be
distinguished by using the selective antagonist
pirenzepine (3). Each of these subtypes is considered to occur in two interconventible conformational states as shown by the low and high
affinity agonist binding sites.
c) The interconversion of the high affinity
agonist binding site into the low affinity agonist binding site can be achieved by guanine
nucleotides, thus suggesting the occurence of
a GTP-binding protein which might be associated
with the muscarinic receptor.
d) Indirect evidence clearly demonstrates, that
the muscarinic receptor transmits signals to
Ca^{2+} and K^{+}-ionophores, the adenylate cyclase
and the phosphoinositol metabolism. Unfortunately, the molecular mechanism of the coupling
is still unknown. Furthermore, is seems that the
muscarinic receptor exists in different coupling
states in different tissues.
 The aim of the present study is to contribute
to the development of a unifying model of

Proceedings of the 16th FEBS Congress
Part B, pp. 501–508
© 1985 VNU Science Press

structure and function of muscarinic receptors.
This is mainly done by the comprehensive analysis of solubilized muscarinic receptors with
different biochemical and pharmacological properties which are first described in this report.
The experiments were extended to the use of
model membranes.

2. SOLUBILIZED NATIVE MUSCARINIC RECEPTORS
   WITH DIFFERENT BIOCHEMICAL PROPERTIES

Native muscarinic receptors can be solubilized
by mild nonionic detergents such as digitonin/
gitonin or CHAPS but also by lysolecithin.
In extension of systematic studies about the
solubilization of muscarinic receptors by
digitonin/gitonin mixtures, we found that the
receptor is solubilized by the micellar form
of the detergent. That means, that at a fixed
detergent concentration the amount of free
detergent can be reduced below the critical
micelle concentration by increasing the protein
content in the sample. Using synaptosomal membranes, an optimal receptor solubilization
(yield 70 %) is achieved by 1 % (w/v) digitonin/
gitonin at a concentration of 8 mg protein/ml,
whereas no muscarinic receptors are solubilized
at 23 mg protein/ml. The latter conditions
were used for extraction of peripheral membrane
proteins before muscarinic receptor solubilization in a second step at 14 mg protein/ml.
    Seven lectins (lotus lectin, ricinus lectin,
phytohaemagglutinin, soja lectin, concanavalin
A, lentil lectin and wheat germ agglutinin
(WGA))were covalently bound to Sepharose 6 B
and used for affinity chromatography of muscarinic receptors which were solubilized by the
one step procedure. The receptors were only
bound to WGA and could be specifically eluted
with N-acetyl glucosamine. The binding of the
receptors (80 % of the total amount) could be
completely abolished either by treatment with

neuranimidase or by extraction of peripheral membrane proteins before muscarinic receptor solubilization (two step procedure).

This permits the following conclusions: a) The sugar moiety is not covalently bound to the receptor. b) The muscarinic receptor is coupled to wheat germ agglutinin via N-acetyl neuraminic acid which binds also to WGA, although with lower affinity than N-acetyl glucosamine.

WGA-binding and not WGA-binding preparations of solubilized muscarinic receptors from pig striatum were prepared by either the one step or the two step procedure. The ligand binding kinetics of both preparations was examined by ^{3}H-QNB competition experiments. The data of three independent preparations were fitted by a non-linear curve fitting procedure according to a two independent site model. Agonists, partial agonists and antagonists were included in this study. The most striking results of the analysis are: a) Two agonist binding sites (for example oxotremorine: $K_{D1}=2.4\pm0,6$ µM (60 %), $K_{D2}=50.0\pm0$ µM (40 %) and one antagonist binding site (for example atropine: $K_D= 0.6$ nM) could be detected in both receptor preparations. b) The affinity of the low affinity agonist binding site is increased five-fold either by the presence of GTP or the removal of the WGA-binding moiety from the solubilized receptor.

Although these results are not quantitatively identical with those which were obtained with synaptosomal membranes, they focus the interest to the hypothetical WGA-binding glycoprotein, which might bind GTP and can be dissociated from the muscarinic receptor by a selective solubilization procedure as described here.

3. COMPUTER ASSISTED ELEKTROPHORETIC ANALYSIS OF NATIVE AND DENATURATED SOLUBILIZED MUS-CARINIC RECEPTORS

Based on the results which were described in

the previous section, we analysed whether a
noncovalent association of the receptor with a
(regulatory?) glycoprotein could be detected.
Preparations of the solubilized WGA-binding and
not WGA-binding receptors were run in the tris/
glycinate electrophoresis at optimum conditions.
Therefore, 70–80 % of the specifically bound
^{3}H-QNB remained bound to the receptor during the
electrophoresis. This permits the identification
of a single sharp receptor peak in the sliced
gel. The Rf-values were plotted according to
Ferguson (5). The slope of the resulting line
(K_R) and its intercept with the y-axis (Y_o) were
calculated by weighted regression analysis by
the aid of the computer program RFT 1 (5).

Since the differences between the WGA-binding
and not WGA-binding receptors appear rather
small (Fig. 1a), an identity test was performed
by superimposition of the 95 % coinfidence limits
for K_R and Y_o. The resulting joint coinfidence
envelopes (Fig. 1b) permit the following conclusions: a) Both receptor– detergent complexes
are significantly $(p < (0.05)^2 = 0.0025)$ different.
b) The coinfidence envelopes are displaced
along the y-axis, thus demonstrating that both
complexes differ in charge and not in respect
to the size (5).

The molecular net charge of the receptor-
detergent complexes can be determined from the
Y_δ-values. This computation is based on a number of assumptions (5) and results in a
valence of 9.28 net protons/molecule for the
WGA-binding receptor and 11.25 for the receptor
which does not bind to WGA (program CHARGE).

The following conclusions might be drawn:
a) The occurence of a regulatory G-protein in
the WGA-binding receptor-detergent complex can
be excluded since the molecular weight of the
receptor (65 000 D, see below) and the presently
known G-proteins (45 000 + 35 000 D) would
exceed the roughly calculated molecular weight
of the receptor-detergent complex (116 000 D).

However, it cannot be excluded, that a low mole·
cular weight glycoprotein is associated with th₁
receptor, thus substituting a certain amount of
detergent, so that the overall molecular size
of the complex remains unchanged.
b) The other alternative might be the occurence
of gangliosides (source of NANA?) within the
WGA-binding receptor-detergent complex. The not
WGA-binding receptor might have lost these gangliosides during the first extraction step, but
should contain significantly more other charged
components (phospholipids?) according to its
higher net charge.

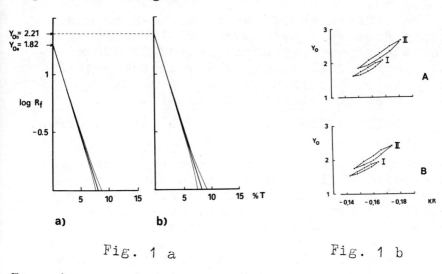

Fig. 1 a   Fig. 1 b

Fig. 1
a) Weighted regression analysis of Ferguson
plots from tris/glycinate electrophoresis of
WGA-binding (a) and not WGA-binding (b) muscarinic receptors (program RFT 1; % T= 4, 5, 6, 7;
n = 6; redrawn from the computer output).
b) Joint 95 % coinfidence envelopes for K_R and
Y_o, indicating that the significant differences
between the WGA-binding (I) and not WGA-binding
(II) receptor are due to charge differences.
This is not dependent on the mode of Rf-deter-
mination (compare A and B).

Since the previous molecular weight determinations of the covalently labelled (^{3}H-PrBCM) muscarinic binding site were based on SDS-electrophoresis at only one gel concentration, we performed these experiments on the basis of Ferguson plot analysis which is considered to permit a higher accuracy (5). These Ferguson plots (6 standard proteins; % T = 5,7,8,9,10; n = 3) were analysed by weighted regression (program RFT 1). Based on the regression line for the K_R values of the standard proteins and their molecular weight, the molecular weight for the muscarinic receptor was computed (program RADKR, 5).

The difference of the results which was obtained by this procedure (65 128 D) to the previously reported data (around 80 000 D) is not due to proteolysis, the weighted regression analysis or the front marker as shown by different series of control experiments.

4. MUSCARINIC RECEPTORS IN ARTIFICIAL MEMBRANE SYSTEMS

Comprehensive experiments were performed in order to develop a first approach to the reconstitution of functional muscarinic receptors into artificial membrane systems. Since all approaches to direct incorporation of native solubilized receptors into a planar BLM failed, we examined the previous incorporation into liposomes. The highest yield of incorporated receptors was obtained by reconstitution into phosphatidyl choline liposomes during their generation by a detergent removal method (20.2 %) However, successful fusion of these liposomes with a planar brain lipid BLM could not be achieved (6). Therefore brain lipid liposomes (maximal yield of incorporated receptors: 4 %) were used. The fusion of these liposomes with the planar BLM could be clearly documented by the elektrical properties of the BLM (6).

However, no conductivity change could be induced
in the BLM either by muscarinic agonists or antagonists. No response could be obtained also after
fusion of synaptosomes with a planar brain lipid
BLM using similar techniques.

These obviously preliminary experiments indicate, that the muscarinic receptor itself might
be not an ionophore.

In order to examine the influence of the biophysical properteis of the lipid membrane on
the stability of muscarinic receptors, we formed
monolager structures from enriched synaptosomal
membranes. These films were characterized by
recording of the continously varied surface
pressure and surface potential. This technique
permitted the quantitative determination of
muscarinic receptors by ^{3}H-QNB binding in the
films which were sucked off after removal of
the free ligand from the subphase buffer.

After correction of the dissociation rate,
a decrease of the specific binding could be
found neither after formation of a true monolayer nor after expansion of the monolayer to
a surface pressure of 0 dyn/cm (7). It might
be concluded, that the native conformation of
the muscarinic receptor is not dependent on an
ordered structure of the lipid membrane.

Summarizing the following picture of the
molecular structure of the muscarinic receptor
might be drawn: Contrary to others we found
a molecular weight of 65 000 D and an isoelectric
point of 4.4 (4). No indications for smaler
subunits or larger aggregates could be
found in our experiments using either native
or denaturated receptors. Heterogenous agonist
binding sites are not due to subunit assembly
since they were found in both receptor preparations. An association of the receptor with
one of the known G-proteins is rather unlikekly.
A different lipid (especially ganglioside)
composition in the receptor-detergent complex

a well as in the membrane might be of striking
importance for the receptor conformation, althoug:
the stability of the receptor is not dependend
on on ordered lipid layer.

There is no indication for a sugar component
(containing NANA) of the muscarinic receptor,
since the WGA-binding moiety is not covalently
linked to the muscarinic binding site. This
component is not responsible for the heterogeneity of agonist binding.

It is likely, that the receptor transmits
a presently unknown signal to calcium and
potassium ionophores but is not an ionophore
itself.

Acknowledgements

The author gratefully acknowledges the valuable
contributions of Drs. M. Schmitt, J. Gaál and
A. Chrambach to this study.

References

1. Venter, J.C. (1983) J. Biol. Chem. 258,
   4842-4848.
2. Avissar, S., G. Amitai and M. Sokolovsky
   (1983) Proc. Natl. Acad. Sci. USA 80, 156-159.
3. Potter, L.T. et al. (1984) TIPS Suppl.
   Jan. 84, 22-31
4. Repke, H. and H. Matthies (1980) Brain Res.
   Bull. 5, 703-709.
5. Chrambach A. and D. Robard (1980) In: Gel
   electrophoresis of proteins: A practical
   approach, B. D. Hames and D. Rickwood,
   (eds.). IRL Press Ltd. London
6. Repke, H., A. Berczi and H. Matthies (1980)
   Acta biol. med. germ. 39, 657-663.
7. Repke H. and I.Szundi (1983) studia biophys.
   97, 165-175.

TIME-AVERAGED PHOSPHORESCENCE STUDIES OF (Ca^{2+}-Mg^{2+})ATPASE ROTATIONAL DIFFUSION.

COLIN J. RESTALL and DENNIS CHAPMAN

Department of Biochemistry and Chemistry,
Royal Free Hospital School of Medicine,
Rowland Hill Street,
London, NW3 2PF
U.K.

The measurement of protein mobility can be used to provide valuble information about membrane dynamics and can potentially yield data relating the structure and movement to enzymatic function. However, the traditional methods of measuring protein rotational diffusion involve the use of complex and expensive apparatus. In an effort to make protein rotational diffusion measurements available to a greater number of laboratories we have recently described a new technique, termed time-averaged phosphorescence polarization, for qualitatively measuring the rotational diffusion of intrinsic proteins in biological membranes [1]. This technique has the dual advantages of being both quick and easily performed on a commercially available luminescence spectrometer.

A prerequisite for the measurement of rotational diffusion using phosphorescence emission techniques is the presence of a suitable phosphor linked to the molecule of interest. Typically, this is a compound such as erythrosin isothiocyanate. Excitation of this compound with a brief pulse of light under appropriate conditions results in transient emission of phosphorescence at wavelengths greater than 650nm [1,2]. When the

Proceedings of the 16th FEBS Congress
Part B, pp. 509–514

excitation beam is plane polarized, the phosphorescence emission is also polarized and the time for which the emitted light remains polarized is dependent upon the degree of movement that the phosphor is allowed. The greater the freedom or rate of movement, the faster the phosphorescence emission becomes depolarized. The degree of polarization is usually measured by monitoring the level of light emission both parallel (I_{VV}) and perpendicular (I_{VH}) to the vertically polarized excitation beam and then calculating the emission anisotropy $R = (I_{VV} - I_{VH})/(I_{VV} + 2I_{VH})$.

The technique of time averaged phosphorescence polarization relies upon exciting the sample with a flash of plane polarized light and then integrating the intensities of phosphorescent light emitted both parallel and perpendicular to the polarization plane of the exciting light. The integration is performed over a preset time interval corresponding to the time over which the anisotropy is expected to decay and then using these integrated intensities, the anisotropy is calculated as described earlier.

We have recently used the technique of time-averaged phosphorescence to study the interaction of calcium ions and ATP with the calcium-dependent adenosine triphosphatase ((Ca^{2+}-Mg^{2+})ATPase) in sarcoplasmic reticulum membranes. Earlier studies have indicated how the binding of calcium ions to the (Ca^{2+}-Mg^{2+})ATPase affects both the level of the intrinsic tryptophan fluorescence and the fluorescence yield of fluorescein isothiocyanate covalently bonded to the protein [3,4]. Other studies have, in turn, shown how these effects are coupled with changes in the availability of sulphydryl and carboxyl groups [6,7] leading to the idea that a conformational change in the protein structure was occurring. The advantage of using methods such as phosphorescence polarization to investigate interactions like calcium ions with the $(Ca^{2+}-Mg^{2+})$ATPase is that they directly monitor the protein mobility. This is in contrast with other methods which infer a conformational change based upon the observation of a secondary effect.

Our studies have shown that the addition of excess calcium ions to erythrosin isothiocyanate-labelled $(Ca^{2+}-Mg^{2+})$ATPase results in a lowering of the phosphorescence emission anisotropy by about 20%. Reducing the free calcium level once more by the addition of excess ethyleneglycol-bis-(β-aminoethyl ether)N,N'-tetraacetic acid (EGTA) restored the anisotropy to its initial value. The reduction in the emission anisotropy caused by calcium ions was found to be completely abolished by the presence of 1mM n-ethyl maleimide. This is in accord with the earlier studies on the tryptophan and fluorescein fluorescence [3,4].

Time averaged phosphorescence alone cannot distinguish between a simple change in mobility and a conformational change in the protein structure. Therefore, to examine in more detail the nature of the changes observed when calcium ions are added to the $(Ca^{2+}-Mg^{2+})$ATPase, time-resolved phosphorescence polarization was used. This technique differs from the simpler time-averaged method in that following excitation of the sample with a light pulse, the emission anisotropy is followed with time by rapid sampling (every μs) over a discrete interval. A complete time-course of the emission anisotropy is therefore obtained.

The detailed analysis of time-resolved phosphorescence polarization measurements is capable of yielding much information about

511

molecular dynamics [8]. In this study however, the complex segmental movement of the $(Ca^{2+}-Mg^{2+})$ATPase was analysed in terms of an equation comprising two exponential terms plus a constant. The results of such an analysis revealed that the apparent relaxation times of the protein had changed very little and that the decrease in anisotropy was caused by a change in the pre-exponential terms. Since these terms are governed by the angular displacement of the probe as it reorients, it follows that a change in the conformation of the protein must have occurred such that the portion of the protein on which the probe is located has now assumed a new orientation.

The effect of ATP on the time-averaged phosphorescence polarization was also investigated. Up to 10μM ATP, no effects were observed but at levels of 1 and 5mM, a decrease in the anisotropy of about 15% was observed. Since the $(Ca^{2+}-Mg^{2+})$ATPase has both a high affinity, catalytic site (Kd about 10μM) and a low affinity, regulatory site (Kd in the millimolar range), [9] the results suggest the ATP is interacting with the low affinity site in these studies. When ATP is added, giving a final concentration of 5mM, to a system in which excess Ca^{2+} are already present, a further decrease in the anisotropy is observed. This cumulative effect is also apparent if excess Ca^{2+} are added to a system containing 5mM ATP. Furthermore, the total decrease in anisotropy obtained after the addition of both Ca^{2+} and ATP appears to be independent of the order in which the ligands are added.

Consideration of the reaction sequence of the $(Ca^{2+}-Mg^{2+})$ATPase proposed by de Meis and Vianna [10] leads us to conclude that the two forms of the enzyme responsible for the high and low anisotropy terms are most likely to be

512

the E_2 and E_1 forms respectively. Since the E_1 to E_2 step is believed to be responsible for calcium translocation it is possible that phosphorescence emission polarization may be able to provide insights into how proteins pump ions across membranes.

References

1. Murray, E.K., Restall, C.J. and Chapman, D. (1983). Monitoring membrane protein rotational diffusion using time-averaged phosphorescence. Biochim. Biophys. Acta 732, 347-351.
2. Garland, P.B. and Moore, C,H. (1979). Phosphorescence of protein-bound eosin and erythrosin. A possible probe for measure-ments of slow rotational mobility. Biochem. J. 183, 561-572.
3. Dupont, Y. (1976). Fluorescence studies of the sarcoplasmic reticulum calcium pump. Biochem. Biophys. Res. Commun. 71, 544-550.
4. Pick, U. and Karlish, S.J.D. (1980). Indications for an oligomeric structure and for conformational changes in sarcoplasmic reticulum Ca^{2+}-ATPase labelled selectively with fluorescein. Biochim. Biophys. Acta 626, 255-261.
5. Pick, U. (1981). Dynamic interconversions of phosphorylated and non-phosphorylated intermediates of the Ca-ATPase from sarco-plasmic reticulum followed in a fluorescein-labeled enzyme. Biochim. Biophys. Acta 123, 131-136.
6. Murphy, A.J. (1976). Sulfhydryl group modification of sarcoplasmic reticulum mem-branes. Biochemistry 15, 4492-4496.
7. Pick, U. and Racker, E. (1979). Inhibition of the (Ca^{2+})ATPase from sarcoplasmic reticulum by dicyclohexylcarbodiimide: Evidence for location of the Ca^{2+} binding

513

site in a hydrophobic region. Biochemistry 18, 108-113

8. Restall, C.J., Dale, R.E., Murray, E.K., Gilbert, C.W. and Chapman, D. (1984). Rotational diffusion of the calcium-dependent ATPase in sarcoplasmic reticulum - A detailed study. Biochemistry (in press).
9. Verjovski-Almeida, S. and Inesi, G. (1979). Fast-kinetic evidence for an activating effect of ATP on the Ca^{2+} transport of sarcoplasmic reticulum ATPase. J. Biol. Chem. 254, 18-21.
10. de Meis, L. and Vianna, A. (1979). Energy interconversions by the Ca^{2+}-dependent ATPase of the sarcoplasmic reticulum. Ann. Rev. Biochem. 48, 275-292.

REORGANIZATION OF INNER MITOCHONDRIAL MEMBRANE AND REVERSIBLE PROTEIN TRANSLOCATION.

ALBERT WAKSMAN[a], GERARD CREMEL[b], PIERRE HUBERT[c], CHRISTINE MUTET and CLAUDE BURGUN.
Centre de Neurochimie du CNRS - 5, rue Blaise Pascal - 67084 Strasbourg Cedex - France.
[a]Maître de Recherche au CNRS - [b]Chargé de Recherche à l'INSERM - [c]Attaché de Recherche à l'INSERM.

INTRODUCTION

Biological membranes can be defined either :
- as structures separating in space the different cellular and subcellular compartments and which possess the opposite property to unify specifically these compartments by conveying information and transporting matter from one side to the other of the membrane ;
- as spacio temporal structures endowed with self assembly properties and whose cohesion is insured by non covalent bonds.
This last approach leads to the view that the temporal localization of any membrane component is ruled by its chemical potential as modulated by the nearby inter-acting forces, which are the electrostatic and the hydro-phobic forces.
The question that follows is whether in the course of the constant remodelling of the membrane occuring under the pressure of these ever varying forces some of the membrane components could be brought to change comport-ment or to move across the membrane altogether (1).
Protein translocation across biological membranes has been associated with diverse physiological functions including protein secretion, protein turnover, receptor expression and modulation, action of toxins, ligand transport, etc... (2,3,4,5).
We shall report in this paper the experimental evidence for one of the mechanisms proposed for protein translo-cation through inner mitochondrial membrane : environmen-tally-induced reversible translocation. We shall focus

Proceedings of the 16th FEBS Congress
Part B, pp. 515–525
© 1985 VNU Science Press

more particularly our attention on the reversible translocation of two enzymes : aspartate aminotransferase (AAT) which is to be found on the inner face, of the inner mitochondrial membrane in a mitochondria isolated in isotonic sucrose, and malate deshydrogenase (MDH) which is under similar conditions a matrix enzyme. Translocation occurs in presence of molecules such succinate, fumarate, oxalacetate, pyruvate, phenylsuccinate... substances that we shall call movement effectors. Well defined and controlled techniques are available to separate the different submitochondrial compartments which makes the mitochondria a perfectly suited tool for the proposed studies (6,8) (Fig. 1).

MATERIAL AND METHODS

were those described in (1,6,7,8)

Reversible protein translocation through inner mitochondrial membrane

The following observations confirm the view that changes in exogenous environment mediate perimembranal relocalization of membrane or perimembrane proteins.

Movement effectors provoke release or translocation of matrix proteins or proteins bound to the inner face of the inner membrane into the intermembrane space. When mitochondria were isolated in 0.25 M sucrose and incubated (5 min at 37°C) in the presence of succinate (0 to 50 mM), translocation of up to 75 % of aspartate aminotransferase (AAT) from the inner face of the inner membrane where it was localized initially to the intermembrane space could be observed. Likewise up to 50 % of the malate deshydrogenase (MDH) initially present in the matrix relocalized in the intermembrane space. It was found also that the total protein concentration in the intermembrane space increased in the presence of succinate ; however, this was not a general phenomenon since cytochrome oxidase, as might be expected for an intrinsic protein of the inner membrane, did not move (8).

Figure 1 - Environmentally-induced aspartate aminotransferase movement within the mitochondria (Methodology).
Step 1 : Succinate 50 mM (or less) provokes externalization of AAT into intermembrane fluid (10 % AAT = ∗). 0.8
mg of digitonin per 10 mg protein removes outer membrane.
Mitoplasts were separated from intermembrane fluid by
differential centrifugation.
Step 2 : Fluid containing externalized protein was dialyzed, concentrated and reincubated with the above mitoplasts, leading to vesicles where AAT reinternalized.
AAT activity in presence of non permeant substrate, accessibility to specific antibodies or accessibility of 125I
AAT to protease were tested on such vesicles.
Step 3 : Corresponding inside out vesicles were prepared
and tested for AAT accessibility using the same methods
as for mitoplasts (see step 2).

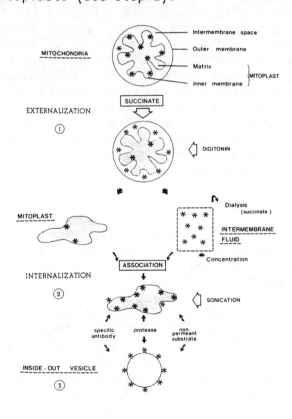

Before these results could be interpreted in terms of protein translocation across the inner membrane proof was provided that the integrity of the mitoplast was preserved during the incubations (7).

Aspartate aminotransferase and other externalized proteins resume their initial localization upon removal of the externalizing movement effectors. Data supporting this statement are best summarized by the following experiments.
Upon removal of the movement effector (succinate) 70 % of the previous released AAT, rebinds to mitoplast (Fig. 2) of which 60 % loses accessibility to non-permeant substrate as well as to controlled proteolytic digestion (Fig. 2) and to specific 125I labeled antibody on its outer face whereas it gains accessibility on its inner face as shown by the accessibility of bound AAT in inverted vesicles. The method used to explore both faces of the mitoplast is described in Figure 1. The results clearly show that although 70 % to 80 % of AAT rebound to the mitoplast, never more than 30 % of that bound activity was accessible on the outer face of this vesicle. However, by preparing the corresponding inside-out vesicles, the missing 70 % of the enzyme was now accessible and was detected by the three methods outlined above. Thus, approximately 70 % of the rebound enzyme had traversed the inner membrane (6).

Specificity of translocation

If one expects this phenomenon to play a physiological role, its two major properties would be reversibility and specificity. Reversibility was demonstrated above, what about specificity ?

Movement effectors provoke protein redistribution in membrane and perimembrane compartments. This is shown in a qualitative way by comparing electrophoretic protein patterns in the intermembrane fluid after incubation of mitochondria in the presence of different movement effectors. Polyacrylamide gel electrophoresis

Figure 2 - After rebinding to mitoplast AAT loses accessibility to non permeant cofactor NADH (coupled reaction), and thus becomes latent, and to antibody. ^{125}I labelled AAT loses accessibility to protease (6). Whereas total enzyme presence can be detected by the above three methods after thorough sonication of the particles. Moreover AAT rebound to inside out vesicles becomes accessible with regards to the three methods used ($*$ = 10 % AAT).

ACCESSIBILITY OF **AAT** AFTER INTERNALIZATION

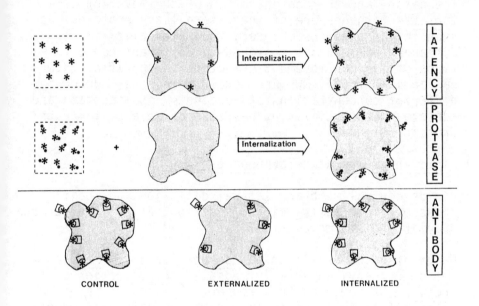

CONTROL   EXTERNALIZED   INTERNALIZED

of the fluids obtained from mitochondria exposed to sucrose alone, sucrose plus pyruvate, 2-oxoglutarate or malate showed that, although there were common protein bands, the pattern differed with each movement effector (8,11). Some of the protein bands that were present in the intermembrane compartment of sucrose-incubated mitochondria disappeared when pyruvate or 2-oxoglutarate was added, suggesting that a more general reorganization of the perimembranal compartments occured upon modification of the environment. This was further confirmed

519

by testing the influence of different movement effectors on the specific repartition of AAT between intermembrane, inner membrane and matrix.
The latter results revealed specific patterns of repartition of AAT between these compartments, bringing up more evidence for the translocation of AAT across the inner membrane, and showing that the localization of the enzyme in each compartment is a function of the environment of the mitochondria (7).

The nature and the concentration of the movement effector affect the nature of the externalized proteins. As seen in the previous chapter, the externalization of different proteins as provoked by different concentrations of various movement effectors is specific. Externalization of AAT, MDH and total protein as induced by different concentrations of succinate, oxaloacetate and acetate, showed different patterns of release for each protein (8).

Lipid and temperature dependancy

Lipids control membrane lateral diffusion, do modifications of their fatty acid composition, affect the perpendicular protein movements ?

Fatty acid compositition of the phospholipid fraction influences environmentally mediated translocation of protein. We compared "environmentally-induced" protein externalization in mitochondria whose fatty acid compositions had been modified either as a consequence of diet or hibernation. In addition, it is known (12) that the fatty acid composition of mitochondria is different in nerve cell bodies and their corresponding nerve endings. Thus, these differences in mitochondria from the same cell family were also exploited to study their effects on protein translocation.
Comparison of the break point of Van t'Hoff curves for externalization, for theoretical melting points and for ratio of saturated fatty acids to polyunsaturated fatty acids showed that, the more "fluid" the membrane, in

terms of the lateral diffusion of lipids, the lower the temperature of the break in the Van t'Hoff curve for externalization of proteins (12). In the case of hibernators, the seasonal variation of the break of the Van t'Hoff curve compared to the variation in concentration of the most polyunsaturated fatty acid : docosohexanoïc acid (22:6), showed that the lower the concentration of this fatty acid, the higher the temperature of the break of the Van t'Hoff curve for protein externalization. This shows a relationship between fluidity and protein translocation but also suggests that a specific microenvironment might play a role in reversible protein movement (13).

Succinate and phenylsuccinate which provoke protein externalization also induce a greater fluidity of the lipid matrix at the membrane polar interface. Both fluorescence anisotropy measurements and EPR spectra obtained from succinate (or phenylsuccinate) incubated mitochondria and control mitochondria suggested a "fluidization" at the polar interface of the inner membrane of the incubated mitochondria. Thus if an increase of fluidity favors the externalization of AAT, MDH and total protein from mitoplast towards intermembrane space (see previous chapter), movement effectors which induce externalization of AAT, MDH and total protein, increase in turn the fluidity at the polar interface of the inner mitochondrial membrane. Doing so, they could promote more favorable (9) conditions for externalization to occur (Table 1). Furthermore, using paramagnetic probes which bind covalently to SH groups of the inner mitochondrial membrane it was possible to reveal the existence of two pools of sites, weakly and strongly immobilized. The later pool looses part of its accessibility to the SH probe MAL 6, when the mitochondria are incubated in presence of succinate (or phenylsuccinate) compared to control mitochondria exposed to sucrose alone (10).
These results suggest   change in protein configuration, leading to the partial "burial" in the membrane of these SH groups. This occurs simultaneously to an increase of fluidity of the bilayer at its polar interface.

Table 1 - Order parameters and correlation times of CDTAB, 5NMS, 12NMS and 16NMS in control-mitoplasts and in succinate-mitoplasts.

Label	Control mitoplasts		Succinate mitoplasts	
	S	τC(NS)	S	τC(NS)
CDTAB	0.69 (± 0.01)	-	0.62 (± 0.01)+	-
5NMS	0.72 (± 0.01)	-	0.69 (± 0.01)++	-
12NMS	0.54 (± 0.01)	-	0.50 (± 0.01)++	-
16NMS	-	1.82 (± 0.09)	-	1.76 (± 0.09)

S : order parameter ; τC : rotational correlation time expressed in nanoseconds ; + : P<0.005 ; ++ : P<0.01. CTAB : hexadecyl N,N dimethyl 4 amino 2,2-6,6 tetramethyl-pydine ; NMS : doxylstearic methylester-5,12,16 : position ofdoxylgroup.

Fluorescence anisotropy and rotational correlation time for the fluorescent probes : TMA-DPH and DPH in control-mitoplasts and in succinate-mitoplasts.

Label	Control mitoplasts		Succinate mitoplasts	
	τ(NS)	ρ(NS)	τ(NS)	ρ(NS)
DPH	7.9 (± 0.1)	20.7 (± 0.35)	7.9 (± 0.1)	20.1 (± 0.35)
TMA-DPH	4.1 (± 0.1)	17.4 (± 0.6)	4.0 (± 0.1)	15.5 (± 0.6)

τ is the life time expressed in nanoseconds ; ρ is the rotational relaxation time expressed in nanoseconds. DPH : diphenylhexatriene ; TMA-DPH : trimethyl-amonium-DPH.

Driving force

What drives reversible environmentally-induced protein translocation ? This phenomenon does not require energy derived from oxidative phosphorylation, nor the modification of the primary structure of the protein to be translocated. a) Reversible translocation does not seem to require oxidative phosphorylation. To test this hypothesis reversible translocation of AAT was assayed in presence of antimycin A, rotenone, 2,4-dinitrophenol, FCCP, amytal and atractylate, all inhibitors either of electron flux, or energy coupling. Under these conditions, the reversible movement of AAT still occured (8). Furthermore, phenylsuccinate, a non-permeant, non-metabolizable analogue of succinate also triggered externalization of the enzyme (8).
b) Translocation does not require the modification of primary structure of "mobile" AAT. After externalization, AAT was purified, labeled with $125I$ and internalized into mitoplasts ; after which it was re-externalized by addition of succinate. In these three situations (out, in and out of the mitoplast), molecular weight of AAT was compared by gel electrophoresis. The results clearly show no difference of apparent molecular weight. A configurational modification induced by the environment might thus be responsible for the reversible movement of protein (14).
c) The driving force for this protein movement may possibly be the chemical potential of the interacting membrane components and translocating protein as modulated by the presence or absence of movement effectors (specific molecules, salts, pH, etc...). This is illustrated by the experiment of Furaya, Yoshida and Tagawa (15) in which it was shown that mitochondrial AAT becomes latent and non-accessible to proteases, and thus probably internalized, when incubated in the presence of negatively charged liposomes but not in the presence of positively charged ones (15).

CONCLUSION

The above results and those we published elsewhere
(1,6,7,8) clearly show that proteins are able to cross
reversibly the inner mitochondrial membrane as a result
of membrane reorganization occuring under the influence
of the environment.

ACKNOWLEDGEMENTS

The work described in this review has been supported by
funds of the "Institut National de la Santé et de la
Recherche Médicale", n° 80.30.22, the "Fondation pour la
Recherche Médicale Française", n° 50.91.31.

REFERENCES

Waksman, A., Hubert, P., Crémel, G., Rendon, A. and
    Burgun, C. (1980). Translocation of proteins through
    biological membranes. A critical view. Biochim.
    Biophys. Acta 604, 249-296.
Palade, G.E. (1975). Intracellular aspects of the process
    of protein synthesis. Science 347-358.
Blobel, G. and Dobberstein B. (1975). Transfer of proteins
    across membranes. II-Reconstitution of functional
    rough microsomes from heterologous components. J.
    Cell. Biol. 67, 852-862.
Schatz, G. (1979). How mitochondria import proteins from
    cytoplasm. FEBS Lett. 103, 203-211.
Gill, D.M. (1978). Seven toxic peptides that cross cell
    membranes. In : Bacterial Toxins and Cell Membranes,
    J. Jeljaszewics and T. Walström (eds). Academic Press,
    New York, pp. 291-332.
Hubert, P., Crémel, G., Rendon, A., Sacko, B. and Waksman
    A. (1979) Direct evidence for internalization of mito-
    chondrial aspartate aminotransferase into mitoplasts.
    Biochemistry 18, 3119-3126.
Waksman, A., Rendon, A., Crémel, G., Pellicone, C. and
    Goubault de Brugière, J.F. (1977) Intramitochondrial
    intermembranal reversible translocation of aspartate

aminotransferase and malate dehydrogenase through the inner mitochondrial membrane. Biochemistry 16, 4703-4707.

Waksman, A. and Rendon, A. (1974). Intramitochondrial intermembranal large amplitude protein movements. I-A possible novel aspect of membrane fluidity. Biochimie 56, 907-924.

Mutet, C., Duportail, G., Crémel, G. and Waksman, A. (1984). Increase of the fluidity of the lipid bilayer of the inner mitochondrial membrane by succinate and phenylsuccinate : a study by EPR and fluorescence. Biochem. Biophys. Res. Comm. 119, 854-859.

Mutet, C., Crémel, G. and Waksman, A. (1984). Succinate and phenylsuccinate as modifiers of sulfhydryl groups of inner mitochondrial membranal protein. Study by EPR. Biochem. Biophys. Res. Comm. In press.

Goubault de Brugière, J.F. and Waksman, A. (1977). Relargage réversible de protéines dans la mitochondrie hépatique de rat : analyse par électrophorèse sur gel de polyacrylamide. Biochimie 59, 627-635.

Crémel, G., Rebel, G., Warter, J.M., Rendon, A. and Waksman, A. (1976). Reversible intramitochondrial release of protein related to unsaturated fatty acids of membranes. Arch. Biochem. Biophys. 173, 255-263.

Crémel, G., Rebel, G., Canguilhem, B., Rendon, A. and Waksman, A. (1979). Seasonal variation of the composition of membrane lipids in liver mitochondria of the hibernator Cricetus cricetus. Relation to intramitochondrial intermembranal protein movement. Comp. Biochem. Physiol. 63A, 159-167.

Waksman, A., Crémel, G., Hubert, P., Mutet, C. and Burgun, C. (1984). Large amplitude protein movement. What functions ? Biochem. Soc. Trans. 12, 378-381.

Furuya, E., Yoshida, Y. and Tagawa, K. (1979). Interaction of mitochondrial aspartate aminotransferase with negatively charge lecithin vesicles. J. Biochem. (Tokyo) 85, 1157-1163.

STRUCTURE AND FUNCTION OF PURE RENAL Na,K-ATPase

Peter Leth Jørgensen
Institute of Physiology
Aarhus University
8000 Aarhus C, Denmark

The goal of our studies is to solve the structure and mechanism of the Na,K-pump of mammalian kidney. An important aspect of the function of the Na,K-pump in both proximal and distal nephron segments is the coupling with carriers that mediate secondary active, μNa^+-driven transport of nutrients like glucose and aminoacids, of metabolites such as citrate or succinate, of medicamina like penicillin or the loop diuretics furosemide and bumethanide, and of ions like protons, calcium, phosphate or chloride [1]. In the thick ascending limb of Henle, transcellular NaCl transport consists of primary active transport of Na^+ across the basolateral membrane and secondary active transport of Cl^- across the lumen membrane. Correct understanding of this transport requires not only knowledge of Na,K-pump structure but also the isolation and characterization of the Na,K,Cl-cotransport system that mediates secondary active Cl-transport across the lumen membrane in coupling with transport of Na^+ along its gradient. This cotransport system is the receptor for the most potent loop-diuretics furosemide and bumethanide.

The purpose of this talk is to discuss recent developments in elucidation of Na,K-pump structure arising from analysis of two-dimensional membrane crystals and soluble preparations of fully active $\alpha\beta$-units. We will also pursue structure-function relationships between conformational transitions in the α-subunit and binding, occlusion and translocation of Na^+ and K^+.

Purification of the Na,K-pump and the Na,K,Cl-cotransporter

The red outer medulla of rabbit or pig kidney provided the

Proceedings of the 16th FEBS Congress
Part B, pp. 527–534

starting material for the first successful procedures of purification of the Na,K-pump or Na,K-ATPase [2]. In this tissue the
basolateral cell membranes of the TAL are tigthly packed with
Na,K-pump sites in a concentration exceeding 40 million sites
per cell as estimated by [^{3}H]-ouabain binding [3]. The Na,K-pump
remains embedded in the membrane throughout the purification
procedure and retains its assymmetric orientation in the
membrane. Formation of two-dimensional crystals suitable for
image analysis can be induced by incubation in vanadate or
phosphate solution. The pure preparation is an ideal object for
studying organization of the protein in the membrane and for
establishing structure-function relationships.

In contrast to the detailled information about Na,K-pump
structure and function little is known about the structure of the
Na,K,Cl-cotransport system. As shown in Fig. 1 the initial steps

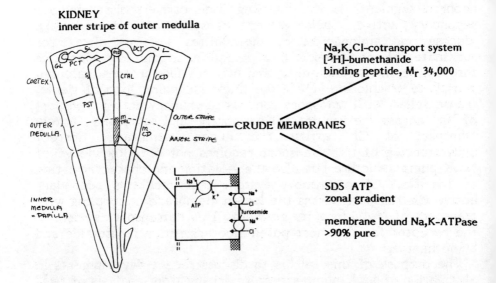

Figure 1
Summary of procedures for purification of Na,K-ATPase in
membrane bound form as described in Ref. 2 and for initial steps
of purification of the Na,K,Cl-cotransport system as described in
Ref. 4.

for purification of the Na,K-pump from the basal membrane
have proven of good value for isolation of the Na,K,Cl-cotrans-

porter from the lumen membrane. Recently we have identified a component of this transport system with M_r 34,000 by covalent binding of [^{3}H]-bumethanide after direct photolysis at 345 nm, a wavelength where the fluorescent bumethanide has an absorbtion maximum [4]. This technique for covalent labeling with [^{3}H]-bumethanide will be usefull for identifying the system both in membrane-bound and in soluble preparations. A procedure for reconstitution of the cotransport protein into phospholipid vesicles [5] has been developed to allow studies of structure-function relationships for the cotransport protein. Assay of transport in reconstituted vesicles is also required to ensure that the entire cotransport system has been isolated in a given purification scheme.

Preliminary centrifugation data and experiments with detergent extraction show that the bumethanide binding protein is associated with cytoskeleton components suggesting that these associations are important for regulation of the transcellular transport processes [4].

Shape and structure of the Na,K-pump in membrane crystals

The Na,K-pump molecules are tightly packed in the lipid bilayer of the discs-shaped membrane fragments of the pure preparation. The average concentration of α-subunit in the lipid phase amounts to 6-8 mM corresponding to almost 1 gram protein per ml of lipid phase. In these conditions of supersaturation, the protein associates rather easily in two dimensions and forms crystalline arrays [6]. Already within hours after start of incubation in vanadate or phosphate medium formation of linear polymers, some of them dimeric is observed in the membranes. Later these polymers associate laterally to form two-dimensional arrays.

Computer based image prossessing of electron micrographs of the negatively stained crystals shows that the unit cell contains one αβ-unit, Fig. 2 and that the symmetry in the vanadate crystal is p1. The part of the particle protruding above the plane the bilayer is a compact structure with diameter close to 50 Å without evidence for a two-fold rotational symmetry between particles Fig. 2. These observations show that the αβ-unit is the minimum asymmetric unit of Na,K-ATPase in the membrane [6].

The unit cell in the arrays grown in phosphate medium contains two strong positive regions. These regions are subdivided into one large and one smaller peak possibly corresponding to α-subunits and β-subunits, respectively. The symmetry is p21 and two αβ-units can easily occupy one unit cell. Using the same techniques, the Ca-ATPase from sarcoplasmic reticulum also forms two-dimensional crystals [8]. In parallel with the 40% larger molecular weight of Na,K-ATPase due to the presence of the β-subunit the a-lattice dimensions of Na,K-ATPase is 40% larger than that of Ca-ATPase.

Computer reconstruction of negatively stained two-dimensional crystals thus gives a diameter of 5 nm for the protein portion protruding from the membrane surface. It should be remembered

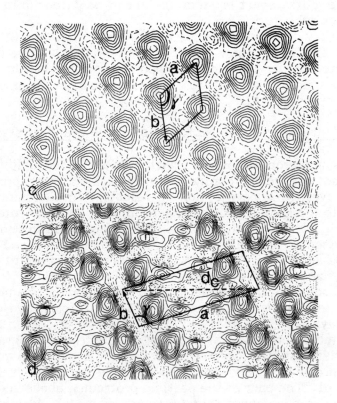

Figure 2.
Computer reconstructed images of two dimensional crystals of Na,K-pump protein formed in vanadate as described before in Refs. 6 and 7.

530

that negative staining only reveals external hydrophilic surface components while details within the lipid bilayer and the protein molecule remain obscure. Information about these features of the Na,K-pump structure requires more extensive and regular crystals and preferably the preparation of three-dimensional crystals.

Subunit structure of soluble renal Na,K-ATPase

The analysis of the crystal lattices shows that the $\alpha\beta$-unit is the minimum asymmetric unit in the membrane, but the observation of two crystal structures clearly presents the problem of the subunit structure of Na,K-ATPase. If the pump consists of only one $\alpha\beta$-unit, the pathway for cations must pass through the structure of the $\alpha\beta$-unit. If formation of oligomer $(\alpha\beta)_2$-units is required for transport, the cation pathway may be formed in the interface between two subunits.

We currently try two apprachs to this problem. One is to obtain a 3 demensional structure by electron diffraction analysis, but the resolution of 20-25 Å in the crystals currently available may not be sufficient to identify structural detail.

The other approach is biochemical and hydrodynamic studies of the pump protein. Soluble and fully active Na,K-ATPase is prepared by incubation of the pure membrane-bound Na,K-ATPase with $C_{12}E_8$ in ratio 2-3. The soluble and fully active Na,K-ATPase has M_r 140.000-170.000 and $S_{20,w}$ is 7.0-7.3 [9,10]. The analysis show that there is one site for binding of ATP [11] and phosphorylation per $\alpha\beta$-unit both in the membrane bound enzyme and after solubulization in $C_{12}E_8$. The $\alpha\beta$-unit is therefore also the minimum active protein unit of soluble Na,K-ATPase.

Conformational transitions in soluble $\alpha\beta$-units

One requirement for accepting the $\alpha\beta$-unit as the transport system is that it can undergo the conformational transitions between E_1 and E_2 that can be associated with cation exchange by the membrane bound pump.

The transition from E_1 to E_2 involves motion of 60-100 residues in the α-subunit. This was first demonstrated as a change in pattern of tryptic digestion [12] and by changes in fluorescence from intrinsic tryptophan and exctrinsic probes [13].

531

Both E_1 and E_2 exist in dephosphoforms and in phosphoforms. In E_1-forms cation sites face the cytoplasmic surface. E_1P is a high energy intermediate as it has sufficient energy to react with ADP to form ATP. In absence of ATP E_1 binds K with high affinity and undergoes transition to E_2K. In E_2 -forms cation sites are exposed to the extracellular surface. In presence of K, E_2P reacts with water to release P_i. The rate limiting step in the reaction cycle is the transition from E_2K to E_1. The rate is determined by the cytoplasmic concentration of ATP, Na and K.

Analysis of proteolytic cleavage and fluorescence responses show that the conformational transitions in the α-subunit are the same for the soluble αβ-unit as in the membrane bound system. From this point of view the αβ-unit is therefore competent as a transport system and α-α subunit interaction need not be involved in the conformational transitions.

Localization of the conformational transition within the α-subunit

The alternating exposure of bonds within the α-subunit to proteolytic cleavage is illustrated in Fig. 3.

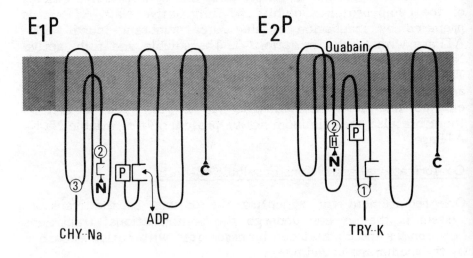

Figure 4.
Model for arrangement of the α-subunit in E_1P and E_2P forms of Na,K-ATPase. The encircled numbers mark the sites of primary tryptic cleavage in KCl (1) or chymotryptic cleavage in NaCl (3).

The potentially most interesting part of the α-subunit is localized between bond 1 and 3 since it contains the aspartyl phosphate. Selective cleavage of these two bonds can be used to examine structure-frunction relationships of this protein. We have isolated this segment and are currently examining its structure.

Examination of Na/Na or K/K-exchange reactions after selective cleavage with trypsin or chymotrypsin demonstrates the tight coupling of conformational transition to cation binding and exchange. Selective cleavage of bond 3 with chymotrypsin abolish the motion of the protein and stabilizes the protein in the E_1-form without interfering with ligand binding. This may be due to interruption of cooperation between ionizable group in the N-terminal segment and the phosphorylated part. The split also interrupts cooperation between cation sites and the nucleotide binding area

Analysis of tryptophan fluorescence, labeling from within the lipid bilayer and differential thermal inactivation show that the transitions from E_1P to E_2P involves movement of the segment with molecular weight 18,000 from relatively hydrophilic to hydrophobic microenvironment. Further elucidation of the relationship of this motion in the protein to cation transport requires identification of the cation sites and their structural relationship to the parts of the α-subunit that are engaged in the conformational transition accompanying cation translocation.

ACKNOWLEDGEMENTS: The study was supported by the Danism Medical Research Council and Novo's Foundation

REFERENCES
1. P.L.Jørgensen (1980). Na,K-ion pump in kidney tubules. Physiol. Rev. 60:864-917
2. P.L. Jørgensen (1974) Isolation of Na,K-ATPase. Methods Enzymol. 32B:277-290.
3. G.E. Mernissi and A. Doucet (1984) Quantitation of [^{3}H]-ouabain binding and turnover of Na,K-ATPase along the rabbit nephron. Am. J. Physiol. 247:F158-F167
4. P.L. Jørgensen, J. Petersen and W.D. Rees (1984) Identification of a Na,K,Cl-cotransport protein of M_r 34,000 from kidney by photolabeling with [^{3}H]-bumethanide. The protein is association with cytoskeleton components. Biochim. Biophys. Acta, 775:105-110

5. C.E. Burnham, P.L. Jørgensen and S.J.D. Karlish (1984) Reconstitution of Na,K,Cl-cotransporter and a barium sensitive K-channel from luminal membranes of rabbit outer renal medulla. Proc. 8th Int. Biophysics Contress, Abstract.

6. H. Hebert, P.L. Jørgensen, E. Skriver and A.B. Maunsbach (1982) Crystallization patterns of membrane-bound Na,K-ATPase. Biochim. Biophys. Acta 689:571-574

7. P.L. Jørgensen, E. Skriver, H. Hebers and A.B. Maunsbach (1982) Structure of the Na,K-pump: Crystallization of pure membrane-bound Na,K-ATPase and identification of functional domains of the α-subunit. Ann. New York Acad. Sci. 402:207-225

8. L. Dux and A. Martonosi (1984) Membrane crystals of Ca-ATPase in sarcoplasmic reticulum of fast and slow skeletal and cardiac muscles. Eur. J. Biochem. 141, 43-49

9. J.R. Brotherus, J.V. Møller and P.L. Jørgensen (1981) Soluble and active renal Na,K-ATPasse with maximum protein molecular mass 170,000+9,000 daltons; formation of larger units by secondary aggregation. Biochem. Biophys. Res. Commun. 100:146-154

10. J.R. Brotherus, L. Jacobsen and P.L. Jørgensen (1983) Soluble and enzymatically stable Na,K-ATPase from mammalian kidney consisting predominantly of protomer αβ-units. Preparation assay and reconstitution of active Na,K-transport. Biochim. Biopphys. Acta 731:290-303

11. J. Jensen and P. Ottolenghi (1983) ATP binding to solubilized Na,K-ATPase. The abolition of subunit-subunit interaction and the maximum weight of the nucleotide-binding unit. Biochim. Biophys. Acta 731:282-289

12. P.L. Jørgensen (1975) Purification and characterization of Na,K-ATPase. V. Conformational changes in the enzyme. Transitions between the Na-form and the K-form studied with tryptic digestion as a tool. Biochim. Biophys. Acta 401:399-415

13. S.J.D. Karlish and D.W: Yates (1978) Tryptophan fluorescence of Na,K-ATPase as a tool for study of the enzyme mechanism. Biochim. Biophys. Acta 527:115-130

INVESTIGATION OF MEMBRANE PROTEINS OF HALOBACTERIA, LACTOBACILLI AND MICROCOCCI

D. N. OSTROVSKY

A. N. Bakh Institute of Biochemistry, Moscow, USSR

Any membrane protein is an object of great interest and presents a puzzle for researchers. A story I am going to tell you is centered round the radiation inactivation approach to some specific features of selected membrane enzymes in three representatives of bacterial world (1). They are:

1. What are the molecular dimensions of some key enzymes od bacterial energetics which resist purification (e.g. enzymes in Halobacteria membranes) ?
2. Do the subunits of oligomeric enzymes (e.g. those of Lactobacillus casei ATP-ase) function in a cooperative manner or independently?
3. What is the mechanism of interaction of a multi-enzyme complex components (e.g. the respiratory chain components in Micriciccus luteus membranes) ?

The rationale for this is that in spite of well documented phenomenon of dicyclohexilcarbodiimide sensitivity of ATP synthesis in Halobacteria, we could not find in the literature direct evidence of H^+-ATP-ase presence in the membrane preparations.

Two explanations were put forward: 1) there is no ATPase in Halobacteria membranes at all because it is replaced by DCCD-sensitive pyrophosphatase notorious for its ability to synthesize macroergic pyrophosphate bond in certain bacteria and even in mitochondria, 2) There are some pecularities in the structure of halobacterial ATP-ase and then it would be of interest to compare it with another example of the very unusual H^+ATP-ase recently discovered in our laboratory in Lactobacillus casei.

So, we isolated Halobacterium halobium membranes by centrifugation of cells broken in Hughes press and

Proceedings of the 16th FEBS Congress
Part B, pp. 535–543
© 1985 VNU Science Press

found out that they contained the largest porion of
the cell'NADH-dehydrogenase and less than 0.1% of the
total pyrophosphatase activity and all but very weak
ATP-ase (2).

Membrane samples and cell free homogenates were frozen in the small glass tubes and irradiated with the
fast electrones in vertical electrone accelerator.

As one can see on Fig. 1, where $-\ln A/A_o$ (activity
at certain dose to initial activity) is given as a
function of the radiation dose, the sensitivity of the
three enzymes is quite different, ATP-ase being much
more susceptible to radiation inactivation than Pyrophosphatase and NADH-dehydrogenase.

Molecular masses of the enzymes can be calculated
from the empirical equation of Hutchinson and Pollard
$M = 0.72 \times 10^{12}D_{37}$ where D_{37} is a dose at which only
37% of initial activity is discovered (3).

Thus according to the data presented molecular masses
approximately are 300.000 for ATPase, 160.000 for
Pyrophosphatase and 20.000 for NADH dehydrogenase.

Those enzymes from others sources, e.g. from E.coli,
are comparable in size (E.coli ATP-ase M=382.000,
pyrophosphatase M=120.000 and NADH dehydrogenase M=
47.000) but E.coli NADH dehydrogenase is twice as large
as that in H.halobium (Table 1., (4-9)).

Halobacterial enzymes are quickly inactivated in
solutions of low ionic strength, and immunochemical
analysis is hardly applicable in this case. However,
we were lucky to detect NADH dehydrogenase on agarose
plates after electrophoresis of the Triton X-100 solubilized cell antigens through the space, containing
rabbit antibodies raised against the whole cells.

Brown line (Fig. 2) of reduced electrone acceptor
tetra nitroblue tetrasolium reveales the position of
the dehydrogenase while blue lines appear after Coumassie staining.

Fig. 2 shows that NADH dehydrogenase is not visualized
by staining with Coumassie only and Fig. 2d illustrates
crossed (two dimensional) immunoelectrophoresis of the
same material.

This finding provided us with a necessary tool for the determination of the subunit composition of the dehydrogenase. After in vivo labeling with ^{14}C-amino acids and rocket immunoelectrophoresis (Fig. 2c) we cut out the dehydrogenase band and reelectrophoresed it in the polyacrylamide gel with SDS containing buffer and determined the position of radioactivity in the gel. In this experiment heavy (H) and light (L) chains of immunoglobulins served as intrinsic standards of molecular mass (Fig. 3). So, the target size of H.halobium NADH-dehydrogenase for radiation inactivation is close to the dimensions of this subunit ($M_r \neq 25.000$).

It is of interest to note that some other halobacterial enzymes are smaller than their analogs from other bacteria. E.g. alcaline phosphatase according to Fitt and Peterkin (7) constitutes one fifth of E.coli enzyme while ketoacid oxidase complex is only 1/10 th of that in E.coli (Table 1.).

To finish the story about Halobacteria I must confess that ATP-ase though very specific to nucleotide, is not inhibited either by DCCD or by vanadate, so its involvement in the bacterial energetics is still under question (2).

In this respect H$^+$ATP-ase of L.casei is more reliable fellow. It is recently shown in joint research of our Laboratory and Moscow University that H$^+$ATP-ase of this anaerobic bacterie can be purified as a hexamer of equal subunits, 43 KDa each (10), thus significantly differing from H$^+$ATP-ases from other sources usually composed of 9 subunits of 5 different types.

This poses the question: is the structural simplification of L.casei ATP-ase accompanied with simplified functional mode, in other words: do the subunits work in cooperative fashion or independent. Radiation inactivation data may help to touch the problem. On Fig. 4 one can see inactivation curves for L.casei and M. luteus ATP-ase in comparison. Calculated molecular dimensions correspond to >70% of actual molecular size, the deflection being possible due to inaccuracy in the dose determination.

Thus all the subunits are needed for the H$^+$-ATP-ase functioning, no matter are they equal in size or not.

The next problem for discussion is the mechanism of interactions within a multienzyme system - M.luteus respiratory chain. In order to make a choise between the diffusion limited and stable assembly mediated process we compared the radiation sensitive target sizes of intact and crosslinked respiring membranes (11).

Professor Y. Kagawa was the first to notice that the respiratory chain target size was very small and comparable with that of individual components (12). We confirm this for M.luteus membranes because inactivation of NADH dehydrogenase and NADH oxidase follow the same law which correspond molecular mass about 47.000. We consider this to be a good indication of no stable respiratory assembly.

On the other hand, crosslinking of proteins with glutar-aldehyde which makes free diffusion of proteins impossible does not inhibit respiration completely. We register 50% of initial O_2 consumption that means that a stable respiratory assembly does function. Also the radiation inactivation curves indicate that target size of respiration increased more than 3 times (to $M_r = 150.000$) (11).

So at the moment we are apt to think that the respiratory chain in bacterial membranes is an equilibrium between free and assembled electrone carriers revealed consequently with radiation inactivation and crosslinking methods.

Main points again:

1. Equal subunits of the unusual H^+-ATP-ase from L.casei function in a cooperative manner as well as H^+-ATP-ases from other organisms.
2. M.luteus respiratory chain exists as a dynamic assembly with a short life span.
3. NADH dehydrogenase of H.halobium was shown to be half as large as that in other bacteria, while dimensions of pyrophosphatase and ATP-ase do not fall off the line.

REFERENCES

1. Kempner, E. and Schlegel, W. (1979).
   Analyt. bioch. 92, N1, 2-10.
2. Zhukova, I., Chekulaeva, L., Kapreliants, A.,
   Mileikovskaya, E., Nikultseva, T. and Ostrovsky, D.
   (1984). Biol. Membrany 1, N7, 684-690.
3. Hutchinson, F. and Pollard, E. (1961). In: Mechanisms in Radiobiology, M. Errera and A. Forssberg
   (Eds). Acad. Press, N. Y., 1, p. 71.
4. Poulis, M., Shaw, D., Campbell, H. and Young, I.
   (1981). Biochemistry 20, 4178-4185.
5. Wong, S., Hall, D. and Josse, J. (1970).
   J. Biol. Chem. 245, 4335-4342.
6. Futai, M. and Kanazawa, H. (1983).
   Microbiol. Rev. 47, N3, 285-312.
7. Fitt, P. and Peterkin, P. (1976).
   Biochem. J. 157, 161-167.
8. Reynolds, I. and Schlessinger, M. (1969).
   Biochemistry 8, 588-592.
9. Kerscher, L., Nowitzki, S. and Oesterhelt, D.
   (1982). Europ. J. Biochem. 128, 223-230.
10. Biketov, S., Kasho, V., Kozlov, I., Mileikovskaya,
    E., ostrovsky, D., Skulachev, V., Tikhonova, G.
    and Tsyorun, V. (1982). Europ. J. Biochem. 129,
    241-250.
11. Zinov'eva, M., Kapreliants, A. and Ostrovsky, D.
    (1983). Molec. and Cell Biochem. 55, 141-144.
12. Kagawa, Y. (1967). Biochim. et biophys. acta 131,
    586-588.

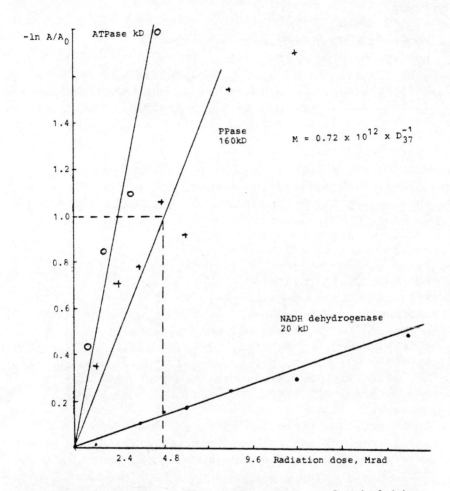

FIGURE 1. Radiation inactivation curves of H.halobium enzymes (2), used for calculation of their M_r.

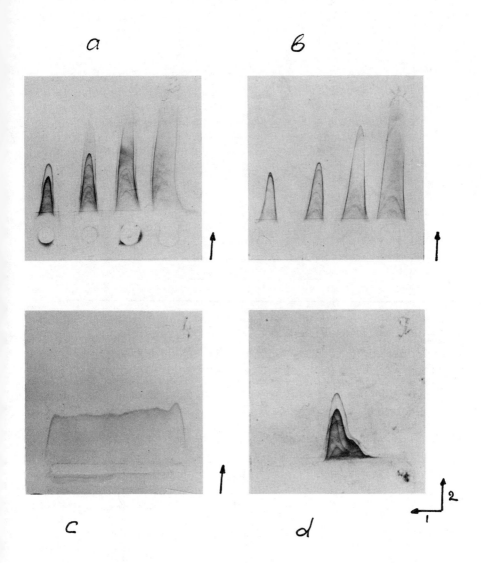

FIGURE 2. Rocket (a-c) and crossed immunoelectrophoresis of H.halobium proteins. Arrows indicate the
position of NADH-dehydrogenase (reduced tetranitro-
blue tetrazolium chloride), other bands are revealed
with Coumassie G-250 staining.

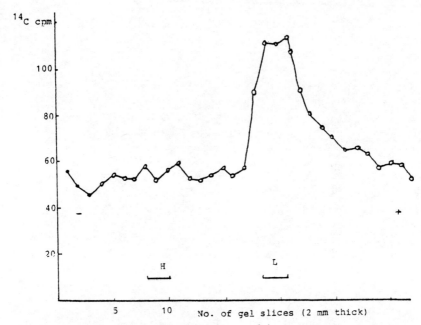

FIGURE 3. Electrophoresis of the ^{14}C-labeled NADH-
-dehydrogenase-antibody complex in SDS containing
polyacrylamide gel. H and L - heavy and light subunits
of immunoglobulins.

TABLE 1. Molecular masses of some bacterial enzymes

	H. halobium	E. coli
NADH-Deh.	22.000[a]	47.000 (4)
P⌒P-ase	145.000	120.000 (5)
ATP-ase	300.000	382.000 (6)
Alcaline phosphatase[b]	15.000 (7)	86.000 (8)
Ketoacid oxidase	$2 \cdot 10^5 - 3 \cdot 10^5$ (9)	$30 \cdot 10^5 - 70 \cdot 10^5$ (9)

a) ± 15%
b) H.cutirubrum

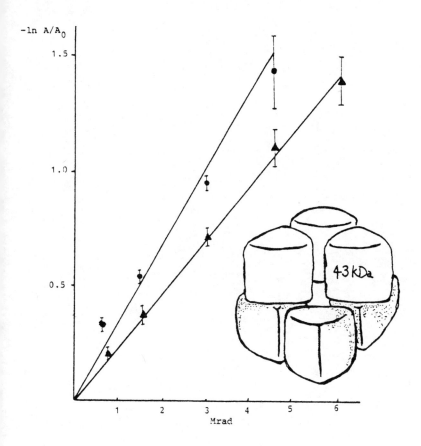

FIGURE 4. Radiation inactivation curves of L.casei
ATPase (1), M.luteus ATPase (2) and schematic drawing
of L.casei ATPase (3) consisting of six equal subunits.

ISOLATION AND PROPERTIES OF THE MAJOR PROTEINS OF THE BRAIN MYELIN.

P. RICCIO and E. QUAGLIARIELLO
Istituto di Chimica Biologica, Facoltà di Scienze, Università di Bari, and Centro di Studio sui Mitocondri e Metabolismo Energetico, CNR, Via Amendola 165/A, 70126 Bari, Italy.

INTRODUCTION

Myelin, the insulating sheath of nerve axons, has the function to facilitate rapid and efficient impulse conduction (1). Disturbance of this function is related to such diseases as multiple sclerosis. Central to the understanding of this pathological process is the knowledge of the functional roles of the major proteins of the myelin membrane. These proteins are the encephalitogenic basic protein, which accounts for about 30% of total myelin proteins, and the proteolipid protein, which accounts for about 50% of the total. Purification of either the basic protein (2,3) or the proteolipid (4, 5) is presently based on different methods which appear overly drastic and furnish denatured proteins. We describe here a new procedure for the isolation of both proteins in the non-ionic detergent n-octylpolydisperse oligooxyethylene (octyl-POE). Purified proteins exhibit properties which could indicate that the proteins are obtained in a state close to the native.

MATERIAL AND METHODS

Octyl-POE, with an average of 5 oxyethylene units, was

Proceedings of the 16th FEBS Congress
Part B, pp. 545–550
© 1985 VNU Science Press

a generous gift of Prof. J.P.Rosenbusch. Myelin was prepared from bovine brain white matter according to (6). Protein content was determined with the BIO-RAD reagent using the microassay procedure and BSA as a standard. Polyacrylamide gel electrophoresis was performed on 15% acrylamide gels as described (7).

RESULTS

The new method for the isolation of both basic protein and proteolipid has been developed starting from bovine brain myelin. The procedure outlined in Table I is based on extraction with the detergent octyl-POE, column chromatography on hydroxyapatite and finally, gel filtration. The whole purification procedure has been carried out at room temperature and at pH 8.5.
Myelin extract contains mostly basic protein and proteolipid (Fig.1, lane B). The two proteins are separated in the first purification step on hydroxyapatite: the basic protein is not adsorbed and is recovered in the pass-through fractions (Fig.1, lane D), while the proteolipid remains bound to the column and is found in the fractions eluted by phosphate. The basic protein and the proteolipid are subsequently isolated by one or by two gel filtrations on Ultrogel AcA 34 respectively.
Isolated basic protein is electrophoretically pure (Fig. 1, lane E). As detected by analitical ultracentrifugation studies the protein is present in a monomeric homogeneous form, but it is showing a tendency to give fragments. Aminoacid composition corresponds to that described (8). The N-terminus is blocked. Only one tryptophane is present. The C-terminus is Ala-Arg, different from the expected Ala-Arg-Arg. Our basic protein is identical to that prepared in the conventional way (3), as established by the immunoblotting technique

546

TABLE I. SCHEME OF THE ISOLATION OF MAJOR MYELIN PROTEINS

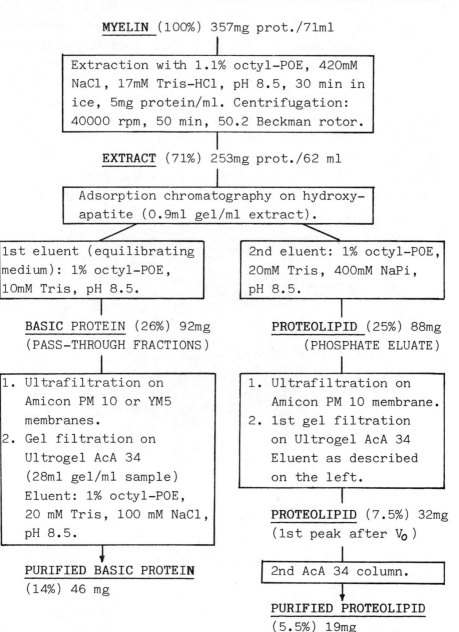

MYELIN (100%) 357mg prot./71ml

Extraction with 1.1% octyl-POE, 420mM
NaCl, 17mM Tris-HCl, pH 8.5, 30 min in
ice, 5mg protein/ml. Centrifugation:
40000 rpm, 50 min, 50.2 Beckman rotor.

EXTRACT (71%) 253mg prot./62 ml

Adsorption chromatography on hydroxyapatite (0.9ml gel/ml extract).

1st eluent (equilibrating
medium): 1% octyl-POE,
10mM Tris, pH 8.5.

2nd eluent: 1% octyl-POE,
20mM Tris, 400mM NaPi,
pH 8.5.

BASIC PROTEIN (26%) 92mg
(PASS-THROUGH FRACTIONS)

PROTEOLIPID (25%) 88mg
(PHOSPHATE ELUATE)

1. Ultrafiltration on
   Amicon PM 10 or YM5
   membranes.
2. Gel filtration on
   Ultrogel AcA 34
   (28ml gel/ml sample)
   Eluent: 1% octyl-POE,
   20 mM Tris, 100 mM NaCl,
   pH 8.5.

1. Ultrafiltration on
   Amicon PM 10 membrane.
2. 1st gel filtration
   on Ultrogel AcA 34
   Eluent as described
   on the left.

PROTEOLIPID (7.5%) 32mg
(1st peak after V_0)

PURIFIED BASIC PROTEIN
(14%) 46 mg

2nd AcA 34 column.

PURIFIED PROTEOLIPID
(5.5%) 19mg

using antibodies of the traditional preparation. From another point of view our preparation still differs from the conventional one. In fact, our basic protein is not water soluble, it contains high amounts of bound lipids and has a secondary structure, whereas the conventional preparation is water soluble, does not bind lipids and is largely unfolded. In our preparation every basic protein molecule binds about 22 molecules of phospholipids (phosphatidylethanolamine, phosphatidylserine and either phosphatidylcholine or phosphatidylinositole), 5 molecules of cholesterol, and finally both cerebrosides and sulfatides. Two other lipids have been

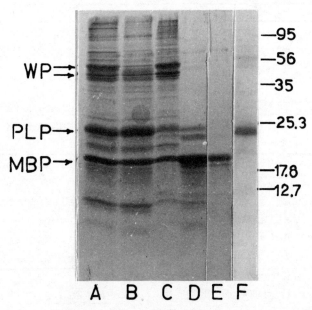

Fig.1 Polyacrylamide gel electrophoresis in sodium dodecylsulfate of myelin proteins at different steps of purification. From left to right, the sample are: (A) myelin proteins; (B) myelin extract; (C) non extracted material; (D) hydroxyapatite non adsorbed fractions; (E) purified basic protein; (F) purified proteolipid.

detected but not identified. By using circular dichroism we found that the basic protein obtained by our procedure contains about 45-50% of β-structure and 6-10% of α-helix. With regard to the proteolipid the yield is not high because of the tendency of proteolipid to form aggregates. Purified proteolipid is electrophoretically pure (Fig.1, lane F). A second band in the higher MW region is only due to a dimeric form of the same protein. The proteolipid appears to be in a delipidated oligomeric form. On the basis of a subunit molecular weight of 25 KDa, following sedimentation equilibrium experiments, purified proteolipid appears to be present in the form of trimers. Instead, in recent preparations of the proteolipid in deoxycholate or Triton X-100 the presence of lipid-free hexamers has been established (9). Further characterization of both myelin proteins is in progress.

REFERENCES

1. Gregson,N.A. (1983). The Molecular Biology of Myelin. In: Multiple Sclerosis, Pathology, Diagnosis and Management, J.F.Hallpike, C.W.M.Adamy and W. Tourtellotte, (eds.) Chapman and Hall, London, pp. 1-27.
2. Oshiro,Y. and Eylar,E.H. (1970). Allergic Encephalomyelitis: Preparation of the Encephalitogenic Basic Protein from Bovine Brain. Arch. Biochem. Biophys. 138, 392-396.
3. Deibler, R.G., Martenson,R.E. and Kies,M.W. (1972). Large Scale Preparation of Myelin Basic Protein from Central Nervous Tissue of Several Mammalian Species. Prep. Biochem. 2, 139-165.

4. Tenenbaum,D. and Folch-Pi,J. (1966). The Preparation and Characterization of Water-soluble Proteolipid Protein frm Bovine Brain White Matter. Biochim. Biophys. Acta 115, 141-147.
5. Agrawal,H.C., Randle,C.L. and Agrawal,D. (1982). In Vivo Acylation of Rat Brain Myelin Proteolipid Protein. J. Biol. Chem. 257, 4588-4592.
6. Norton,W.T. (1974). Isolation of Myelin from Nerve Tissue. Methods Enzymol. 31, 435-444.
7. Laemmli,U.K. (1970). Cleavage of Structural Proteins During the Assembly of the Head of Bacteriophage T4. Nature 227, 680-685.
8. Eylar,E.H., Brostoff,S., Hashim,G., Caccam,J. and Burnett,P. (1971). Basic A1 Protein of the Myelin Membrane. The Complete Amino Acid Sequence. J. Biol. Chem. 246, 5770-5784.
9. Smith,R., Cook,J. and Dickens,P.A. (1984). Structure of the Proteolipid Protein Extracted from Bovine Central Nervous System Myelin with Nondenaturing Detergents. J. Neurochem. 42, 306-313.

PENICILLIN-BINDING PROTEINS AND CELL DIVISION IN Escherichia coli.

A. Rodríguez-Tébar, R. Prats, J. Díaz, V. Arán, J.A. Barbas and
D. Vázquez.
Instituto de Biología Molecular, C.S.I.C., Cantoblanco, Madrid-34, Spain.

INTRODUCTION

Penicillin-binding proteins (PBPs) are located in the cell envelope of
bacteria. They catalyze the last steps of peptidoglycan biosynthesis.
PBPs act on the peptide moieties of peptidoglycan modifying its structure, in order that the bacterial sacculus can be adapted to the dynamic
changes of the bacteria along the cell cycle. Thus, some of the PBPs are
engaged in the process of cell elongation and, at least one, PBP 3, is
involved in the formation of septal peptidoglycan which is needed for
the separation of the daughter cells after division (see 1 for a recent
review). The mode of action of β-lactams has been elucidated to a great
extent in the last twenty years. The structure of a β-lactam resembles
the conformation of the peptide peptidoglycan substrate when bound to
the PBP in the activated state of the enzymic reaction (2). Indeed β-lac
tams are competitive inhibitors of peptide substrates for PBP enzymes.
The enzymic reaction consists, according to its simplest mechanism, of
two steps. In the first step, acylation, the PBP enzyme exerts a nucleophylic attack on the carboxyl carbon of the terminal D-alanyl-D-alanine
amide bond located in the peptide moiety of peptidoglycan. In the second
step, the peptidyl-PBP complex is deacylated and the PBP enzyme regenerated. Usually deacylation is faster than acylation and, therefore, the
enzyme-substrate intermediate complex does not accumulate and cannot be
trapped (1). β-lactams are also substrates for the PBP enzymes. These en
zymes perform a nucleophylic attack on the C_5 of the penicillin ring
that results in acylation of the PBP. However, the deacylation step is
usually very slow and, therefore, the PBP is not regenerated and loses
its ability to catalyze further reactions. When a radioactive β-lactam is
incubated with either whole cells or purified cell envelopes, the antibiotic binds to some (or all) PBPs. These labelled PBPs can be further
chromatographed in polyacrylamide gel electrophoresis and detected by
autoradiographical means as we will see below.

In the present communication we shall restrict our attention to two
interrelated topics chosen among the vast field of PBPs. First point
deals with the structure and location of PBPs and the second one will
deal with the mechanism of cell septation conducted by PBP 3.

Proceedings of the 16th FEBS Congress
Part B, pp. 551–563
© 1985 VNU Science Press

LABELLING OF PBPs BY RADIOACTIVE β-LACTAMS.

PBPs are minoritarian proteins in the cell envelope of E. coli. They can be detected by autoradiography when labelled with radioactive β-lactams. PBPs from B. subtilis were first labelled by Blumberg and Strominger (3) using benzyl(^{14}C)penicillin. This technique was later applied and standardized for E. coli by Spratt (4). Several proteins can be labelled with benzyl (^{14}C)penicillin, are named PBPs 1a, 1b, 2, 3, 4, 5, 6, 7, 8a and 8b. PBP 8a has been often named unduely as PBP 7 while PBP 8b was frequently named simply PBP 8. Actually the real PBP 7 (around 38 kDa) only appears in some E. coli strains. PBPs 8a and 8b are two forms of the same protein with identical affinity for β-lactam antibiotics (P.M. Lacal, unpublished).

Some other radioactive β-lactams have been synthesized recently. These β-lactams, because of their higher specific radioactivity, allow a more rapid autoradiographical detection of PBPs. A radioiodinated Bolton and Hunter derivative of ampicillin (^{125}I-ampicillin, see Figure 1, compound I) was first synthesized by Schwarz et al (5). An improved method for the preparation of this β-lactam has been carried out in our laboratory (6). Figure 2, lane A, shows the pattern of PBPs labelled with ^{125}I-ampicillin in which one additional protein (PBP 1c) is also elicited.

Other β-lactams of high specific radioactivity have been also prepared in our laboratory, such as (^{3}H)hydroxymethylphenoxyacetamidopenicillanic acid (in short, HAPA, see its structural formula indicated as II in Figure 1) and (^{3}H)hydroxymethylphenoxyacetamido(N)ampicillin (HAMPI, Figure 1, III). The patterns of PBPs yielded by these two β-lactams can be seen in Figure 2, lanes B and C respectively and show that HAPA failed to label PBP 1a.

The binding of nonradioactive β-lactams can be studied by competition with a radioactive antibiotic. The incubation of either cells or cell envelopes with increasing concentrations of the unlabelled β-lactam is followed by further incubation with saturating concentrations of the radioactive β-lactam, which will bind to the empty binding sites not filled by the first antibiotic. By these means, the binding properties of dozens of β-lactam antibiotics have been studied.

Not all β-lactams are capable to bind to all PBPs. Generally speaking, cephalosporins bind poorly to low molecular weight PBPs from E. coli. On the other hand, other antibiotics display a remarkable selectivity for one PBP. When this case occurs, it is possible to know, at least at a phenomenological level, the role of a PBP in the physiology of the cell, such as its effects on cell growth, morphology, etc. For example, the β-lactam mecillinam only binds to PBP 2 from E. coli and, concomitantly, produces ovoid-shaped cells. The rod of PBP 2 in the maintenance of the bacterial rod form can be readily inferred. Furthermore, the blockade of PBP 3 from E. coli by cephalexin, furazlocillin or azthreonam prevents the synthesis of septal peptidoglycan and produces filamentous cells (4). The importance of PBP 3 in septation was established accordingly.

SPECIAL β-LACTAMS AS PROBES FOR IDENTIFICATION AND CHARACTERIZATION OF PBPs.

As described above, β-lactams can be useful tools for peptidoglycan studies and also for the investigation of some crucial events in the cell cycle. Unfortunately, nearly all β-lactams have been prepared because of their pharmaceutical interest and not for purposes of basic reseach. The introduction of special chemical groups into the β-lactam molecule can be very useful for characterization of PBPs.

Any PBP is labelled by a β-lactam provided that: i) the antibiotic dis plays enough affinity to bind to the PBP; ii) the intermediate PBP-antibiotic complex is accumulated to some extent; iii) the covalent bond lin king the β-lactam and the PBP in the intermediate state is properly stabilized. The conditions ii) and iii) may be fulfilled with the use of photoreactive derivatives of β-lactams. The photoreactive head can form an irreversible covalent bond linking the β-lactam and the PBP on one hand. On the other hand, the half life of the light activated state is, by far, much shorter than that of the intermediate β-lactam-PBP complex. We have developed two families of photoreactive derivatives of β-lactams (7, 8). One group consists of nitroguaiacol derivatives and a second one of arylazide derivatives. Figure 1 (IV) shows the chemical formula of one of the β-lactams of the latter group. Figure 2, lane D, shows the pattern of PBPs from E. coli labelled with compound IV with illumination of the reaction mixture. It can be observed that this compound not only labelled most of the standard PBPs, but also protein bands of 170, 146 and 89 kDa. The bond formed by chemical labelling can be destroyed by the nucleophilic agent hydroxylamine whilst the covalent bond formed upon illumination cannot be destroyed by this procedure.PBPs 2, 3, 8a and 8b were not chemically labelled, while the 170, 146 kDa were chemically labelled, at least partly. However, all proteins were fully labelled upon illumination. This is a clear demonstration that pho toaffinity labelling was a useful approach for detection of PBPs that otherwise would have remained undetected with chemical labelling (see Figure 3, lane D).

We have also synthesized a photoactivable derivative of peptidoglycan.

554

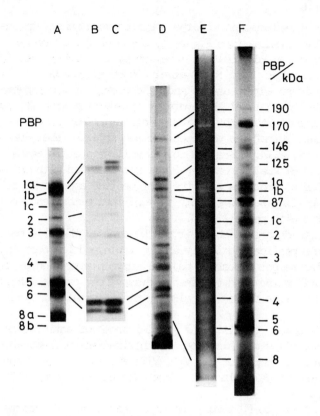

Figure 2: Patterns of PBPs from purified E. coli envelopes labelled with radioactive compounds. All antibiotics were used at saturating concentrations. Lanes: A) 125I-ampicillin; B) HAPA; C) HAMPI; D) compound IV of Figure 1; E) compound V of Figure 1; F) compound IX of Figure 1.

Figure 1 (forerun page): Chemical structures of radioactive acyl-D-Ala-D-Ala analogues used for labelling of PBPs. Compounds: I, 125I-ampicillin; II, HAPA; III, HAMPI; IV, a photoreactive antibiotic; V, a photoreactive derivative of the peptidoglycan substrate analog; VI, VII, VIII and IX, some compounds of the bis-β-lactam group.

This is an arylazide derivative of the peptidoglycan substrate analogue L-lysyl-D-alanyl-D-alanine (see Figure 1, compound V). It was interesting to see whether any PBP could be labelled by this substrate. The substrate analogue had been used for D-alanine carboxypeptidase and peptido glycan transpeptidase enzyme assays and, therefore, it was expected that the photopeptide should label the proteins interacting with it, due to the short halflife of its light activated state. Indeed it can be seen in Figure 2, lane E, that the photopeptide was able to label PBPs 1a, 1b (very efficiently), 2, 4, 6, 8a and 8b, as well as protein bands of 190, 170, 146, 125 and 87 kDa whereas PBP 3 was not labelled with this substrate. Labelling of proteins with the photopeptide appears to be specific, because labelling was completely impeded when membranes were previously incubated with penicillin G.

From the results described above it can be deduced that: i) most PBPs interact with the peptide-peptidoglycan substrate, and ii) protein bands of high molecular weight appear to be real enzymes acting on peptidoglycan . These proteins that had remained undiscovered, can be labelled by our photo-β-lactam (see above) and also by bis-β-lactam antibiotics as described below.

Indeed, bis-β-lactams constitute a special group of antibiotics (8,9). Some of the antibiotics of this group synthezised in our laboratory can be seen in Figure 1, compounds VI, VII, VIII and IX. They are symmetrical or nearly symmetrical β-lactams, first designed for cross-linking studies of PBPs.

Bis-β-lactams bind to PBPs more strongly than normal β-lactams (9). As studied by Le Pecq et al (10), using acridine dimers as DNA-intercalating agents, the free energy of the binding of each reactive part of the molecule will add up and the resulting affinity of the bis-β-lactam may increase several orders of magnitude (9). This may be the reason why bis β-lactam can label the high molecular weight PBPs (see Figure 2, lane F). The bis-β-lactams also produce homologous cross-linking of PBPs 1b, 1c and 3, demonstrating the multimeric structure of these proteins (9).

LOCATION OF PBPs.

PBPs are located in the cell envelope of bacteria. However, when envelopes from E. coli are prepared by breaking the cells either with a French press or by sonication, substantial amounts of PBPs are apparently solubilized. Since PBPs 8a and 8b are particularly more solubilized, most workers did not pay much attention to these PBPs. Nearly all PBP material (including PBPs 8a and 8b) remains in the envelope when cells are broken mildly such as using a very short pulse of sonication after spheroplasts formation.

In Gram-negative bacteria, it has been considered that PBPs are located in the inner membrane (4). This point was established on the basis of the solubility of PBPs in sodium lauroyl sarcosinate (Sarkosyl). By that time it was considered that the inner membrane (IM) was 100% solubilized by this detergent while the outer membrane (OM) was 100% insoluble (11). Recent work established that, although most proteins in the IM are Sarkosyl soluble, some minor proteins from the OM are solubilized by the detergent as well (12, and our unpublished work). Actually, even some major OM proteins, like OmpA, are partially but significantly solubilized by 1% Sarkosyl. Thus, IM and OM from E. coli must not be further distinguished from each other on the basis of their Sarkosyl solubility. Separation of IM and OM is today accomplished by taking advantage of the different bouyant density of both membranes. The OM is heavier than the IM due to its content in lipopolysaccharide. Thus, both membranes can be separated in sucrose gradients.

We have used the method of Osborn et al (13) for the separation of both membranes. Labelling of both membranes with ^{125}I-ampicillin reveals that all PBPs, except PBP 3, are also contained in the OM as clearly shown in Figure 3. It may occur that PBPs are not 'intrinsic' OM proteins and that they remain associated to this membrane through peptidoglycan unbroken during spheroplasts formation from the cells. Our studies on biosynthesis of PBP 8b reveal that this protein is first found in the IM and then part of it is incorporated into the OM. It must be born in mind that enzymic reactions on peptidoglycan are not energy dependent and therefore, a PBP can be located outside the IM in a nonenergized environment. We believe that some PBPs are located in the OM, might be in order to achieve a better accesibility to some peptide moieties of peptidoglycan. Indeed, recent studies on peptidoglycan structure reveal that peptide moieties are protruding either innerwards or outerwards from the plane of the glycan chains (14).

LOCATION OF PBP 3.

All, or nearly all, PBP 3 molecules are found in the IM (see Figure 3). PBPs are engaged in the building of peptidoglycan septa (4). Undoubtedly, the formation of this new surface must be templated by the IM, as the completion of the OM does not take place until the septum is formed. This may be the reason for PBP 3 to be found in the IM.

PBP 3 is possibly the final target of the complex machinery of cell division. The division is the final result of a long series of events

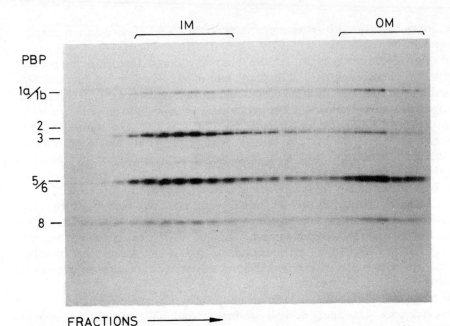

Figure 3: PBPs in the IM and OM from E. coli. Inner and outer membranes were separated by isopycnic centrifugation in a sucrose gradient (13). Gradients were analyzed into fractions. Markers for IM (succinate dehydrogenase and β‑NADH oxidase) and for OM (lipopolysaccharide and visualization of OM proteins in polyacrylamide gels) were studied. Cross‑contamination of both membranes was less than 3%. PBPs from each fraction were labelled with ^{125}I‑ampicillin.

that take place in the cell. Over two hundred genes have been identified as related to division. Some of them are located at the minute 2.5 of the standard E. coli map (15). One of these genes is pbpB that encodes for PBP 3 (16). This region also contains some genes that are engaged in peptidoglycan synthesis. Additionally, this zone also contains a cluster of three genes, namely, ftsA, ftsZ and ftsQ that are involved in cell division. ftsZ gene product plays a role in the SOS‑mediated filamentation (17).

In spite of a great deal of genetic information, not much is known about the biochemical events that take place in the making of the separating wall. Anyhow, the acting processes should be synchronized to occur at the division period of the cell cycle. We shall focus our attention to some features related to PBP 3 such as its activity on one hand, and the modulation of this activity, on the other hand.

558

REGULATION OF PBP 3 ACTIVITY.

PBP 3 appears to be synthesized at a given moment of the cell cycle. How ever, previous data showed that the PBP levels remained constant along the cell cycle. Hence we have used a different approach for these studies. E. coli cells (PAT 84 strain, ftsZ) were grown at 30°C up to an $A_{550} = 0.2$. Then azthreonam (1 µg/ml) was added to the culture. This concentration of the antibiotic ensures the filling of 97% of PBP 3 binding sites. The binding of azthreonam to PBP 3 is irreversible and no protein is regenerated. Cells were allowed to filament until no change of absorbance was detected ($A_{550} = 1.0$). Then, the antibiotic was filtered off from the culture and cells were allowed to divide. Samples were collected and the appearance of PBP 3 was followed in whole cells. Results can be seen in Figure 4, A. It can be observed that, within the first ten minutes after removal of the β-lactam there is a burst of PBP 3 synthesis which is maintained constant during the time of the cycle. A second burst is produced when, supposedly, the second septation is going to occur.

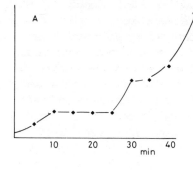

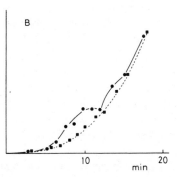

Figure 4: A) Synthesis of PBP 3: The amount of PBP 3 in the cell was estimated by labelling with ^{125}I-ampicillin (ordinates in arbitrary units). Cells were then electrophoresed and the radio activity of PBP 3 was measured in a γ-counter. B) Labelling of peptidoglycan: After azthreonam was filtered off, filaments were transfered to fresh culture medium: ∎---∎ without azthreonam, ●——● with azthreonam (1 µg/ml). Cells were labelled with (^{3}H)diaminopimelic acid (1 µCi/ml) Aliquots were taken and the cells were treated with 2% hot SDS. The insoluble radioactivity was collected by filtration and the radioactivity of the filters was measured (ordinates in arbitrary units). Further details are given in the text.

When azthreonam is removed from the culture, and, simultaneously, peptidoglycan is labelled with (^{3}H)diaminopimelic acid, the first septum can be detected as clearly shown in Figure 4, B. There is, after azthreonam removal, a synchrony in cell septation, probably maintained for two cycles. It can be noticed that de novo PBP 3 is synthesized within ten minutes after restoration of permissive conditions and septum is formed immediately. These data suggests that PBP 3 is synthesized at one moment of the cell cycle and, therefore some regulation of the expression must exist, so that the protein appears just before septation. We put forward the hypothesis that only a certain fraction of the PBP 3 found in normal cells is involved in the formation of a new septum. This part is just synthesized before performing its function and properly located in pre-septal zones. After septation PBP 3 molecules probably migrate to other parts of IM and are not reused in building new septa. This hypothesis contains some experimental support, such as the data described above and our further observation that inhibition by azthreonam of 40–45% of PBP 3 is sufficient to cause filamentation.

However, there must be other mechanisms regulating septum formation. One of these is the regulation of enzyme activity, and the second one may be the availability of the substrate used by PBP 3. Concerning the later point, we have carried out transpeptidase studies on other treated cells using as precursors both UDP-N-acetylmuramylpentapeptide and UDP-N-acetylmuramyltripeptide. Transpeptidase assays were carried out as in ref. 17. When using the pentapeptide we could not demonstrate any activity for PBP 3, unlike previously reported data (18). Azthreonam inhibits very slightly and not reproducibly the transpeptidase activity, under conditions where this antibiotic only blocks PBP 3. On the other hand, the β-lactam cefsulodine, under conditions where PBPs 1a, 1b and 1c are blocked and nearly all PBP 3 is free, inhibits 100% transpeptidase activity, using the pentapeptide precursor. However, we have demonstrated transpeptidase activity for PBP 3 when using the tripeptide as a precursor. Results are summarized in Table I. It can be observed that transpeptidation is 70% inhibited by azthreonam. Therefore, PBP 3 must be a reverse transpeptidase that perform its activity using substrates containing terminal D-Ala-D-Ala previously incorporated into macromolecular peptidoglycan. We believe that PBP 3 activity is also modulated by the availability of UDP-N-acetylmuramyltripeptide. This molecule might be either the nascent natural precursor or, otherwise, the emerging pentapeptide precursor might be degraded to tripeptide by the action of carboxypeptidase.

Finally the activity of PBP 3 is modulated by other proteins. Somehow, there is a physiological link between the ftsZ gene product and the activity of PBP 3. When E. coli PAT 84 (ftsZ) strain is grown at 42°C (non permissive conditions) there is a filamentation of the cells. Under these conditions, the levels of PBP 3 decrease about 60–70%. This fact may be the ultimate cause of the filamentation process. Furthermore, the activity of PBP 3 from filaments is zero when transpeptidase assays are carried out at 42°C. However, transpeptidation due to PBP 3 is elicited when the assay is done at 30°C. These data suggest that there is a close relationship between ftsZ protein and PBP 3. The ftsZ protein might modulate the activity of PBP 3 probably taking part of a multimeric enzyme complex.

TABLE I

Transpeptidase activity in ether–treated E. coli PAT 84 cells *

Conditions	Temperature of the assay	Antibiotic used	Enzyme activity **
Normal cells grown at 30°C	30°C	– – – –	906
	30°C	azthreonam (1 µg/ml)	322
	30°C	cefsulodine (50 µg/ml)	900
	30°C	teichoplanin (1 µg/ml)	0
	42°C	– – – –	698
	42°C	azthreonam (1 µg/ml)	350
Filaments grown at 42°C	30°C	– – – –	24
	30°C	azthreonam (1 µg/ml)	9
	42°C	– – – –	4
	42°C	azthreonam (1 µg/ml)	0

* Assays were carried out as in ref. 17. UDP–N–acetylmuramyl–L–Ala–D–Glu–Dap was used as peptidoglycan precursor.
** One unit corresponds to 1 pmol of radioactive precursor incorporated into SDS–insoluble peptidoglycan per mg cell protein per hour.

REFERENCES

1. Waxman, D.J. and Strominger, J.L. (1983). Penicillin-binding proteins and the mechanism of action of β-lactam antibiotics. Ann. Rev. Biochem. 52, 825-869.
2. Tipper, D.J. and Strominger, J.L. (1965). Mechanism of action of penicillins in a proposal based on their structural similarity to acyl-D-alanyl-D-alanine. Proc. Natl. Acad. Sci. USA 54, 1133-1141.
3. Blumberg, P.M. and Strominger, J.L. (1972). Five penicillin-binding components occur in Bacillus subtilis membranes. J. Biol. Chem. 247, 8107-8113.
4. Spratt, B.G. (1977). Properties of the penicillin-binding proteins of Escherichia coli K12. Eur. J. Biochem. 72, 341-352.
5. Schwarz, U., Seeger, K., Wengenmayer, F. and Strecker, H. (1981). Penicillin-binding proteins of Escherichia coli identified with a 125I-derivative of ampicillin. FEMS Microbiol. Letters 10, 101-109.
6. Rojo, F., Ayala, J.A., Rosa, E. de la, Pedro, M. de, Arán, V., Berenguer, J. and Vázquez, D. (1984). Binding of ^{125}I-labelled β-lactam antibiotics to the penicillin-binding proteins of Escherichia coli. J. Antibiotics 37, 389-393.
7. Arán, V., Rodríguez-Tébar, A. and Vázquez, D. (1983). Labelling of penicillin-binding proteins from Escherichia coli with photoreactive derivatives of β-lactam antibiotics. FEBS Letters 153, 431-437.
8. Arán, V., Rodríguez-Tébar, A. and Vázquez, D. (1983). Labelling and cross-linking of E. coli with bis-β-lactams and photoreactive derivatives of β-lactam antibiotics. In: The Target of Penicillin, R. Hakenbeck, J.-V. Höltje and H. Labischinski (eds.) Walter de Gruyter. Berlin, New York, pp. 433-438.
9. Rodríguez-Tébar, A., Arán, V. and Vázquez, D. (1984). Labelling and crosslinking of Escherichia coli penicillin-binding proteins with bis-β-lactam antibiotics. Eur. J. Biochem. 139, 287-293.
10. Le Pecq, J.B., Le Bret, M., Barbet, J. and Roques, B. (1975). DNA polyintercalating drugs: DNA binding of diacridine derivatives. Proc. Natl. Acad. Sci. USA 72, 2915-2919.
11. Filip, C., Fletcher, G., Wulff, J.L. and Earhart, C.F. (1983). Solubization of the cytoplasmic membrane of Escherichia coli by the ionic detergent sodium lauroyl sarcosinate. J. Bacteriol. 115, 717-722.
12. Chopra, I. and Shales, S.W. (1980). Comparison of the polypeptide composition of Escherichia coli outer membranes prepared by two methods. J. Bacteriol. 144, 425-427.
13. Osborn, M.J., Gander, J.E., Parisi, E. and Carson, J. (1972). Mecha-

nism of assembly of the outer membrane of <u>Salmonella typhimurium</u>.
J. Biol. Chem. 247, 3962–3972.

14. Barnickel, G., Naumann, D., Bradaczek, H., Labischinski, H. and Gies
    bretch, P. (1983). Computer aided modelling of the three dimension
    al structure of peptidoglycan. In: The Target of Penicillin, R. Ha
    kenbeck, J.-V. Hölje and H. Labischinski (eds.). Walter de Gruyter.
    Berlin, New York, pp. 61–66.

15. Bachmann, B. J. (1983). Linkage map of <u>Escherichia coli</u> K–12. Micro-
    biol. Rev. 47, 180–230.

16. Lutkenhaus, J.F. (1983). Coupling of DNA replication and cell divi-
    sion: <u>sulB</u> is an allele of <u>ftsZ</u>. J. Bacteriol. <u>154</u>, 1339–1346.

17. Mirelman, D., Yashouv-Gan, Y. and Schwarz, U. (1976). Peptidoglycan
    biosynthesis in a thermosensitive mutant of <u>Escherichia coli</u>. Bio-
    chemistry 15, 1781–1790.

18. Botta, G.A. and Park, J.T. Evidence of involvement of penicillin-bin
    ding protein 3 in murein synthesis during septation but not during
    elongation. (1981). J. Bacteriol. 145, 333–340.

IMMUNOTARGETED CHEMOTHERAPY IN CANCER RESEARCH

RUTH ARNON
Department of Chemical Immunology, The Weizmann
Institute of Science, Rehovot 76100, Israel

Chemotherapy constitutes a major therapeutic approach
for the treatment of cancer. Its major drawback is that
anti-cancer drugs, although destructive to the tumor cells
are also toxic to normal cells. A possible way to overcome this difficulty is by employing affinity targeting
to chemotherapy e.g. with drug-antibody conjugates.
Therapy by antibodies against tumor-associated antigens
alone has as a rule not been successful, probably since
such antibodies, though capable of recognizing the cells,
are not cytotoxic in vivo. However, the combination of
antibody therapy and chemotherapy could be useful, since
the antibody would selectively deliver the cytoxic drug
to the target cell.

In our studies, as summarized in several recent reviews
(1-3), we attempted to use conjugates, in which drugs
were linked chemically to the antibody carrier, for
immunotargeting in several experimental tumor systems.
We have attached drugs such as daunomycin, adriamycin,
cytosine arabinoside, 5-fluorouridine and methotrexate
to the various antitumor antibodies, usually via a poly-
meric "bridge". In addition, we have used derivatives in
which platinum was complexed to the antibodies in an
attempt to reconstruct cis-platinum structure on antibody
conjugates. As carriers, we used both polyclonal and
monoclonal antibodies. The monoclonal ones have the
advantage of monospecifity towards tumor specific antigenic determinants. The prerequisite in these studies
was to retain the activities of both the antibodies and
the drugs, and consequently the resultant conjugates
were effective both in vitro and in vivo against the
respective tumors.

The results we achieved with various experimental
tumors systems, using the different drug-antibody

Proceedings of the 16th FEBS Congress
Part B, pp. 565–570
© 1985 VNU Science Press

conjugates, are described in the following.

The Yac lymphoma

The Yac lymphoma is a Moloney virus-induced tumor (4)
growing in ascitic or subcutaneous form in A/J mice. In
early experiments with this tumor system we used daunomycin conjugates with polyclonal affinity-purified antibodies that were prepared in goats against membrane
antigen obtained from the tumor cells by papain digestion.
These antibodies were specific towards Yac cells as
determined by comlement-mediated cytotoxicity, but were
nevertheless able to bind to normal splenocytes as well.
In therapy studies (10^5 tumor cells transplanted i.p. or
s.c. and the treatment given two days later i.v.), dauno-
mycin-dextran-anti-Yac at high doses was more effective
than either free drug or antibodies alone. A similar
effect, however, was sometimes obtained by using the drug
conjugated to normal Ig or just to dextran. At lower drug
doses, the specific conjugate was more effective than the
non-specific conjugate but the free drug was also quite
effective, preventing the development of the tumor in 60%
of the mice.

In view of these results it was envisaged that antibodies with higher specificity might improve the efficacy
of the drug antibody conjugate. Monoclonal antibodies
were prepared for this purpose by hybridization of spleen
cells from BALB/c x A/J F_1 mice immunized with whole tumor
cells. These antibodies, designated KH_{3-4}, which were of
the IgM class, bound to Yac cells 10-50 fold better than
to normal spleen cells and did not react with normal
thymocytes or with lymph node cells. Yet, the effectivity of the KH_{3-4} dextran-daunomycin conjugate (containing 500 mol of daunomycin per mol antibody) in vivo was
not higher than that of the polyclonal goat anti-Yac conjugate. The latter was very effective and at a low dose
(12 mg/kg), it led to 100% long-term survival (5). The
higher efficacy of the conjugates of the polyclonal antibodies is probably due to their higher avidity, that could
be the result of their specificity towards many determinants on the tumor cells. These results might represent

566

a general phenomenon, except when the monoclonal antibodies are directed towards a particularly abundant antigen on the tumor cells.

The Lewis lung carcinoma (3LL)

Lewis lung carcinoma is originally a spontaneous tumor (6) which is maintained in C57BL mice. It grows at the transplantation site subcutaneously as a local primary tumor and 2-3 weeks later, develops as visible metastatic foci in the lungs. Enhanced metastasis was obtained by injecting the tumor into the footpad and amputation of the tumoric leg (7) or by injecting the tumor intravenously. In this system as well, experiments were performed with drug conjugates of both polyclonal (rabbit and syngenic mice) and monoclonal antibodies, The polyclonal antibodies prepared against the primary tumor were found to react with the primary and metastatic tumor cells to the same extent and showed almost no reactivity with normal syngeneic cells. Furthermore, their daunomycin conjugates demonstrated prominent in vitro efficacy on both types of tumor cells. However, in vivo these antibodies showed a relatively low specific distribution factor (less than 2 fold) in the lungs as compared to other organs. The monoclonal antibodies (denoted 6B), on the other hand, which reacted in vitro almost exclusively with the 3LL cells, showed much more effective homing. These antibodies showed strong anti-lung tissue reactivity, and therefore accumulated in the lungs of normal mice as well. All the same, their specific accumulation factor in the metastatic lungs of tumor-bearing mice was approximately 30, as compared to all other organs (8).

These monoclonal antibodies served as carriers for attachment of daunomycin, adriamycin and methotrexate. These drugs are effective inhibitors of the 3LL cells in vitro, but are uneffective against the 3LL tumor or its metastases in vivo. We hoped that in view of the very high specific accumulation of the monoclonal antibodies in the lungs, the localization of their drug conjugates at the tumor site may increase their efficacy. However, the conjugates, although highly inhibitory to the 3LL cells in vitro, were not significantly effective in vivo. It must therefore be concluded that this tumor is resistant to these drugs and their delivery to the site did not overcome this resistance.

Anti-α-fetoprotein (AFP) reactive against rat hepatoma

Rat hepatoma (AH 66) is an AFP-producing hepatoma maintained in Donryu rats (9). In the case of this tumor system as well, we prepared drug conjugates of both polyclonal and monoclonal antibodies, that can be comparatively evaluated. Horse polyclonal antibodies against rat AFP were shown to recognize the tumor cells vitro and to localize on them in vivo. Monoclonal antibodies to rat AFP (312) were prepared in BALB/c mice, and also showed a high affinity towards AFP. Both types of antibodies served as carriers for linking of daunomycin via dextran T 10. In their specific cytotoxicity towards the hepatoma cells in vitro, the conjugates of daunomycin with the horse anti-AFP and the monoclonal antibodies were of similar activity, both demonstrating 4-5 fold higher efficacy than free daunomycin (10).

The most important aspect of this study was to evaluate the chemotherapeutic effectivity of the drug antibody conjugates on tumor bearing rats. For that purpose, rats challenged i.p. with 10^4 AH66 cells were treated with a multiple dose of the specific drug-antibody conjugates and with the various controls. The treatments were given 5 times, from the third day after the tumor injection, on alternate days, and were administered either i.v. or i.p.

The in vivo efficacy of the monoclonal anti-AFP and its drug conjugate was similar to that of conventional horse anti-rat AFP and its drug derivative. Both conjugates were much more effective than the free drug and antibody, which caused only slight delay in the median survival time by both routes of treatment. An interesting finding is that the i.v. treatment was much more effective than the i.p. and led to remarkable life prolongation as well as to 60% long-term survival. This high efficacy may indicate specific homing of the conjugates to the target cells at the tumor site. The presumable high abundance of the tumor-spcific antigen AFP on the hepatoma cell is probably a decisive parameter which facilitates an efficient immunotargeting in this case.

Antibodies as carriers for the chemotherapeutic drug cis platinum

Cis platinum is an effective inhibitor of DNA synthesis of tumor cells and is currently being used in the treatmet of several human tumors. However, its high toxicity often limits the effectivity of treatment by this drug. In our studies we attempted to bind Pt to anti-tumor antibodies (immunoglobulin (Ig) fractions or monoclonal anti-antibodies) in order to render the drug less toxic and more specific towards the tumor cells.The Pt salt K_2PtCl_4 was complexed to Ig either directly or via diamine acceptor molecules bound to dextran T 10. The resulting Pt-Ab complexes retained their antibody activity, as well as their respective activity in vitro against 3 different tumor cell lines (leukemia 38C, Yac, lymphoma, and Lewis lung carcinoma 3LL. At high Pt concentrations and short incubation periods (24 hr) the free Pt salt was sometimes more effective than either complex, but cis-Pt had a toxic effect. However, at low drug concentrations, Pt inthe specific complexes had a clear advantage over free Pt (5-25 folds), or Pt diamine-dextran complexes with non-specific Ig. In cultures incubated for 48 hr, the relative efficiency of Pt-complexes, especially in the specific complexes increased as compared to free Pt which often exerted poor activity after prolonged incubation. Preliminary in vivo studies have also demonstrated significant beneficial effect of the specific Pt-dextran-antibody complexes. These results suggest that antibodies indeed may serve as carriers for targeting of cis-Pt and similar drugs.

The main conclusions from these studies are that antibodies may indeed serve as carriers for anti-cancer drugs for the purpose of immunotargeting. The monoclonal antibodies have both advantages and disadvantages over the polyclonal ones. They are advantageous since they can be readily obtained by immunization with the whole tumor cells including neoplasms which do not bear a known tumor marker; they can also be prepared from naturally existing antibody-producing peripheral blood lymphocytes by in vitro culturing procedures, thus leading to human-human hybridomas; they are uniformly specific, and if directed against an abundant antigen - may show very high efficiency. Their uniformity can be of a disadvantage if they are directed towards a scarce antigen on the tumor cell, or if the drug-binding modification leads to loss of their reactivity. In such cases polyclonal antibodies may be superior. It is thus apparent that both polyclonal and monoclonal antibodies should be considered in future efforts towards immunotargeted chemotherapy of cancer.

REFERENCES

1. Arnon, R., and Sela, M. (1982) Immunol. Rev. 62, 5-27.
2. Arnon, R., and Sela, M. (1982) Cancer Surveys 1 429-449.
3. Arnon, R., Hurwitz, E. (1983) in: "Targeted Drugs" (ed. E.P. Goldberg) Wiley, N.Y., p.23-25.
4. Klein, E. and Klein, G. (1964) J. Natl. Cancer Inst. 32 547-568.
5. Arnon, R. and Hurwitz, E. (1984) in Drug and Enzyme Targeting, R. Baldwin Ed. Academic Press. In press.
6. Sugiura, K. and Stock, C.C. (1955) Cancer Res. 15, 38-51.
7. Gorelik, E., Segal, S. and Feldman, M. (1978) Int. J. Cancer 21, 617-625.
8. Eshhar, Z, Hurwitz, E. and Hadas, E. (1980) in: New Developments with Human and Vetinary Vaccines, Alan R. Liss, N.Y. 357-365.
9. Isaka, H., Umehara, S., Yoshii, H., Tsukada, Y. and Hirai, H. (1976) GAAN 67, 131-135.
10. Tsukada, Y., Hurwitz, E. Kashi, R., Sela, M. Hibi, N., Hara, A. and Hirai, H. (1982) Proc. Natl. Acad. Sci. USA 79, 7896-7899.

RAPID LASER-FLASH PHOTOAFFINITY LABELING OF ACETYLCHOLINE RECEPTOR FUNCTIONAL STATES

A.FAHR, P.MUHN, L.LAUFFER AND F.HUCHO

Freie Universität Berlin, Institut für Biochemie und Institut für Atom- und Festkörperphysik, Abt. Biophysik, Arnimallee 14, 1000 Berlin 33

Introduction

The nicotinic acetylcholine receptor (AChR) is activated by the physiological neurotransmitter acetylcholine or other agonists. Its action consists of several elementary steps: a) binding of the ligand to the receptor b) channel opening, c) channel closing and d) dissociation of the ligand-receptor complex. Additional steps as e.g. receptor desensitization and rapid channel closing and opening have been observed. The molecular mechanisms of these elementary steps are largely unknown. So far their kinetics have been investigated by various biophysical methods: ligand binding, a diffusion controlled process, can be analyzed by means of fluorescent agonists. Channel opening and closing is observed by the patch clamp method, desensitization and other conformational changes of the receptor protein can be monitored by changes of intrinsic or extrinsic fluorescence changes or by alteration of SH-group reactivity. For a recent review see ref. 1.

Several rapid methods are available for measuring the cation flow through the agonist-gated ion channel of the receptor (2,3). But despite these many kinetic data very little is known as to the structural changes underlying AChR activity. The reason for this lack of information may be found in the fact that most direct biochemical methods are dealing with the receptor statically fixed

Proceedings of the 16th FEBS Congress
Part B, pp. 571–576
© 1985 VNU Science Press

in one or the other state or at best with a population of receptor molecules in a given equilibrium of states.

Our aim was to develop a direct biochemical method to investigate the dynamics of AChR activity. We propose a photoaffinity labeling technique for labeling irreversibly transient receptor states with a physiologically relevant time resolution. This method is applied to detect the protein moieties involved in regulating the ion permeability of the ion channel (6).

The photolabel used, ^{3}H-triphenylmethylphosphonium, (TPMP$^+$) has been shown previously to be a specific non-competitive antagonist, i.e. a true ion channel blocker (4). If the TPMP$^+$-receptor complex is irradiated with uv-light, TPMP$^+$ is covalently linked to several polypeptide chains in the receptor protein. The amount of TPMP$^+$ linked to the various chains seems to depend on the physiological status of the receptor protein, indicating structural changes within the receptor protein, correlated with hitherto unidentified events such as desensitation and possibly channel gating.

Stopped-flow apparatus for photoaffinity labeling

In order to monitor these changes in the physiological time scale, we combined a modified stopped-flow apparatus (Fig. 1) with a high energy pulsed laser (wavelength 266 nm, pulse energy 15 mJ, pulse duration 4 ns).

The regular mixing chamber was replaced by a thermoresistant chamber made of german silver. The reaction chamber volume is about 22 µl, the dead time of the stopped-flow apparatus about 2.4 ms. The laser is triggered by a pre-stop-switch, mounted at the moving pistons of the stopped-flow apparatus. The time between mixing and laser pulse can be adjusted.

After irradiation the sample (about 30 µl) can be removed from the mixing chamber with a Hamilton air-locked syringe.

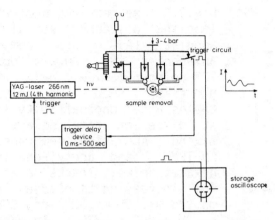

Fig.1: Schematic drawing of the main components of the stopped-flow apparatus

Photoaffinity labeling of the AChR
One syringe of the stopped-flow apparatus contained receptor-rich membranes (1mg/ml) from Torpedo marmorata, as described elsewhere (5). The other syringe contained ^{3}H-TPMP$^+$ (0.4 µM) and either 0.1 mM acetylcholine (or other agonists e.g. carbamoylcholine) or 0.1 mM hexamethonium (or other antagonists e.g. flaxedil), all in Ringer solution at room temperature.

After photoaffinity labeling we performed SDS gel electrophoresis on the irradiated samples. Autoradiography and radioactivity determination of the labeled receptor peptides can be done in the usual manner.

Results
In both cases, using agonist and antagonist, we could find an immediate labeling of the α-polypeptide chains of the AChR after mixing, as we can see in the autoradiograms (Fig. 2).

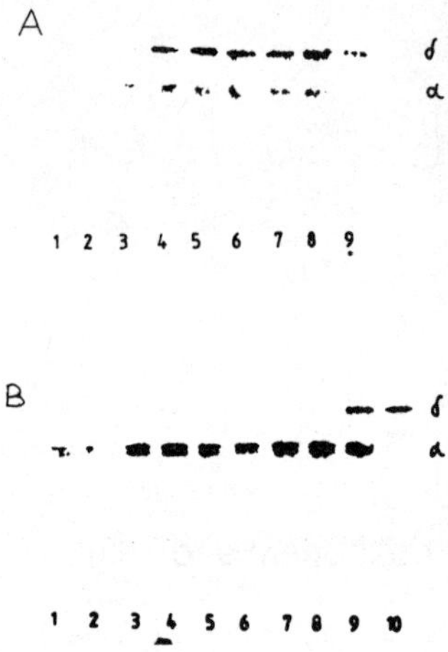

Fig.2: Time resolved photoaffinity labeling of AChR, stimulated by agonist (A) or a competitive antagonist (B). Autoradiogram of SDS-polyacrylamide gel electrophoresis shows AChR-polypeptide chains after photoaffinity labeling at different time delays after mixing AChR-rich membranes with ^{3}H-TPMP$^+$ and acetyl-choline or hexamethonium. Tracks are ordered for increasing timelapses (A): 8 ms, 23 ms, 50 ms, 200 ms, 500 ms, 2 s, 5 s, 50 s, 330 s. In experiment (B) the time lapses were identical as in (A), but tracks 7 and 8 are identical (5 s). Other conditions see text.

The agonist acetylcholine shifts the reaction site to the δ-chain in time. At about 500 ms after mixing the labeling of the δ-chain is halfmaximal.

Kinetics in the presence of the antagonist hexamethonium however are quite different. Here, the δ-polypeptide chain becomes labeled several seconds after mixing.

In order to evaluate the results in a more quantitative manner, we excised in the following experiments the bands of the gels and determined their radioactivity by liquid scintillation counting.

Carbamoylcholine, an agonist, if mixed simultanously with AChR-rich membranes and ^{3}H-TPMP$^+$ promotes the δ-reactive state in a similar manner as acetylcholine; halftime being about 500 msec. In contrast, after preincubation with carbamoylcholine, the halftime rises to 10 sec (Fig.3a). Labeling of the α-chain remains more or less the same or decreases slightly.

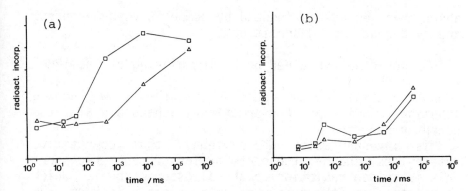

Fig.3: Photoaffinity labeling kinetics of the δ - polypeptide chain with ^{3}H-TPMP$^+$ stimulated by carbamoylcholine (a) or flaxedil (b), respectively. -☐-☐-☐- 0.1 mM carbamoylcholine (a) or 0.1 mM flaxedil (b) added to receptor-rich membranes simultaneously with the photolabel, -△-△-△- Receptor-rich membranes preincubated with the respective effector.

All tested competitive antagonists also stimulated labeling of the δ-chain, but the time constants of this process are in the order of ten seconds (Fig.3b). Preincubation of the receptor protein with antagonists did not alter significantly the time constant of labeling.

Discussion

The laser-flash photoaffinity labeling method can covalently mark protein structures involved in receptor functions.

a) The labeling of the α-chain indicates, that the receptor is either in the active or in the resting state.

b) labeling of the δ-chain with a time constant of 500 ms represents the agonist induced state.

c) labeling of the δ-chain with a time constant of

about ten seconds is induced by competitive antagonists and by desentitizing conditions.

This could be explained by a slow binding of the TPMP$^+$ to the δ-chain.

Another explanation would be that the slow δ-chain labeling indicates conformational changes of the receptor protein.

This interpretation would mean, that competitive antagonists change the conformation of the receptor. This is in contradiction to the allosteric model, which postulates as the action of antagonists a lock of the resting state of the receptor protein, e.g. no conformational change in comparison to the resting state.

The next step in this research has to be the localizing of the TPMP$^+$-label in the different polypeptide chains by fingerprint analysis. This should give a more detailed view of the structural changes of the ACh-receptor protein during its function.

References

1. Maelike, A., (1984) Angew. Chem. 96, 193-216
2. Hess,G.P., Cash,D.J. and Aoshima,H. (1979) Nature 282, 329-331
3. Moore,H.-P.H., and Raftery,M.A. (1979) Biochemistry 18, 1862-1867
4. Lauffer,L., and Hucho,F. (1982) Proc.Natl.Acad.Sci. USA 79, 2406-2409
5. Schiebler,W. and Hucho,F. (1978) Eur.J.Biochem. 85, 55-63
6. Muhn,P., Fahr,A., and Hucho,F. (1984) Biochemistry 23, 2725-2730

THE ROLE OF PROTON COUPLING IN NUTRIENT TRANSPORT IN YEASTS

A. KOTYK
Institute of Microbiology, Czechoslovak Academy of
Sciences, 142 20 Praha-Krč, Czechoslovakia

Like in bacteria and in plants, most nutrient transports in various yeast species are believed to be driven by the electrochemical potential gradient of protons across the external plasma membrane. The evidence
for this [1-4] derives (a) from the transient alkali-
fication of the external medium (or a decrease of its
titration acidity) observed upon adding an H^+-sympor-
ted solute to the suspension, (b) from the depolarization of the membrane when such a solute is transported
(Fig. 1).

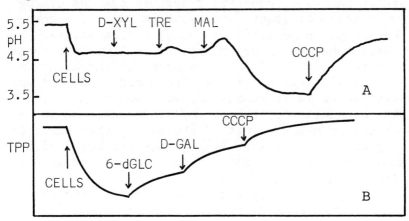

FIG. 1. Extracellular pH of *Saccharomyces cerevisiae*
(A) and extracellular tetraphenylphosphonium concentration (reflecting inversely the membrane potential)
in *Rhodotorula glutinis* (B) as various sugars and the
proton conductor carbonylcyanide m-chlorophenylhydrazone are successively added to the suspension. The
time span of the abscissa is 40 min. The maximum membrane potential measured in this case was -85 mV although the value may be only approximate.

Proceedings of the 16th FEBS Congress
Part B, pp. 577–582
© 1985 VNU Science Press

Unfortunately the evidence is only rarely convincing, presumably owing to the rapid response of the H^+-extruding machinery of the cell which compensates for the uptake of H^+ concomitant with the transport of the solute in question. Still, the view draws strong teleonomic support from the fact that the cell uses several mechanisms to create the electrochemical potential difference or, at any rate, a pH difference across the membrane (a H-ATPase, a K^+/H^+ exchange, a leak of organic acids and a leak of CO_2/H_2CO_3) and hardly anyone will now contest its general validity.

However, the actual molecular mechanism remains unclear and disturbing data appeared particularly in quantitative assessments of the accumulation ratio of the H^+-symported solute. Kinetics and thermodynamics permit one to make predictions in this respect. Changes in the concentration of H^+ either outside or inside the cells and of the membrane potential result in changes of the half-saturation constants, the maximum rate of uptake and the accumulation ratio of the symported solute. From their type the actual molecular mechanism of transport can be assessed [5]. In the present communication the accumulation ratio will be considered in detail and inconsistencies in its behaviour will be shown.

1. The dependence of the accumulation ratio on pH – predicted from measurements of the electrochemical potential gradient of protons $(\Delta\tilde{\mu}_H^+)$ does not agree with the observed dependence both in qualitative and in quantitative terms (Fig. 2).

2. The temperature dependence is also inconsistent with the prediction made on the basis of $\Delta\tilde{\mu}_H^+$ (Fig. 2).

3. Addition of salts, such as KCl, depolarizes the membrane as expected from a permeant ion but it does not affect much the accumulation ratio.

The question arises whether the $\Delta\tilde{\mu}_H^+$ is at all relevant in our considerations. For instance,

1. an artificial creation of high ΔpH by acidifying the external solution does not increase accumulation in cells if the membrane extrusion of H^+ is impaired, such as in some yeast protoplasts;

2. under anaerobic conditions in *Saccharomyces cere-*

visiae, when both ΔpH and Δφ (the membrane potential) are high so that a protonmotive force of some 200 mV is generated, no accumulation of amino acids takes place;

3. in strictly aerobic yeasts, such as *Candida parapsilosis* or *Rhodotorula glutinis*, no uptake of sugars or amino acids takes place anaerobically in spite of sizable $\Delta\tilde{\mu}_H$+.

On the other hand, effects of added solutes on pH_{out} and on Δφ support the view that the electrochemical potential gradient of protons is somehow involved in nutrient transport in yeast.

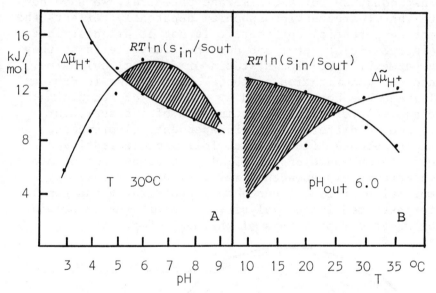

FIG. 2. Dependence of the electrochemical potential gradient $\Delta\tilde{\mu}_H$+ of protons in *R. glutinis* on external pH (A) and on temperature (B). The $\Delta\tilde{\mu}_H$+ was computed from measured values of its component terms, the membrane potential and the ΔpH. This is compared here with the actual accumulation ratio of 6-deoxy-D-glucose expressed in identical units. The shaded areas correspond to the situation where the actual accumulation of the sugar exceeds the one predicted theoretically on the basis of tight coupling of transport with the $\Delta\tilde{\mu}_H$+.

All this leads to the conclusion that the macroscopic values of ΔpH and/or Δφ are irrelevant and that we should rely on values in or near the membrane.

What are now the chances of obtaining such reliable values ?

The membrane potential has only rarely been measured directly with microelectrodes in single cells. In *Neurospora crassa,* Slayman s laboratory [6] obtained values of -200 mV or so, in *S. cerevisiae* we reached -50 mV at best [7 and unpublished]. In fact, most values are derived from indirect measurements of distribution of tetraphenylphosphonium [8], presumably according to the Nernst equation for the membrane potential. We have now data that tetraphenylphosphonium apparently reflects the membrane potential but that it is not at all distributed in intracellular water and does not leave cells as they are permeabilized with nystatin or dimethyl sulfoxide. Hence the quantitation of these observations is dubious.

The ΔpH has been measured by a number of techniques; the one we prefer is the estimation of intracellular pH based on differential, pH-dependent, fluorescence of dyes, such as fluorescein, following excitation at two different wavelengths [9-11]. It gives instantaneous, concentration-independent, results and, moreover, by a combination of fluorescence microphotography and computer-assisted image analysis, it permits us to obtain real pH-topographic maps of the cell (Fig. 3).

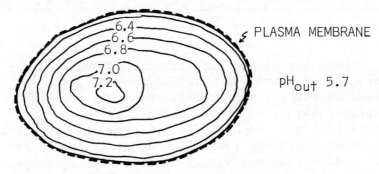

FIG. 3. pH contour lines of a *S. cerevisiae* cell suspended in distilled water. The resolution of the pH estimation in this case was 400 nm.

If now a pH profile is drawn across the cell boundary it is apparent that the pH drop across the plasma membrane is negligible, particularly so in water or in a weak buffer. Thus it appears that even at low external pH, when the potential is near zero [3], the ΔpH is also near zero and still, the accumulation of H^+-symported solute may be quite substantial.

If the H^+-driven transport idea is to be saved one must assume highly localized and globally insignificant domains in the membrane where both the potential and the difference in pH are preserved and where the secondary transport can be effected.

Our speculation, supported by considerable, even if indirect, evidence, is that such domains must exist near the H^+-extruding plasma membrane ATPase. Moreover, this ATPase appears to function only when activated, say, through glucose metabolism - e.g., in yeast protoplasts we have practically no uphill transport of substances and it is here, too, that the ATPase cannot be suitably activated [12].

References

1. Misra, P.C. and Höfer, M. (1975). An energy-linked proton extrusion across the cell membrane of *Rhodotorula glutinis*. FEBS Lett. 52, 95-99.
2. Aldermann, B. and Höfer, M. (1981). The active transport of monosaccharides by the yeast *Metschnikowia reukaufii*: Evidence for an electrochemical potential gradient of H^+ across the cell membrane. Exptl. Mycol. 5, 120-132.
3. Hauer, R., Uhlemann, G., Neumann, J. and Höfer, M. (1981). Proton pumps of the plasmalemma of the yeast *Rhodotorula glutinis*. Their coupling to fluxes of potassium and other ions. Biochim. Biophys. Acta 649, 680-690.
4. van den Broek, P.J.A., Christianse, K. and van Steveninck, J. (1982). The energetics of D-fucose transport in *Saccharomyces fragilis*. The influence of protonmotive force on sugar accumulation. Biochim. Biophys. Acta 692, 231-237.

5. Kotyk, A. (1983). Coupling of secondary active transport with $\Delta\tilde{\mu}_H$+. J. Bioenerget. Biomembr. 15, 307-320.
6. Sanders, D., Slayman, C.L. and Pall, M.L. (1983). Stoichiometry of H^+/amino acid cotransport in *Neurospora crassa* revealed by current-voltage analysis. Biochim. Biophys. Acta 735, 67-76.
7. Vacata, V., Kotyk, A. and Sigler, K. (1981). Membrane potentials in yeast cells measured by direct and indirect methods. Biochim. Biophys. Acta 643, 265-268.
8. Boxman, A.W., Barts, P.W.J.A. and Borst-Pauwels, G.W.F.H. (1982). Some characteristics of tetraphenyl-phosphonium uptake into *Saccharomyces cerevisiae*. Biochim. Biophys. Acta 686, 13-18.
9. Slavík, J. (1982). Intracellular pH of yeast cells measured with fluorescent probes. FEBS Lett. 140, 22-26.
10. Slavík, J. (1983). Intracellular pH topography: determination by a fluorescent probe. FEBS Lett. 156, 227-230.
11. Slavík, J. and Kotyk, A. (1984). Intracellular pH distribution and transmembrane pH profile of yeast cells. Biochim. Biophys. Acta, in press.
12. Kotyk, A., Michaljaničová, D., Stružinský, R., Baryshnikova, L.M. and Sychrová, H. (1985). Absence of glucose-stimulated transport in yeast protoplasts. Folia Microbiol., in press.